Functional Imaging in Nephro-Urology

Functional Imaging in Nephro-Urology

Edited by

Alain Prigent MD

Professor of Physiology and Biophysics
Faculté de Médecine Paris-Sud
Le Kremlin-Bicêtre
France

Chief of the Department of Biophysics and Nuclear Medicine
CHU Bicêtre
Le Kremlin-Bicêtre
France

Amy Piepsz MD

Professor of Pediatrics and Nuclear Medicine
Free University of Brussels
CHU St Pierre
Department of Radioisotopes
B-1000 Brussels
Belgium

CRC Press
Taylor & Francis Group
Boca Raton London New York

CRC Press is an imprint of the
Taylor & Francis Group, an **informa** business

CRC Press
Taylor & Francis Group
6000 Broken Sound Parkway NW, Suite 300
Boca Raton, FL 33487-2742

First issued in paperback 2019

© 2006 by Taylor & Francis Group, LLC
CRC Press is an imprint of Taylor & Francis Group, an Informa business
Typeset by Scribe Design Ltd, Ashford, Kent, UK

No claim to original U.S. Government works

ISBN-13: 978-1-84184-511-1 (hbk)
ISBN-13: 978-0-367-39127-0 (pbk)

Visit the Taylor & Francis Web site at
http://www.taylorandfrancis.com

and the CRC Press Web site at
http://www.crcpress.com

Contents

Contributors

M Donald Blaufox
Albert Einstein College of Medicine
Montefiore Medical Park
NY 10461
USA

Stephen CW Brown
Department of Urology
Stepping Hill Hospital
Stockport
Cheshire
UK

Michel Claudon
Service de Radiologie
CHU Nancy Brabois-Hôpital d'Enfants
54511 Vandoeurve Cedex
France

Jean-Nicolas Dacher
Departement Central d'Imagerie Médicale
CHU de Rouen-Hôpital Charles Nicolle
76031 Rouen
France

Thomas Dissing
Institute of Clinical Medicine
Aarhus University Hospital – Skejby
DK-8200 Aarhus N
Denmark

Emmanuel Durand
CHU de Bicêtre
Faculté de Médecine Paris-Sud
Department of Biophysics and Nuclear Medicine
94275 Le Kremlin-Bicêtre Cedex
France

Anni Eskild-Jensen
Department of Clinical Physiology and Nuclear Medicine
Aarhus University Hospital – Skejby
DK-8230 Aarhus N
Denmark

Julie Ferzli
Départment Central d"Imagerie Médicale
CHU de Rouen-Hôpital Charles Nicolle
76031 Rouen
France

Jørgen Frøkiær
Department of Clinical Physiology and Nuclear Medicine
Aarhus University Hospital – Skejby
DK-8230 Aarhus N
Denmark

Isky Gordon
Great Ormond Street Hospital for Children
London
UK

Nicolas Grenier
Service de Radiologie
Groupe Hospitalier Pellegrin
33076 Bordeaux Cedex
France

Jean-Pierre Guignard
Division of Pediatric Nephrology
Centre Hospitalier Universitaire Vaudois
1011 Lausanne
Switzerland

Hamphrey Ham
Department of Nuclear Medicine
Academic Hospital
University of Ghent
9000 Ghent
Belgium

Sverker Hansson
The Queen Silvia Children's Hospital
Pediatric Uronephrologic Centre (PUNC)
Göteborg University
Göteborg
Sweden

Olivier Hauger
ERT CNRS 'Imagerie Moléculaire et Fonctionnaell
Université Victor Ségalen-Bordeaux 2
Groupe Hospitalier Pellegrin
33076 Bordeaux Cedex
France

Laurent Juillard
Department of Nephrology and Hypertension
Hôpital Edouart-Herriot
Lyon Cedex 03
France

Stephen A Koff
Pediatric Urology
Children's Hospital
Education Building
Ohio 43205
USA

Maurice Laville
Department of Nephrology and Hypertension
Hôpital Edouard Herriot
Université Claude Bernard Lyon 1
Lyon Cedex 03
France

Lilach O Lerman
Division of Nephrology and Hypertension
Mayo Clinic College of Medicine
Rochester
Minnesota 55905
USA

Damien Mandry
Service de Radiologie
CHU Nancy Brabois-Hôpital d'Enfants
54511 Vandoeuvre Cedex
France

William B Mathews
Division of Nuclear Medicine
Johns Hopkins University
Nelson Building
Baltimore
MD 21287
USA

Joseph V Nally
Department of Nephrology and Hypertension
Cleveland Clinic Foundation
Cleveland
Ohio 44195
USA

Amy Piepsz
CHU St Pierre
Department of Radioisotopes
B-1000 Brussels
Belgium

Alain Prigent
Faculté de Médecine Paris-Sud
Department of Biophysics and Nuclear Medicine
94275 Le Kremlin-Bicêtre Cedex
France

Patrick H O'Reilly
Department of Urology
Stepping Hill Hospital
Stockport
UK

Michael Pedersen
Magnetic Resonance Centre
Institute of Clinical Medicine
Aarhus University Hospital – Skejby
DK-8200 Aarhus N
Denmark

Monica A Rossleigh
University of New South Wales
Department of Nuclear Medicine
The Prince of Wales and Sydney Children's Hospitals
Randwick NSW 2031
Australia

Zsolt Szabo
Johns Hopkins Outpatient Center
Baltimore
MD 21287
USA

Andrew Taylor
Division of Nuclear Medicine
Emory University School of Medicine
Atlanta
GA 30322
USA

Preface

In 1967, a first international symposium on radionuclides in nephro-urology was held in Liège (Belgium). The purpose of this symposium was to bring together a group of people with a common interest in the application of radionuclides in nephro-urology. Internists, radiologists, urologists, physiologists and others representing the basic and clinical sciences were brought together for intensive discussions. Since that time, similar meetings were organized by the International Scientific Committee of Radionuclides in Nephrourology (ISCORN) in New York (1971), Berlin (1974), Boston (1978), London (1981), Lausanne (1986), Williamsburg (1989), Chester (1992), Santa Fé (1995), Copenhagen (1998), Monterey (2001) and La Baule (2004). The final purpose of these meetings was the application of the radionuclide techniques in clinical fields such as hypertension, renal transplantation, hydronephrosis and infection. At the same time, a huge amount of methodological studies had given rise to new developments in nuclear medicine. It has been the role of ISCORN to chair consensus conferences, which resulted in a better standardization of radionuclide methods in fields such as measurement of renal clearance, evaluation of renal transit and drainage, application of captopril renography to renovascular disease, cortical scintigraphy in urinary tract infection in children and management of renal transplants.

The meeting, held in May 2004 in La Baule (France), was a kind of achievement. It was the feeling of the Committee that the time had come to bring together the different specialities involved in the strategy of uro-nephrological diseases and to evaluate the potential place of various techniques in the management of patients. The basic structure of the symposium was therefore centred on a series of clinical topics, all of them characterized by a significant number of controversial matters: determination of renal function in child and in adult, antenatally detected hydronephrosis, renal obstruction in adults, renovascular hypertension, renal infection in childhood. Radiologists, nuclear medicine physicians, physiologists, paediatric and adult nephrologists, paediatric and adult urologists, all eminent experts in their respective fields, developed the state of the art and constituted then a large panel for long and well-structured discussions with the audience. The most up-to-date developments of the traditional methods were presented by the different speakers, while new techniques, such as functional and molecular imaging with MR, CT and PET appeared as promising approaches. What came out of these multidisciplinary sessions is remarkably similar for all topics, namely a critical appraisal of the traditional strategies of management and a series of potential new directions which might, in the near future, significantly change the clinical management of the patient.

It appeared therefore that the moment was well chosen to reassemble this huge amount of information within a book under the general title of 'The Role of Functional Imaging in Nephro-urology'. The chapters correspond to the five clinical sessions and for each topic, the contributors provided a detailed and referenced overview of their expertise, completed by a rich iconography.

This book, by its multidisciplinary approach, is a 'première' and will provide outstanding information to radiologists working on child and adult, to nuclear medicine physicians, to internists and paediatricians, to nephrologists and urologists specialized in child and adult.

We want to express our sincere thanks for help to the other members of the ISCORN committee: Donald Blaufox (New York, USA), Keith Britton (London, UK), Eva Dubovsky (Birmingham, USA), Belkis Erbas (Ankara, Turkey), Jörgen Frökiaer (Aarhus, Denmark), Joseph V. Nally (Cleveland, USA), Patrick O'Reilly (Stockport, UK), Pilar Orellana (Santiago, Chile), Monica Rossleigh (Sydney, Australia), Michael Rutland (Auckland, New Zealand) and Andrew Taylor (Atlanta, USA). Thanks also to the experts of all specialities who contributed by their outstanding presentations to the success of this multidisciplinary event. Their lectures were the starting materials for the different chapters of this book. All of this would not have been possible without the help of the organizing committee (Joseph Lecloirec, MD and Mrs Maïté Lepelletier) who did a great job in making this conference one of the most exciting meetings ISCORN has ever experienced. Finally sincere thanks to Tyco France and Tyco USA whose role in sponsoring the meeting has been essential.

Alain Prigent, Paris, France
Amy Piepsz, Brussels, Belgium
Editors

Measurement of renal function in health and disease

1   Introduction

Alain Prigent

Operational definition of renal function

The level of the glomerular filtration rate (GFR) is generally accepted as the best overall index for the complex functions of the kidney in health and disease.[1] This agreement holds on to functional, pathological, clinical and prognostic arguments. The functional coupling between GFR and tubular function especially relies upon the 'positive' glomerulotubular balance and the 'negative' tubuloglomerular feed-back, which ensure an integrative regulation of the whole nephron function. Similarly, the GFR decrease correlates with the extent of tubulointerstitial fibrosis and/or tubular atrophy in chronic renal diseases.[2] GFR being reduced prior to the onset of symptoms of renal failure, its assessment enables earlier diagnosis and therapeutic interventions in patients at risk. Thus the level of GFR is a strong predictor of the time of onset of kidney failure as well as the risk of complications of chronic kidney disease.[1] Many techniques, using either chemical or radiopharmaceuticals, exist providing either estimates or true measurements of the global GFR.

In case of asymmetrical renal disease the determination of the individual renal function requires a global GFR measurement to be combined with the assessment of the split renal function (e.g., expressed in percentages of the global function) by a noninvasive imaging modality. Although renal scintigraphy is presently the most often used because of its widespread availability, low cost (compared to the alternative modalities of computed tomography and magnetic resonance imaging), and absence of side effects from the tracers,[3] new applications of computed tomography (e.g., multidetector CT, electron beam computerized tomography) and magnetic resonance imaging appear promising (see Chapters 15 and 17).

The clearances of some tubularly secreted organic anions, such as p-aminohippuric acid (PAH), [131]I- or ^{125}I-ortho-iodohippurate (OIH), or even ^{99m}Tc-mercaptoacetyltriglycine (MAG 3), are referred to as the effective renal plasma flow (ERPF). GFR is related to ERPF by the expression:

$$GFR = ERPF.FF/EF_{oa}$$

where EF_{oa} is the extraction fraction of the used organic anion ($EF_{oa} = ERPF/RPF$, RPF being renal plasma flow), and FF the filtration fraction (FF $=$ GFR/RPF, about 0.20 in normal humans). However, as FF changes occur in certain clinical circumstances (e.g., proteinuric glomerulopathy, ischaemia, postischaemic injury after transplantation, renovascular hypertension, acute urinary obstruction, …), RPF changes do not always parallel GFR changes. Moreover, EF_{oa} varies dramatically and unpredictably in numerous conditions, especially in chronic renal diseases. As an example, the extraction fraction of PAH, considered as the gold standard molecule for ERPF measurement, is 0.92 ± 0.03 (mean $\pm$ SE) in normal volunteers[4] but may decrease to an average of 0.80 in benign essential hypertension,[5] 0.75 in patients treated with cyclosporin,[4] 0.70 in proteinuric glomerulopathies,[6] or to 0.20 in ischaemic acute renal failure and to 0.10 in the recovery period.[7] Moreover, in all these cases the standard deviation of the mean EF_{oa} is about 0.10 to 0.15, indicating a wide range of variation between individual data. In renovascular disease, where the renal function is asymmetrical, EF_{oa} of PAH is about 0.55 and 0.75 in the stenotic and contralateral kidney, respectively, and decreases further to 0.35 and 0.65, respectively, after administration of captopril.[8] Even with the most sophisticated curve-fitting procedures most methods are too imprecise for accurate prediction of EF_{oa} in a given individual.[4]

Renal function in health

Notwithstanding the great variability of GFR even in healthy individuals due to many physiological factors (e.g., body size, gender, age, salt and dietary protein intakes, diurnal variations), normal ranges of GFR have been reported. This variability can be reduced by taking into account body surface area ('normalization' to 1.73 m^2). When using the 'classical' gold standard of inulin clearance,[9] the mean values of GFR in young adults are 127 ml/min/1.73 m^2 in men and 118 ml/min/1.73 m^2 in females with a standard deviation of approximately 20 ml/min/1.73 m^2, while when using ^{51}Cr EDTA (ethylenediaminetetraacetic acid) plasma clearance,[10] the normal mean ($\pm$SD) GFR is 105 ($\pm$25) ml/min/1.73 m^2 (no gender difference after correction for BSA). With regards to transversal studies,[10–13] GFR linearly decreases by approximately 1.0 ml/min/1.73 m^2 per year with large interindividual variation even among 'healthy' individuals. Indeed, regarding longitudinal studies,[14] one-third of the healthy elderly subjects has no absolute change, another third has a progressive but small decline, and in the last third of elderly GFR declines to 50–70% of the maximum GFR value. In one-month aged neonates,[15,16] the mean GFR is about half the adult value (55 ml/min/1.73 m^2) and increases progressively until 18 months–2 years. Between 2 and 17 years of age, expressed as ml/min/1.73 m^2, the GFR remains constant, with a mean value of 114 ml/min/1.73 m^2 (SD: 24 ml/min/ 1.73 m^2), similar to the value in adults.

In normal individuals, the reactive increase in GFR (120–140% of the baseline value) within the 2 hours following an oral protein load (e.g., 300–500 g of cooked beef) is defined as 'functional renal reserve'.[17] Subsequently, similar increases in GFR were reported[18] with either gluconeogenic amino acids (50–75 g within 3 hours) or dopamine (1.5–2 µg/kg/min for 2 hours) infusion. Although it was initially thought that this 'reserve' was lost in the presence of early renal impairment (i.e., not diagnosed by plasma creatinine test), these findings were not confirmed in many later series. Expressed as a percentage of baseline GFR value, the 'functional reserve' does not decrease in kidney diseases (see reference 19). Apart from this diurnal variation due to meal intake, there is a circadian rhythm of GFR[20] with a maximum around 1 pm, a minimum around 1 am, and a relative amplitude ([max − min]/mean) of about 30% for inulin clearance and 20% for creatinine clearance. The nutritional status also affects GFR,[21] especially dietary intakes of proteins, calories (whatever the nutriments), and sodium (an important determinant of extracellular fluid volume, ECFV). For an example, GFR increases to about 140% of its baseline value during pregnancy in relation to an increase in ECFV.

At the borderline between health and disease, the compensatory hyperfunction of the remnant kidney in donors restricts, partly the functional lost. Thus GFR (^{125}I-iothalamate urinary clearance measurements) is about 60% (69 ± 4 ml/min/1.73 m^2) and 70% (78 ± 5 ml/min/ 1.73 m^2) of the predonation value (111 ± 6 ml/min/ 1.73 m^2) at about one month and 5 years after the nephrectomy, respectively.[18]

Renal function in disease

The aim of the following chapter is to go through every issue related to the measurement of renal function and to define which methods are adequate for which patients'. However, we agree that no single test of GFR is perfectly suited for every clinical and research application. Thus, the goal should be to propose a specific clinical question (screening, confirming, following, …) the most accurate, precise, safe, convenient and cost-effective (not only the cheapest) method.

Recently, the Kidney Disease Outcome Quality Initiative (K/DOQI) of the National Kidney Foundation (USA) has proposed guidelines,[1] among which one is dedicated to the definition and classification of stages of chronic kidney disease (guideline 1) and another to its evaluation by estimation of GFR (guideline 4).

GFR plays a cornerstone role in the definition of chronic kidney disease (CKD), since CKD is defined on two criteria, one of which being a decreased GFR:

1. **Kidney damage for 3 months at least**, as defined by structural or functional abnormalities of the kidney, with or without decreased GFR, manifest by either pathological abnormalities, or markers of kidney damage (including abnormalities in the composition of the blood or urine, or abnormal imaging tests);
2. **GFR lower than 60 ml/min/1.73 m^2 for 3 months at least**, with or without kidney damage (as defined in criteria 1).

Similarly, the GFR level is used for the stage definition of CKD:

- Stage 1: with normal or increased GFR: GFR ≥ 90 ml/min/1.73 m^2
- Stage 2: GFR between 60 and 89 ml/min/1.73 m^2 (mild)
- Stage 3: GFR between 30 and 59 ml/min/1.73 m^2 (moderate)
- Stage 4: GFR between 15 and 29 ml/min/1.73 m^2 (severe)
- Stage 5: GFR < 15 ml/min/1.73 m^2 (renal failure).

For the 'estimation' (not the measurement) of GFR, the recommendation is to use prediction equations taking into account serum creatinine concentration and some of the variables, which determine the creatinine production, such as age, gender, body size, ethnicity, etc. Estimating GFR by prediction equation based on serum creatinine is more reliable (i.e., more accurate and more precise) than measuring 24-hour creatinine clearance, mainly because of inter-patient and intrapatient variability in creatinine tubular secretion and inability of most patients to accurately collect timed urine samples.[22–24] The day-to-day coefficient of variation of creatinine clearance has been reported as high as 27% in a routine clinical setting.[25]

The two recommended formulae for predicting either creatinine clearance or GFR are, for adult patients, the Cockroft–Gault equation[26] and the 'abbreviated' MDRD study equation (MDRD for Modification of Diet in Renal Disease), respectively and in children, the Schwartz[27] and Counahan–Baratt[28] equations, respectively (Table 1.1). However, these recommendations do not answer the question 'which methods for which patients' since the guideline about *estimation* of GFR only states that 'all four formulae reviewed provide a marked improvement over serum creatinine alone' for clinical assessment of kidney disease. Moreover, K/DOQI guidelines acknowledge, firstly that 'estimation of GFR and creatinine clearance from serum creatinine is critically dependent on calibration of the serum

Table 1.1 Equations recommended by the National Kidney Foundation (NKF/DOQI) to predict creatinine clearance and GFR based on serum creatinine

Adult

Cockcroft–Gault[26] $\quad C_{CR}$ (ml/min) $= \dfrac{(140 - age) \times weight}{72 \times S_{CR}} \times$ (0.85 if female)

Abbreviated MDRD[78] $\quad$ GFR (ml/min/1.73 m^2) $= 186 \times (S_{CR})^{-1.154} \times (age)^{-0.203} \times$ (0.742 if female) $\times$ (1.210 if African-American)

$\qquad\qquad\qquad\qquad\qquad\quad = \exp(5.228 - 1.154 \times L_n [S_{CR}] - 0.203 \times L_n (age) - (0.299 \text{ if female}) + (0.192 \text{ if African-American}))$

Children

Schwartz[27] $\quad C_{CR}$ (ml/min) $= \dfrac{0.55 \times length}{S_{CR}}$

Counahan–Barratt[28] $\quad$ GFR (ml/min/1.73 m^2) $= \dfrac{0.43 \times length}{S_{CR}}$

S_{CR}, serum creatinine in mg/dl (to convert mg/dl to μmol/l multiply by 88); C_{CR}, creatinine clearance; weight in kg; length in cm; age in years.

creatinine assay', and secondly that, 'in certain clinical situations, *clearance measures* may be necessary to estimate GFR'.

Numerous methods are used to measure creatinine, mainly colorimetric (based on Jaffe' reaction) or enzymatic assays. The more commonly used colorimetric methods systematically overestimate creatinine concentrations by about 20% compared to enzymatic measures (lower interference with noncreatine chromogens) and by 20% to 80%, when compared to high-performance liquid chromatography (HPLC) and dilution mass spectrometry measures, which should approximate 'true creatinine'.[1] The College of American Pathologists[29] reported that in laboratories surveyed in 1994, creatinine was overestimated on average by 13% to 17% (0.12–0.17 mg/dl or 11–15 μmol/l). Serum creatinine assays on the same samples were 0.23 mg/dlL (20.3 μmol/l) higher at the White Sands Laboratory (Third National Health and Nutrition Examination Survey, NHANES III) than at the Cleveland Clinic (MDRD study), although both laboratories used Jaffe' reaction-based methods but on different auto analysers.[30]

Without any correction of this bias by a calibration factor (0.81), the prevalence of low GFR (30–60 ml/min/1.73 m^2) in NHANES III would have been erroneously increased fourfold (12.5 versus 3.2%).[31] Recently, the French Society of Clinical Biology assessed interassay variation and accuracy of blood creatinine measurements as well as the effect of the standardization of calibration procedures on interassay variation. Thirty frozen human sera and three certified reference materials were analysed by 17 creatinine assays (12 colorimetric, four enzymatic and one HPLC).[32] Most of the commercially available methods had inaccuracy higher than 10% for serum creatinine lower than 1.7 mg/dl (150 μmol/l). The median dispersion factor was 14% between 0.5 and 1.7 mg/dl (45–150 μmol/l, the range of mild to moderate renal impairment) and 8% between 2.9 and 4.0 mg/dl (250–350 μmol/l). Moreover, the bias was not constant over the clinical range of serum creatinine, enzymatic assays producing lower results than colorimetric ones for low creati-

nine levels, but conversely higher results for high creatinine levels. Due to the lack of a standardized calibration procedure using several concentrations (with at least one between 0.1 and 1.7 mg/dl or 90–150 μmol/l), the intra-assay variation is too high to allow prediction of creatinine clearance or GFR from serum creatinine levels, contrarily to K/DOQI guidelines recommendations. Similar conclusions have been reached by other groups working on the prevalence of low GFR in nondiabetic Americans[31,33] or on the risk factors on renal function (Prevention of Renal and Vascular End-stage Diseases study, PREVEND).[34] Although the K/DOQI working group has chosen an estimated GFR cutoff of less than 60 ml/min/1.73 m^2 for diagnosing chronic kidney disease in the absence of kidney damage, an improvement in estimating GFR from MDRD formula could be to include creatinine assay methods as a covariable in the prediction equation used[30,32] keeping in mind the interlaboratory variation in measurement of serum-creatine.

Since creatinine clearance overestimates GFR, the estimates given by the Cockcroft–Gault and Schwartz formulae are biased too. Thus, in a large sample of more than 500 adults with a wide range of GFR (up to approximately 90 ml/min/1.73 m^2), Cockcroft–Gault formula overestimates GFR, directly measured by ^{125}I-iothalamate urinary clearance, by 23%.[35] With Schwartz formula, the bias increases markedly in children with low GFR, with overestimation up to 32% and 67% for GFR (^{125}I-iothalamate clearance) between 31–50 ml/min/1.73 m^2 and lower than 30 ml/min/1.73 m^2, respectively.[36]

Another issue is the reliability of the claimed statement that the four formulas recommended provide a clinically useful estimate of GFR' in the K/DOQI guidelines. This statement relies on a rather optimistic definition of what is an accuracy sufficient enough for good clinical decision-making. Thus, the accuracy was defined as the percent of GFR estimates within 30% of measured GFR (i.e.; in the 70–130% range of GFR measured by radionuclide tracer, inulin or iohexol clearances). Results of about ten studies (see reference 1) assessing accuracy in adults and children indicated that a quarter of the patients have estimated GFR by Cockcroft–Gault and Schwartz formulae, respectively, out of this large range of uncertainty (about 60% of the measured, 'true' GFR). Although the claimed clinical usefulness of Cockcroft–Gault and Schwartz formulae are questionable regarding such a low accuracy, abbreviated MDRD and Counahan–Baratt formulae are more efficient with only 10% and 15–30% of estimated GFR, respectively, which did not fall into the 30% accuracy range.

Assuming that a GFR prediction formula derived from a patient population will be valid when applied to another population may be erroneous. For example, Cockcroft–Gault formula systematically overestimates GFR in obese[37] or oedematous individuals[38] and is inaccurate in diabetic patients.[39] Similarly, Schwartz formula is not reliable in children with insulin-dependent diabetics mellitus,[40] with liver disease,[41,42] and after liver transplantation.[43] Even the more recent abbreviated MDRD formula was recently reported as inaccurate for GFR estimation in healthy potential kidney donors,[11,44] a conclusion not so surprising since the patients included to derive the MDRD formulae had GFR up to 90 ml/min/1.73 m^2 only. The same conclusion is predictable for the early stage of CKD in diabetic patients, where GFR may be normal or even increased.[45] Therefore, measurements of GFR are needed to identify early decline or increase in kidney function, especially in patients at high risk for renal functional impairment (e.g., diabetes, renal transplant rejection, systemic lupus erythematosus, etc.).[1,46,47]

In clinical situations in which the average rate of production of creatinine is unpredictable from the variables used in the prediction formulae, GFR measurements by clearance methods are mandatory. Estimates will be unreliable in severe malnutrition, obesity, prolonged parenteral nutrition, corticotherapy (e.g., chronic kidney and liver disease and transplantation), neuromuscular diseases, paraplegia or quadriplegia and vegetarian diet (low creatinine dietary intake). More problematic, the fundamental assumption of the MDRD formula that age, gender, ethnicity and blood urea nitrogen (BUN) account for creatinine production, is invalid in patients with advanced renal failure, and the use of MDRD formula in these patients might introduce biases.[48]

Even if the prediction equations to estimate GFR had been validated by tests in adults (or children), elderly, diabetics and nondiabetics, high-risk patients (e.g., for CKD or cardiovascular disease), transplant recipients and among different ethnicities (and not only African/Mexican/Caucasian/American), their clinical use would be limited. The most important hurdle remains that they were derived from adjustment variables (e.g. age, gender, height and body weight) more effective for detecting interpatient differences than intrapatient time changes. Consequently, and as specified in the K/DOQI guidelines, 'estimates of GFR based on serum creatinine will only enable the detection of substantial progression (>25% to 50% decline) … and will lead to false measures of lower degrees of progression'. In this context, it should be recalled

that the coefficient of variation (CV) of inulin clearance measured on different days in the same individual (with invasive bladder catheterization, no data using spontaneous voiding) is approximatively 7.5%,[49] the median intertest (3 months interval) CV of ^{125}I-iothalamate urinary clearance (spontaneous voiding) is 6.3%,[50] and the total day-to-day CV of ^{51}Cr-EDTA plasma clearance (no urinary collection) is 4.1% and 11.5% in patients with a GFR > or ≤ 30 ml/min, respectively.[25]

In 1989, Andrew S. Levey, the first author of many papers published by the MDRD study working group, had already concluded in a review about the use of GFR measurements to assess the progression of renal disease[49] that 'estimation of GFR from renal clearance of radioisotope-labeled filtration markers, using a bolus infusion and spontaneous bladder emptying, is accurate, precise, and more convenient than the classical inulin clearance techniques, and that measurements of GFR should be included in clinical research'.

The next chapters will analyse the chemical and radio-nuclide techniques available to measure GFR in adults and children and propose answers or suggestions for the selection of the most appropriate methods in different clinical settings both in adults and children.

Besides prediction formulae based on serum creatinine, Joe Nally will discuss serum cystatin C, which has been suggested for detecting early changes in GFR especially in children, liver disease and kidney transplant, where creatinine-based formulae are inaccurate. However, sample sizes are limited and results are still conflicting.[51–55] The use of iodine contrast media (e.g., iohexol) as a nonradioactive substitute in urinary and plasma clearance methods[56–62] has been proposed to measure GFR. However, expensive and time-consuming HPLC is required to allow the use of a small injection dose (unlikely to induce adverse effects except allergic reactions) and accurate measurement of low serum concentrations. X-ray fluorescence method is less sensitive and accurate, and needs a higher sampled blood volume.

Table 1.2 Which methods for which patients

Applications	Clinical settings
Screening	Prevalence of low GFR • general population • high-risk patients (diabetes, CVD, etc.)
Confirming	Inaccurate/doubtful estimated GFR (e.g., chronic rejection), prognostic information (e.g., SLE), need for therapy or additional diagnostic test
Following	Disease progression, therapeutic follow-up, need for dialysis or transplantation (very low GFR)
Investigating	Renal toxicity, renal clearance of drugs to guide dosing, renal functional reserve, normal values (e.g., ageing)

The point of view of the nephrologist and the paediatric nephrologist will be developed by M. Laville and J.P. Guignard, respectively.

Which methods should be used for well-defined clinical conditions? The methods may differ strongly, depending on the type of clinical application concerned. Table 10.2 lists the clinical settings and the corresponding field of application. Answering such questions needs to consider the criteria for the choice, which may have different weights in the decision-making process, depending on the main aim of the test (e.g., screening patients at risk or confirming the need for dialysis or transplantation).

In general, the tests that are most accurate (low bias compared to the standard) and precise (good reproducibility and small difference for a significant change) are also those that are less convenient (simplicity, safety, availability, cost).

E. Durand will present radionuclide clearance methods, either urinary (i.e., either constant infusion or intravenous/subcutaneous single injection) or plasma clearance (i.e., either infusion-equilibrium or single injection) and some external detection based methods, used to measure split renal function, such as the fraction injected dose[63–69] uptake and the functional uptake rate.[70]

A. Piepsz will consider issues more specific to children, especially the advantages and limitations of different plasma clearance techniques (i.e., slope/intercept method, 'only-slope' method,[71,72] one-sample versus two–three sample method, and infusion-equilibrium method[73,74]), the question of normalization/indexation to body surface area (BSA) or extracellular fluid volume (ECFV),[75,76] and the question of the 'switch' from children- to adult-estimated GFR equations in adolescents and young adults.[77]

References

1. K/DOQI clinical practice guidelines for chronic kidney disease: evaluation, classification, and stratification. Am J Kidney Dis 2002; 39(Suppl 1): S1–266.

2. Schainuck LI, Striker GE, Cutler RE, Benditt EP. Structural–functional correlations in renal disease. II. The correlations. Hum Pathol 1970; 1: 631–41.

3. Prigent A, Cosgriff P, Gates GF et al. Consensus report on quality control of quantitative measurements of renal function obtained from the renogram: International Consensus Committee from the Scientific Committee of Radionuclides in Nephrourology. Semin Nucl Med 1999; 29: 146–59.

4. Battilana C, Zhang HP, Olshen RA et al. PAH extraction and estimation of plasma flow in diseased human kidneys. Am J Physiol 1991; 261(Pt 2): F726–33.

5. London GM, Safar ME. Comparaison de l'hémodynamique rénale dans deux types d'hypertension artérielle, essentielle et rénovasculaire, chez l'homme. Implications physiopathologiques. Néphrologie 1988; 9: 21–7.

6. Golbetz H, Black V, Shemesh O, Myers BD. Mechanism of the antiproteinuric effect of indomethacin in nephrotic humans. Am J Physiol 1989; 256 (Pt 2): F44–51.

7. Corrigan G, Ramaswamy D, Kwon O et al. PAH extraction and estimation of plasma flow in human postischemic acute renal failure. Am J Physiol 1999; 277 (Pt 2): F312–18.

8. Wenting GJ, Derkx FH, Tan-Tjiong LH et al. Risks of angiotensin converting enzyme inhibition in renal artery stenosis. Kidney Int Suppl 1987; 20: S180–3.

9. Smith H. Comparative physiology of the kidney. In: Smith H (ed.). The Kidney: Structure and Function in Health and Disease. New York: Oxford University Press; 1951. pp. 520–74.

10. Granerus G, Aurell M. Reference values for 51Cr-EDTA clearance as a measure of glomerular filtration rate. Scand J Clin Lab Invest 1981; 41: 611–16.

11. Rule AD, Gussak HM, Pond GR et al. Measured and estimated GFR in healthy potential kidney donors. Am J Kidney Dis 2004; 43: 112–19.

12. Perrone RD, Madias NE, Levey AS. Serum creatinine as an index of renal function: new insights into old concepts. Clin Chem 1992; 38: 1933–53.

13. Rowe JW, Andres R, Tobin JD et al. The effect of age on creatinine clearance in men: a cross-sectional and longitudinal study. J Gerontol 1976; 31: 155–63.

14. Lindeman RD, Tobin J, Shock NW. Longitudinal studies on the rate of decline in renal function with age. J Am Geriatr Soc 1985; 33: 278–85.

15. Piepsz A, Pintelon H, Ham HR. Estimation of normal chromium-51 ethylene diamine tetra-acetic acid clearance in children. Eur J Nucl Med 1994; 21: 12–16.

16. Rubin M, Bruck E, Rapaport M. Maturation of renal function in childhood: clearance studies. J Clin Invest 1949; 28: 1944.

17. Bosch JP, Saccaggi A, Lauer A et al. Renal functional reserve in humans. Effect of protein intake on glomerular filtration rate. Am J Med 1983; 75: 943–50.

18. ter Wee PM, Tegzess AM, Donker AJ. Pair-tested renal reserve filtration capacity in kidney recipients and their donors. J Am Soc Nephrol 1994; 4: 1798–808.

19. Thomas DM, Coles GA, Williams JD. What does the renal reserve mean? Kidney Int 1994; 45: 411–16.

20. Koopman MG, Koomen GC, Krediet RT et al. Circadian rhythm of glomerular filtration rate in normal individuals. Clin Sci (Lond) 1989; 77: 105–11.

21. Kopple JD, Greene T, Chumlea WC et al. Relationship between nutritional status and the glomerular filtration rate: results from the MDRD study. Kidney Int 2000; 57: 1688–703.

22. Walser M. Assessing renal function from creatinine measurements in adults with chronic renal failure. Am J Kidney Dis 1998; 32: 23–31.

23. DeSanto NG, Coppola S, Anastasio P et al. Predicted creatinine clearance to assess glomerular filtration rate in chronic renal disease in humans. Am J Nephrol 1991; 11: 181–5.

24. Shemesh O, Golbetz H, Kriss JP, Myers BD. Limitations of creatinine as a filtration marker in glomerulopathic patients. Kidney Int 1985; 28: 830–8.

25. Brochner-Mortensen J, Rodbro P. Selection of routine method for determination of glomerular filtration rate in adult patients. Scand J Clin Lab Invest 1976; 36: 35–43.

26. Cockcroft DW, Gault MH. Prediction of creatinine clearance from serum creatinine. Nephron 1976; 16: 31–41.

27. Schwartz GJ, Haycock GB, Edelmann CM Jr, Spitzer A. A simple estimate of glomerular filtration rate in children derived from body length and plasma creatinine. Pediatrics 1976; 58: 259–63.

28. Counahan R, Chantler C, Ghazali S et al. Estimation of glomerular filtration rate from plasma creatinine concentration in children. Arch Dis Child 1976; 51: 875–8.

29. Ross JW, Miller WG, Myers GL, Praestgaard J. The accuracy of laboratory measurements in clinical chemistry: a study of 11 routine chemistry analytes in the College of American Pathologists Chemistry Survey with fresh frozen serum, definitive methods and reference methods. Arch Pathol Lab Med 1998; 122: 587–608.

30. Coresh J, Astor BC, McQuillan G et al. Calibration and random variation of the serum creatinine assay as critical elements of using equations to estimate glomerular filtration rate. Am J Kidney Dis 2002; 39: 920–9.

31. Clase CM, Garg AX, Kiberd BA. Prevalence of low glomerular filtration rate in nondiabetic Americans: Third National Health and Nutrition Examination Survey (NHANES III). J Am Soc Nephrol 2002; 13: 1338–49.

32. Séronie-Vivien S, Galteau MM, Carlier MC et al. Dosage de la créatininémie en 2003: état des lieux analytique et essai de standardisation de l'étalonnage (Groupe de travail de la SFBC "Créatinine" de la section "Assurance Qualité" – Pr G. Férard). Ann Biol Clin 2004; 62: 165–75.

33. Coresh J, Eknoyan G, Levey AS. Estimating the prevalence of low glomerular filtration rate requires attention to the creatinine assay calibration. J Am Soc Nephrol 2002; 13: 2811–12; author reply 2812–16.

34. Verhave JC, Gansevoort RT, Hillege HL et al. Drawbacks of the use of indirect estimates of renal function to evaluate the effect of risk factors on renal function. J Am Soc Nephrol 2004; 15: 1316–22.

35. Levey AS, Bosch JP, Lewis JB et al. A more accurate method to estimate glomerular filtration rate from serum creatinine: a new prediction equation. Modification of Diet in Renal Disease Study Group. Ann Intern Med 1999; 130: 461–70.

36. Seikaly MG, Browne R, Simonds N et al. Glomerular filtration rate in children following renal transplantation. Pediatr Transplant 1998; 2: 231–5.

37. Verhave JC, Balje-Volkers CP, Hillege HL et al. The reliability of different formulae to predict creatinine clearance. J Intern Med 2003; 253: 563–73.

38. Rolin HA 3rd, Hall PM, Wei R. Inaccuracy of estimated creatinine clearance for prediction of iothalamate glomerular filtration rate. Am J Kidney Dis 1984; 4: 48–54.

39. Norden G, Bjorck S, Granerus G, Nyberg G. Estimation of renal function in diabetic nephropathy. Comparison of five methods. Nephron 1987; 47: 36–42.

40. Waz WR, Quattrin T, Feld LG. Serum creatinine, height, and weight do not predict glomerular filtration rate in children with IDDM. Diabetes Care 1993; 16: 1067–70.

41. Papadakis MA, Arieff AI. Unpredictability of clinical evaluation of renal function in cirrhosis. Prospective study. Am J Med 1987; 82: 945–52.

42. McDiarmid SV, Ettenger RB, Hawkins RA et al. The impairment of true glomerular filtration rate in long-term cyclosporine-treated pediatric allograft recipients. Transplantation 1990; 49: 81–5.

43. Berg UB, Ericzon BG, Nemeth A. Renal function before and long after liver transplantation in children. Transplantation 2001; 72: 631–7.

44. Lin J, Knight EL, Hogan ML, Singh AK. A comparison of prediction equations for estimating glomerular filtration rate in adults without kidney disease. J Am Soc Nephrol 2003; 14: 2573–80.

45. Sunder-Plassmann G, Horl WH. A critical appraisal for definition of hyperfiltration. Am J Kidney Dis 2004; 43: 396; author reply 396–7.

46. Kasiske BL, Keane FK. Laboratory assessment of renal disease: clearance, urinalysis, and renal biopsy. In: Brenner BM (ed.). The Kidney. Philadelphia: WB Saunders, 2000: 1129–64.

47. Kasiske BL, Vazquez MA, Harmon WE et al. Recommendations for the outpatient surveillance of renal transplant recipients. American Society of Transplantation. J Am Soc Nephrol 2000; 11 (Suppl 15): S1–86.

48. Beddhu S, Samore MH, Roberts MS et al. Creatinine production, nutrition, and glomerular filtration rate estimation. J Am Soc Nephrol 2003; 14: 1000–5.

49. Levey AS. Use of glomerular filtration rate measurements to assess the progression of renal disease. Semin Nephrol 1989; 9: 370–9.

50. Levey AS, Greene T, Schluchter MD et al. Glomerular filtration rate measurements in clinical trials. Modification of Diet in Renal Disease Study Group and the Diabetes Control and Complications Trial Research Group. J Am Soc Nephrol 1993; 4: 1159–71.

51. Daniel JP, Chantrel F, Offner M et al. Comparison of cystatin C, creatinine and creatinine clearance vs. GFR for detection of renal failure in renal transplant patients. Ren Fail 2004; 26: 253–7.

52. Meier P, Froidevaux C, Dayer E, Blanc E. Cystatin C concentration and glomerular filtration rate. Lancet 2001; 357: 634–5.

53. Swaminathan R. Cystatin for estimation of glomerular filtration rate. Lancet 2001; 357: 143–4.

54. Deinum J, Derkx FH. Cystatin for estimation of glomerular filtration rate? Lancet 2000; 356: 1624–5.

55. Helin I, Axenram M, Grubb A. Serum cystatin C as a determinant of glomerular filtration rate in children. Clin Nephrol 1998; 49: 221–5.

56. Effersoe H, Rosenkilde P, Groth S et al. Measurement of renal function with iohexol. A comparison of iohexol, 99mTc-DTPA, and 51Cr-EDTA clearance. Invest Radiol 1990; 25: 778–82.

57. Gaspari F, Perico N, Remuzzi G. Measurement of glomerular filtration rate. Kidney Int Suppl 1997; 63: S151–4.

58. Frennby B, Sterner G, Almen T et al. The use of iohexol clearance to determine GFR in patients with severe chronic renal failure – a comparison between different clearance techniques. Clin Nephrol 1995; 43: 35–46.

59. Gaspari F, Perico N, Matalone M et al. Precision of plasma clearance of iohexol for estimation of GFR in patients with renal disease. J Am Soc Nephrol 1998; 9: 310–13.

60. Lewis R, Kerr N, Van Buren C et al. Comparative evaluation of urographic contrast media, inulin, and 99mTc-DTPA clear-

ance methods for determination of glomerular filtration rate in clinical transplantation. Transplantation 1989; 48: 790–6.

61. Stake G, Monn E, Rootwelt K, Monclair T. A single plasma sample method for estimation of the glomerular filtration rate in infants and children using iohexol, II: Establishment of the optimal plasma sampling time and a comparison with the 99Tcm-DTPA method. Scand J Clin Lab Invest 1991; 51: 343–8.

62. Brown SC, O'Reilly PH. Iohexol clearance for the determination of glomerular filtration rate in clinical practice: evidence for a new gold standard. J Urol 1991; 146: 675–9.

63. Rehling M, Moller ML, Lund JO et al. 99mTc-DTPA gamma-camera renography: normal values and rapid determination of single-kidney glomerular filtration rate. Eur J Nucl Med 1985; 11: 1–6.

64. Moonen M, Jacobsson L, Granerus G. Gamma camera renography with 99Tcm-DTPA: the impact of variations in input plasma curve on estimated GFR. Nucl Med Commun 1994; 15: 673–9.

65. Moonen M, Jacobsson L, Granerus G et al. Determination of split renal function from gamma camera renography: a study of three methods. Nucl Med Commun 1994; 15: 704–11.

66. Bocher M, Shrem Y, Tappiser A et al. Tc-99m mercaptoacetyltriglycine clearance: comparison of camera-assisted methods. Clin Nucl Med 2001; 26: 745–50.

67. Taylor A Jr, Manatunga A, Morton K et al. Multicenter trial validation of a camera-based method to measure Tc-99m mercaptoacetyltriglycine, or Tc-99m MAG3, clearance. Radiology 1997; 204: 47–54.

68. Inoue Y, Ohtake T, Homma Y et al. Evaluation of glomerular filtration rate by camera-based method in both children and adults. J Nucl Med 1998; 39: 1784–8.

69. Zhao C, Shuke N, Okizaki A et al. Optimization of the uptake method for estimating renal clearance of 99mTc mercaptoacetyltriglycine. Nucl Med Commun 2004; 25: 159–66.

70. Rutland M, Que L, Hassan IM. 'FUR' – one size suits all. Eur J Nucl Med 2000; 27: 1708–13.

71. Peters AM, Henderson BL, Lui D. Comparison between terminal slope rate constant and 'slope/intercept' as measures of glomerular filtration rate using the single-compartment simplification. Eur J Nucl Med 2001; 28: 320–6.

72. Piepsz A, Ham HR. How good is the slope of the second exponential for estimating 51Cr-EDTA renal clearance? Nucl Med Commun 1997; 18: 139–41.

73. Cole BR, Giangiacomo J, Ingelfinger JR, Robson AM. Measurement of renal function without urine collection. A critical evaluation of the constant-infusion technic for determination of inulin and para-aminohippurate. N Engl J Med 1972; 287: 1109–14.

74. van Guldener C, Gans RO, ter Wee PM. Constant infusion clearance is an inappropriate method for accurate assessment of an impaired glomerular filtration rate. Nephrol Dial Transplant 1995; 10: 47–51.

75. Peters AM, Gordon I, Sixt R. Normalization of glomerular filtration rate in children: body surface area, body weight or extracellular fluid volume? J Nucl Med 1994; 35: 438–44.

76. Peters AM. Expressing glomerular filtration rate in terms of extracellular fluid volume. Nephrol Dial Transplant 1992; 7: 205–10.

77. Ham HR, De Sadeleer C, Hall M, Piepsz A. Which single blood sample method should be used to estimate 51Cr-EDTA clearance in adolescents? Nucl Med Commun 2004; 25: 155–7.

78. Levey AS, Greene T, Kusek JW, Beck GJ. A simplified equation to predict glomerular filtration rate from serum creatinine. J Am Soc Nephrol 2000; 11: A0828.

2 Assessment of GFR: chemical techniques and prediction equations

Joseph V Nally

Introduction

The kidney plays a vital role in maintaining total body homeostasis by having both excretory and endocrine functions. The excretory functions are more readily recognized as the kidney rids the body of potential uremic toxins and maintains vascular volume, critical fluid–electrolyte and acid–base balance. The kidney also plays an endocrine role related to the production of such important hormones as renin, 1,25 vitamin D, erythropoietin, etc. Overall, the level of the glomerular filtration rate (GFR) is generally accepted as the best index for the complex functions of the kidney in health and disease.

The Kidney Disease Outcome Quality Initiative (K/DOQI) of the National Kidney Foundation was established to define and classify chronic kidney disease (CKD) to assist the clinician in earlier recognition and treatment of CKD and its complications. These K/DOQI clinical practice guidelines identified GFR as the keystone for the definition and staging of CKD. Table 2.1 lists the two general criteria for defining CKD.[1] In brief, CKD is defined as kidney damage manifest by abnormal renal pathology, urinalysis (albuminuria/haematuria), renal imaging studies or abnormal blood work. In addition, CKD may be defined as a reduction of GFR less than 60 ml/min for at least 3 months – with or without obvious kidney damage. Table 2.2 lists the stages of CKD based upon level of GFR.[1]

Table 2.1 Definition of chronic kidney disease (CKD)

Structural or functional abnormalities of the kidneys for ≥ 3 months, as manifested by either:

1. Kidney damage, with or without decreased GFR, as defined by:
   a. pathologic abnormalities
   b. markers of kidney damage, including abnormalities in the composition of the blood or urine or abnormalities in imaging tests

2. GFR <60 ml/min/1.73 m^2, with or without kidney damage

Table 2.2 Staging of CKD

Stage	Description	GFR (ml/min/1.73 m^2)
1	Kidney damage with normal or increased GFR	>90
2	Mild decrease in GFR	60–89*
3	Moderate decrease in GFR	30–59
4	Severe decrease in GFR	15–29
5	Kidney failure	<15 or dialysis

*May be normal for age.

The K/DOQI report recommends that serum creatinine (SCr) and an estimated GFR (eGFR) derived from prediction equations be reported to the clinician. Hence, a detailed understanding of the methodologies to measure or estimate GFR is vital for today's clinician as GFR is the benchmark for defining and staging CKD.

In order to measure GFR, one must measure the clearance of an agent that is excreted via the kidney by GFR alone. It is important to recognize the characteristics of an ideal agent for measuring GFR. The agent should be safe, nontoxic, and freely filterable at the glomerulus without appreciable tubular reabsorption or secretion. The latter quality separates these GFR agents from effective renal plasma flow (FRPF) agents which are cleared via the kidney by both GFR and active tubular secretion. This chapter will focus on those methodologies that use chemical techniques for assaying those substances in blood and urine which measure or estimate GFR. The reader is referred to Chapter 3 which describes the radionuclide assessments of GFR.

Chemical techniques

Inulin

Inulin has long been regarded as the 'gold standard' of exogenously administered markers of GFR. However, its scarcity and high cost have greatly diminished its usefulness and it is now generally of historical interest only.

Inulin is a fructose polysaccharide (molecular weight 2200 Daltons) found in such tubers as the dahlia, the Jerusalem artichoke and chicory. It possesses the ideal characteristics of a GFR agent as it is inert, freely filtered at the glomerulus and neither reabsorbed nor secreted by the renal tubules. Inulin may be measured in plasma and urine by one of several colorometric assays.

Utilizing inulin to measure GFR was originally developed and championed in the 1930s by Homer Smith, the father of renal physiology.[2] The technique has been used by many investigators over the ensuing decades and has had little modification. The procedure uses a bolus and infusion technique in a water-loaded patient. Urinary clearance was calculated using three to five periods. The coefficient of variation between the clearance periods was 10% and coefficient of variation of inulin clearance measured on different days in the same patient approximate 7.5%.[3]

The urinary clearance techniques were both cumbersome and inconvenient. To avoid problems with collection and/or bladder catheter placement, many investigators turned to plasma disappearance technique using either constant infusion or bolus injection.[4] Nevertheless, the decline in the use of inulin as a GFR marker has been largely attributable to its scarcity, cost and cumbersome methodologies.

Iohexol

Given the difficulty and expense of measuring GFR using inulin infusion clearance techniques, radiological contrast media such as iothalamate diatrizoate and iohexol have been suggested as alternatives which can be measured using chemical techniques. These substances may serve well as GFR markers as they fulfil the ideal characteristics of such agents.

Iohexol has been introduced as nonionic low-osmolar radiologic contrast medium that can be analysed in serum by using HPLC and X-ray fluorescence (Renalyzer) techniques. Over the past two decades, these measurements have opened up the field for use of low-dose iohexol (i.e., 10 ml versus the traditional 100 ml for X-ray purposes) as a GFR marker.[5] Slow intravenous injection with a small dose of iohexol for a clearance procedure is not nephrotoxic as is the case of high-pressure injection of larger amounts of contrast. In a large study of nearly 4000 iohexol clearance measurements, few adverse reactions were noted.[6] Several investigators have found a good correlation with plasma clearance of iohexol with that of inulin, chromium EDTA and technetium DTPA.[7] Furthermore, Brown and O'Reilly made a detailed study utilizing bladder catheterization and the classical continuous infusion techniques and demonstrated an excellent correlation between the renal clearances of iohexol and inulin.[8] These techniques utilize the plasma disappearance methodologies of Brochner–Mortensen, using three to four plasma samples after injection.[9] Other investigators have also

demonstrated acceptable estimates of GFR using the single plasma sample model of Jacobson.[10]

In a cohort of patients with a wide range of kidney function (GFR 14–104 ml/min), Gaspari and colleagues demonstrated a high level of precision of the iohexol plasma disappearance technique using multiple plasma samples measured by HPLC.[11] Overall, the mean intra-individual coefficient of variation and reproducibility was 5.7 and 6.3% – even in patients with GFRs <40 ml/min. Swedish investigators studied iohexol plasma disappearance measured by X-ray fluorescent techniques using the single sample model of Jacobson in patients with renal disease. They concluded that single samples at 4 h for GFR >50 ml/min, 7 h for GFR 20–50 ml/min, and 24 h for GFR <20 ml/min gave values in good agreement with those based upon a four-sample slope clearance of iohexol.[10] In contrast to these patients with impaired kidney function, Australian investigators studied patients with diabetic nephropathy and preserved GFR and suggested that the Brochner–Mortensen modified one compartment model was preferred in patients with GFR >60 ml/min.[12]

In patients with GFR >40 ml/min, Cr^{51}-EDTA was compared to iohexol clearances using two different methods of iohexol analysis, HPLC and X-ray fluorescence, referring both to multisample and single-sample calculations.[7] The single- and multiple-point clearances determined by HPLC and X-ray fluorescence compared to Cr^{51}-EDTA correlated highly (R >0.92 in all). The authors concluded that iohexol and Cr^{51}-EDTA were comparable as GFR markers for multiple point clearance measurements. The single-sample method of GFR for patients with GFR >40 ml/min can be used with high accuracy. The precision and accuracy of X-ray fluorescence analysis of low concentrations of iohexol were less than the more costly HPLC analysis.

In aggregate, many clinical research centres throughout Europe favour the measurement of GFR using either the Cr^{51}-EDTA or iohexol plasma disappearance clearance techniques. Cost may be a factor in the measurement of the latter if the more precise and costly technique using HPLC is used.

Creatinine

SCr is the most widely used assay to measure the presence and progression of CKD.[13] The predictive equations for GFR are also critically dependent on the accuracy and reproducibility of the measurement of SCr.[14] Creatinine is derived from the metabolism of creatine in skeletal muscle. Creatinine is released into the circulation at a relatively constant rate and has a stable plasma concentration in the steady state. Endogenous creatinine production may vary with muscle mass, age, gender, ethnicity and nutritional status of the subject. As noted, creatinine is freely filtered by the glomeruli and it is neither reabsorbed nor metabolized by the renal tubular cells. However, 10–20% of urinary creatinine may be derived from tubular secretion from the proximal tubules by organic cation secretory mechanisms.

The most widely used assay to measure SCr is based on the modified kinetic Jaffe reaction. The Picric-acid–Jaffe reaction has been recognized as overestimating SCr in normal individuals by 20–30% relative to HPLC or mass spectroscopy measurements because of 'noncreatinine chromogens'.[15,16] In contrast, there is a negligible amount of 'noncreatinine chromogens' in urine – which might lead to an underestimate of the creatinine clearance. By coincidence, the overestimation of SCr due to 'noncreatinine chromogens' provides a nearly equal balance for the tubular secretion of creatinine such that the measured creatinine clearance is a good estimate of GFR in healthy subjects. In patients with progressive CKD, the tubular secretion of creatinine is more robust such that the creatinine clearance will overestimate GFR. SCr may be increased in selective circumstances which would not reflect a true reduction in GFR. Certain drugs (e.g., trimethoprim, cimetidine) may increase SCr by decreasing the tubular secretion of creatinine. Other substances or drugs may interfere with the alkaline-picric colorimetric assay as they are recognized as creatinine chromogens (e.g., acetoacetate in diabetic keto-acidosis, cefoxitin, flucytosine, etc.). Endogenous creatinine production may be increased in circumstances such as rhabdomyolysis or catabolic states which might increase SCr.

Precise measurement of SCr is critical in measuring or estimating GFR. Advances in clinical chemistry have led to the development of the modified kinetic rate Jaffe reaction and enzymatic methods which can be calibrated to avoid

measurement of 'noncreatinine chromogens.' In 1994, the College of the American Pathology (CAP) surveyed 700 laboratories and noted that the differences in calibration of SCr assays accounted for 85% of the difference between the SCr measurements.[17] The lab surveys overestimated SCr by 13–17% with considerable interlab variation.

In 2003, a similar survey by CAP of 5624 labs noted significant bias variability related to instrument manufacturer, rather than the type of alkaline picric acid or enzymatic methodologies.[18] In the USA, the National Institutes of Health (NIH)/National Kidney Disease Education Program (NKDEP) recommends that laboratories calibrate their SCr measurements to a Cleveland Clinic Lab standard as it has been the core Renal Function Laboratory in the development of the Modification of Diet in Renal Disease (MDRD) prediction equations for estimating GFR.[18] The precise measurement of SCr is crucial in estimating GFR using predictive equations as a small error in SCr may translate into a more substantial variability in GFR estimates.

Even if creatinine is measured accurately, both SCr and creatinine clearance have significant limitations in estimating true GFR. Equations based on SCr, age, gender and other variables perform much better at predicting GFR than SCr alone. Indeed, from the pioneering days of Homer Smith, the nonlinear (i.e., curvilinear) relationship between increasing SCr and falling GFR was recognized. Creatinine clearance was recognized as a better index of GFR because it takes into account the urinary creatinine which approximates the endogenous production of creatinine based upon muscle mass, age, gender and ethnicity. However, there are two

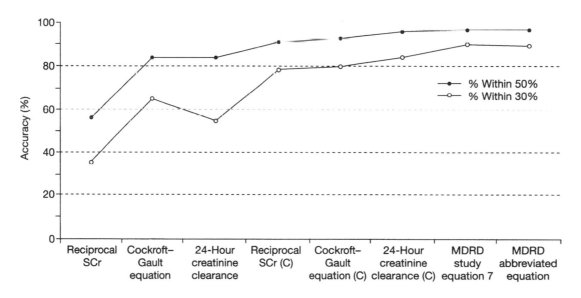

Figure 2.1 Accuracy of different estimates of GFR in adults, expressed as the percentage of estimates within 30% and 50% of the measured GFR in the MDRD Study validation sample (n = 558). Estimates denoted with [C] include a calibration correction of 0.69 for 100/serum creatinine, 0.84 for Cockcroft–Gault equation, and 0.81 for 24-hour creatinine clearance to show performance after bias is eliminated using a multiplicative correction factor. Analysis of MDRD study[14] data prepared by Tom Greene, Ph.D. With permission from reference 1.

major potential errors that limit the accuracy of creatinine clearance: (a) incomplete urine collection, (b) increasing tubular secretion of creatinine – especially with falling GFR – which may overestimate the true GFR. During the K/DOQI process, the investigators examined the accuracy of SCr, creatinine clearance, and the predictive equations vs measured I^{125} iothalamate GFR from the MDRD study cohort.[1] Results from that evaluation can be seen in Figure 2.1. Predictive equations were more reliable estimates of GFR than either SCr or creatinine clearance. Indeed, the day-to-day coefficient of variation of creatinine clearance has been reported as high as 27% by some investigators.[19] The K/DOQI guidelines recommend that a 24-hour urine for creatinine clearance is no longer suggested as an estimate of GFR.

Cystatin C

Given the limitations of SCr, serum cystatin C has been proposed as a screening test in an attempt to improve the detection of a reduction in GFR.[20] Cystatin C is a member of the family of cysteine proteinase inhibitors. It has a low molecular weight (13 kDa) and is produced at a constant rate by all nucleated cells. Cystatin C has been identified as a housekeeping gene whose constant production is independent of age, gender, muscle mass, etc. There are conflicting data as to whether its production may be variable in certain rare malignancies (e.g., metastatic melanoma or colon cancer). Cystatin C is freely filtered by the glomerulus, not secreted by the renal tubules, but is almost entirely reabsorbed and cannibalized by the proximal tubule. The latter characteristic negates the calculation of urinary clearance of cystatin C as a measure of GFR. Since it is completely filtered by the kidney, does not return to the bloodstream, and is not secreted by renal tubules, it has been proposed as an ideal endogenous marker of GFR.

The first radioimmunoassay (RIA) to quantify cystatin C in serum was developed in 1979. Subsequent methods to detect cystatin C were developed using radiofluorescent and enzymatic immunoassays. More recently, automated homogeneous immunoassays using latex or polystyrene particles coated with cystatin C antibodies have been developed and FDA approved.[21,22]

Multiple studies have validated the use of cystatin C as a 'renal marker' in adults, as serum cystatin C correlated with measurement of an impaired GFR. In a recent review, the authors analysed 24 studies that examined the utility of cystatin C versus SCr for detecting an impairment of GFR (usually GFR of less than 80 ml/min, range 60–90 ml/min).[20] Fifteen studies concluded that cystatin C was superior to SCr and nine studies suggested equivalence. In aggregate, these studies consistently demonstrated that cystatin C performed at least as well as SCr as a 'renal marker in adults, in pediatric patients above the age of four, and in selected renal transplant patients'. Importantly, it must be recognized that these initial

studies of cystatin C as a 'marker' of GFR were generally trying to distinguish between 'normal' GFR (greater than 80 ml/min) versus 'impaired' GFR. Cystatin C often had a better diagnostic sensitivity, specificity, negative predictive value and ROC curves than SCr in an adult population for identifying a patient with impaired GFR.[23] However, measurement of serum cystatin C as a *direct* quantification or estimate of GFR has not been well studied. The utility of cystatin C in formulating prediction equations – especially in patients with GFRs greater than 60 – is currently under investigation. Overall, the recent literature suggests that cystatin C may have a role in assessing kidney function in selected patient groups for whom the disadvantages of SCr have become apparent.

Prediction equations

The overall goal of the NKF's K/DOQI Clinical Practice Guidelines was to develop a standard definition and staging of CKD to assist the clinician in early recognition and treatment of CKD and its complications. The Clinical Practice Guidelines recommend GFR as the keystone for the definition and staging of CKD. Given the limitations of SCr and creatinine clearance, the K/DOQI guidelines recommended predictive equations for the estimation (not precise measurement) of GFR based upon SCr measurements. In children, the Schwartz[24] and Counahan–Baratt[25] equations are recommended. For adults the guidelines recommend two formulae: (1) Cockroft–Gault equation, and (2) the abbreviated MDRD study equation. The equations are defined as follows:

Cockroft–Gault:[26]
CCr (ml/min) = (140 – age) × lean body weight (kg)/pCr (mg/dl) × 72

MDRD abbreviated formula:[1]
GFR (ml/min/1.73 m²) = 186.3 × ((SCr) exp [–1.154]) × (age exp [–0.203]) × (0.762 if female) × (1.180 if African American)

Given the greater likelihood of the MDRD equation predicting iothalamate measured GFR, the guidelines favoured the use of the abbreviated MDRD equation in the clinical practice of adult medicine (see Figure 2.1). K/DOQI authors defined the 'accuracy' of eGFR as the percentage of eGFR estimates within 30% of the measured iothalamate GFR (iGFR). In adults, the abbreviated MDRD formula performed better than the Cockcroft–Gault (CG) equation with only 10% of the eGFR falling outside of the 30% accuracy range.

It is critical to appreciate the limitations of the eGFR derived from the predictive equation. First and foremost, one must recognize that these predictive equations are creatinine-based *estimates* (not measurements) of GFR recommended

Figure 2.2 Association of estimated GFR with measured iGFR in outpatients with CKD (circles) and potential kidney donors (squares). Panel A shows the association of iGFR with eGFR-MDRD and panel B with eGFR-CG. Dotted lines subclassify the GFRs based on K/DOQI stages. EGFR is plotted on the horizontal axis and iGFR on the vertical axis. With permission from reference 27.

Secondly, it is also important to recognize that the abbreviated MDRD equation was derived from a stable, outpatient CKD population of approximately 500 patients with iothalamate-measured GFRs ranging from 15–90 ml/min. Hence, the MDRD equation might be expected to provide an adequate estimate of GFR in a clinically similar patient population, but one must not erroneously conclude that the MDRD equation is valid across all patient populations. Recent studies from CCF suggest that the former statement is indeed true at our institution.[27] In comparing eGFRs (MDRD and CG) to iGFR in a stable, outpatient CKD population with GFRs from 15–60 ml/min, a strong performance was noted between eGFR (MDRD) and iGFR; whereas, the performance of eGFR (CG) with iGFR was less robust (Figure 2.2).[27] These findings were applicable in both diabetic and nondiabetic CKD patients. An analysis by these same investigators in stable renal transplant recipients yielded similar observations.[28] In contrast, these investigators report that an eGFR (both MDRD and CG) overestimate iGFR in a hospitalized patient population with stable creatinine.[29] Importantly, they also report that eGFR derived from the MDRD equation is inaccurate in individuals with normal or near normal renal function. Even with reliable calibration, minor imprecision in lower SCr measurements may result in significant variation in eGFRs causing a lack of precision and accuracy of eGFR in a healthy population. Hence, estimating GFR with the MDRD equation in potential renal transplant donors or in patients with early nephropathy (i.e., diabetic hyperfiltration) does not appear to be warranted.

Finally, given the lack of precision of the eGFR, two other considerations are worth noting. First, certain other clinical circumstances exist whereby a patient does not conform to the MDRD study population based upon extremes of age, size, nutrition or comorbid diseases (Table 2.3). In such circumstances, the reliability of eGFR determination is uncertain and a formal *measure* of GFR may be indicated. Secondly, the lack of precision of eGFR, even in appropriate MDRD cohorts, dictates that the eGFR would be an inappropriate clinical tool to measure *precise* reductions in GFR in clinical research trials.

for clinical practice. The predictive equations are based upon SCr and selected variables of endogenous creatinine production such as age, body size, gender, ethnicity, etc. A precise, reproducible measurement of SCr is essential for the eGFR from the predictive equations. As noted previously, the ACP survey reported considerable interlab variations with overestimate of SCr by 13–17% attributable to imprecise creatinine calibrations.[17] For example, creatinine on the same samples were 0.23 mg % higher at the White Sands Laboratory (NHANES III) than the Cleveland Clinic Foundation (CCF) Laboratory (MDRD study), even though both labs used the Jaffe-based methodology.[16] In the USA, the NIH/NKDEP recommended that the labs calibrate their SCr to a standard at the CCF's Lab (MDRD study site) to improve precision in this important determination.

'Which test for which patient?'

In attempting to answer this question, one must define the primary objective regarding the measurement of kidney function. Is the test going to be applied in clinical practice in which an estimate of GFR is adequate? Or, is a precise measurement of GFR required in a clinical research study? In answering these questions, one must balance the accuracy and precision of a test against the important issues of cost and patient convenience (see Table 2.3). As a clinical nephrologist with an interest in clinical research design and analysis, I would offer the following perspective.

Table 2.3 Accuracy, precision, convenience and cost of GFR measurements

Methods	Accuracy	Precision	Convenience	Cost
Inulin clearance	*****	*****	*	N/A
Creatinine				
Serum creatinine	*	*	****	*****
24-h urinary clearance	**	**	*	****
Estimated GFR				
Adults				
CG	***	***	****	*****
MDRD	****	****	****	*****
Children				
Schwartz	****	****	****	*****
Serum cystatin C	****	****	****	***
Iohexol clearance				
HPLC	*****	*****	*	*
X-ray fluorescence	*****	*****	*	**

Clinical practice

Currently, SCr is the most widely used assay worldwide to measure the presence and progression of CKD. However, it is an imprecise measurement of GFR because it does not account for the important variables such as age, gender and ethnicity as they have an impact upon muscle mass and creatinine production. Given this imprecision, the authors of K/DOQI recommend the use of prediction equations for an estimate of GFR. The report recognizes either the MDRD abbreviated equation or the Cockcroft–Gault equation to estimate GFR. Since the detailed report identified less variability with the former, the abbreviated MDRD equation is generally recommended. After a thorough review, the National Institute of Diabetes & Digestive & Kidney Diseases (NIDDK) recommends that clinical laboratories report both the SCr and the estimated GFR (eGFR) to the clinician. This recommendation has been instituted at many leading institutions and commercial laboratories throughout the United States. Given the variability of the estimated GFR in patients with normal kidney function, the NIDDK recommends the

Table 2.4 Clinical situation in which clearance measures may be necessary to estimate GFR

Extremes of age and body size
Severe malnutrition or obesity
Disease of skeletal muscle
Paraplegia or quadriplegia
Vegetarian diet
Rapidly changing kidney function
Liver disease
Prior to dosing drugs with significant toxicity that are excreted
  by the kidneys

eGFR be classified as greater than 60 ml/min, 59–30 ml/min (stage 3 CKD), 29–15 ml/min (stage 4 CKD) and less than 15 ml/min (stage 5 CKD).

In which patient population might eGFR be subject to error? In general, the eGFRs are best applied to stable, CKD patients with expected GFRs between 15–60 ml/min. Implicit in the application of these equations is that the patient must be in the steady state. Application of the eGFR from prediction equations to those patients in a nonsteady state such as acute renal failure is unwarranted. Moreover, special clinical circumstances in 'at-risk' patients (see Table 2.4) will require direct measurement of GFR as the eGFR is unreliable at the extremes of age, weight, malnutrition, liver disease, etc. Furthermore, the MDRD predictive equations were derived from a stable outpatient CKD population. Hence, eGFR is not applicable to a hospitalized population.[27] Finally, estimates of GFR using the MDRD equation are not reliable in patients with near-normal kidney function. Thus, one could not rely upon the eGFR to evaluate potential renal donors or those with early diabetic nephropathy to assess hyperfiltration. New predictive equations using statin C measurements may prove to have clinical utility in these two patient populations in the future.

Clinical research protocols

In order to select the appropriate test for assessing kidney function, one again must address the accuracy of the measurements required. Two general scenarios might be considered.

First, if accurate measurements of GFR over a specified time are required per protocol to identify a renal outcome, then a precise *measurement* of GFR must be used. In clinical trials in the USA, I^{125}iothalamate clearance has been the test of choice; whereas, either Cr^{51}-ETDA or iohexol clearances are the preferred methodologies in Europe. All three methods have been validated against the gold standard of formal inulin urinary clearances and are deemed to be accurate.

Second, if long-term clinical trials in patients with CKD are designed in which the primary clinical outcomes might be related to overall progression of CKD, ESRD, renal transplantation or death, then it may be appropriate to use estimates of GFR. As opposed to the latter three clinical endpoints, the progression of CKD might be defined as a >50% reduction of eGFR. This definition would correlate with the outcome of doubling of SCr used in such pivotal trials as the Captopril Type I Diabetic Nephropathy trial,[30] or the Type II Diabetic Nephropathy Trials using angiotensin II receptor blockers.[31] Utilization of the less precise eGFR in such a clinical trial could result in significant cost savings as compared to using formal GFR methodologies. Furthermore, estimates of GFR have been utilized in some large population studies to estimate risk or outcomes based upon baseline kidney function. For example, stratification of patients by eGFR in over one million patients within the Kaiser Permanente Health Care Plan in northern California demonstrated significant increases in death, cardiovascular mortality and hospitalizations, with lower baseline eGFRs. Similarly, baseline eGFRs in a Veteran's Administration database of nearly 20 000 patients undergoing revascularization of the lower extremities demonstrated postoperative morbidity and mortality increased in patients with lower baseline eGFRs.

In summary, the clinician or the clinical investigator must balance the accuracy and precision of an assessment of kidney function vs. that of patient convenience and cost to select the most appropriate measure of kidney function for their patient population under surveillance.

References

1. K/DOQI clinical practice guidelines for chronic kidney disease: evaluation, classification, and stratification. Kidney Disease Outcome Quality Initiative. Am J Kidney Dis 2002; 39(Suppl 2): S1–246.

2. Kasiske BL, Keane WF. Laboratory assessment of renal disease: clearance, urinalysis and renal biopsy. In: Brenner BM, Rector FC (eds). The Kidney, Vol. 1, 6th edn. Philadelphia: WB Saunders, 2000: 1129–70.

3. Levey AS. Use of glomerular filtration rate measurements to assess the progression of renal disease. Semin Nephrol 1989; 9: 370–9.

4. Florijn KW, Barendregt JN, Lentjes EG et al. Glomerular filtration rate measurement by 'single-shot' injection of inulin. Kidney Int 1994; 46: 252–9.

5. Blaufox MD, Aurell M, Bubeck B et al. Report of the Radionuclides in Nephrourology Committee on renal clearance. J Nucl Med 1996; 37: 1883–90.

6. Nilsson-Ehle P, Grubb A. New markers for the determination of GFR: iohexol clearance and cystatin C serum concentration. Kidney Int Suppl 1994; 47: S17–S19.

7. Brandstrom E, Grzegorczyk A, Jacobsson L et al. GFR measurement with iohexol and 51Cr-EDTA. A comparison of the two favoured GFR markers in Europe. Nephrol Dial Transplant 1998; 13: 1176–82.

8. Brown SCW, O'Reilly PH. Iohexol clearance for the determination of glomerular filtration rate in clinical practice: evidence for a new gold standard. J Urol 1991; 146: 675–9.

9. Brochner-Mortensen J, Jensen S, Rodbro P. Delimitation of plasma creatinine concentration values for assessment of relative renal function in adult patients. Scand J Urol Nephrol 1977; 11: 257–62.

10. Sterner G, Frennby B, Hultberg B, Almen T. Iohexol clearance for GFR-determination in renal failure – single or multiple plasma sampling? Nephrol Dial Transplant 1996; 11: 521–5.

11. Gaspari F, Perico N, Matalone M et al. Precision of plasma clearance of iohexol for estimation of GFR in patients with renal disease. J Am Soc Nephrol 1998; 9: 310–13.

12. Houlihan C, Jenkins M, Osicka T et al. A comparison of the plasma disappearance of iohexol and 99mTc-DTPA for the measurement of glomerular filtration rate (GFR) in diabetes. Aust NZ J Med 1999; 29: 693–700.

13. Levey AS. Measurement of renal function in chronic renal disease. Kidney Int 1990; 38: 167–84.

14. Levey AS, Bosch JP, Lewis JB et al. A more accurate method to estimate glomerular filtration rate from serum creatinine: a new prediction equation. Modification of Diet in Renal Disease Study Group. Ann Intern Med 1999; 130: 461–70.

15. Perrone RD, Madias NE, Levey AS. Serum creatinine as an index of renal function: new insights into old concepts. Clin Chem 1992; 38: 1933–53.

16. Coresh J, Toto RD, Kirk KA et al. Creatinine clearance as a measure of GFR in screenees for the African-American Study of Kidney Disease and Hypertension pilot study. Am J Kidney Dis 1998; 32: 32–42.

17. Ross JW, Miller WG, Myers GL, Praestgaard J. The accuracy of laboratory measurements in clinical chemistry: a study of 11 routine chemistry analytes in the College of American Pathologists Chemistry Survey with fresh frozen serum, definitive methods, and reference methods. Arch Pathol Lab Med 1998; 122: 587–608.

18. Miller WG, Myers GL, Ashwood ER et al. Creatinine measurement: State of the art in accuracy and interlaboratory harmonizations. Arch Pathol Lab Med 2005; 129: 297–304.

19. Walser M. Assessing renal function from creatinine measurements in adults with chronic renal failure. Am J Kidney Dis 1998; 32: 23–31.

20. Laterza OF, Price CP, Scott MG. Cystatin C: an improved estimator of glomerular filtration rate? Clin Chem 2002; 48: 699–707.

21. Newman DJ, Thakkar H, Edwards RG et al. Serum cystatin C

measured by automated immunoassay: a more sensitive marker of changes in GFR than serum creatinine. Kidney Int 1995; 47: 312–18.

22. Finney H, Newman DJ, Gruber W et al. Initial evaluation of cystatin C measurement by particle-enhanced immunonephelometry on the Behring nephelometer systems (BNA, BN II). Clin Chem 1997; 43(Pt 1): 1016–22.

23. Herget-Rosenthal S, Trabold S, Pietruck F et al. Cystatin C: efficacy as screening test for reduced glomerular filtration rate. Am J Nephrol 2000; 20: 97–102.

24. Schwartz GJ, Haycock GB, Edelmann CM Jr, Spitzer A. A simple estimate of glomerular filtration rate in children derived from body length and plasma creatinine. Pediatrics 1976; 58: 259–63.

25. Counahan R, Chantler C, Ghazali S et al. Estimation of glomerular filtration rate from plasma creatinine concentration in children. Arch Dis Child 1976; 51: 875–8.

26. Cockcroft DW, Gault MH. Prediction of creatinine clearance from serum creatinine. Nephron 1976; 16: 31–41.

27. Poggio ED, Wang X, Greene T et al. Performance of the MDRD and Cockcroft-Gault equations in the estimation of glomerular filtration rate in health and in chronic kidney disease. J Am Soc Nephrol 2005; 16: 459–66.

28. Weinstein DM, Augustine JJ, Poggio ED et al. Reliability of the MDRD equation and Cockcroft–Gault in estimating glomerular filtration rate in kidney transplant patients [Abstract]. J Am Soc Nephrol 2003; 14: 435A.

29. Poggio ED, Nef PC, Wong X et al. Performance of the Cockcroft–Gault and MDRD equations in estimating GFR in ill hospitalized patients. Am Kid Dis 2005; 46: 242–52.

30. Lewis EJ, Hunsicker LG, Bain RP, Rhode RD, for the Collaborative Study Group. The effect of angiotensin-converting-enzyme inhibition on diabetic nephropathy. N Engl J Med 1993; 329: 1456–62.

31. Parving HH, Lehnert H, Brochner-Mortensen J et al. The effect of irbesartan on the development of diabetic nephropathy in patients with type 2 diabetes. N Engl J Med 2001; 345: 870–8.

32. Hostetter TH. Chronic kidney disease predicts cardiovascular disease. N Engl J Med 2004; 351: 1344–6.

33. Go AS, Chertow GM, Fan D et al. Chronic kidney disease and the risks of death, cardiovascular events, and hospitalization. N Engl J Med 2004; 351: 1296–305.

3 Measurements of renal function with radionuclide techniques in adults

Emmanuel Durand

Introduction

Assessing such a basic physiological parameter as renal function is not straightforward. Biochemical techniques are easy to use, but they are not reliable in all circumstances. Radio-isotope techniques, either urinary or plasmatic, are presented here. The points addressed comply with the international consensus published in 1996,[1] which is still up to date.

When using any method to measure a physiological parameter, one aims at getting the 'true value'. The first question to answer here is, what is renal function?. This point has already been addressed in Chapter 1: most renal diseases affect both glomerules and tubules, though decoupling may rarely occur. As no ideal tracer provides a precise assessment of tubular function, it is widely considered that renal function is best assessed by glomerular filtration rate (GFR), on which this text focuses. Measuring renal plasma flow (RPF) instead has two drawbacks: first, the tracers used measure effective RPF (ERPF), which is RPF multiplied by extraction fraction (EF); as EF varies in many circumstances, there is no way to determine RPF. Second, even RPF varies much more than GFR under physiological circumstances; indeed, RPF can be considered as an input function to kidneys but it is not a function by itself. For all these reasons, it is probably not a good parameter to measure.[2]

The second question is, how we can assess whether a method gives 'true values', assuming that it can be compared to a gold standard? In fact, there are two answers because two types of errors can be encountered. A method that is 'biased' will give systematic errors so that the average values will not match the reference; such a method may be defined as inaccurate. A method that has strong fluctuations will give variable errors so that the average values might match the reference, but with a wide scattering around the central value; such a method may be defined as 'imprecise'. A good method must therefore be both 'accurate' and 'precise'. (Note that the meaning of accuracy here is different from the definition used by the K/DOQI guidelines referred to in Chapter 1.) Robustness has a slightly different meaning: a method is said to be robust when conditions outside the nominal ones (e.g. sampling errors, time errors, extravasation) result in only small errors.

The purpose of this text is to present the various techniques that can be used to determine the absolute renal function, namely GFR. The relative renal function, namely the percentage of function performed by each kidney, can be determined accurately by means of a gamma-camera.[2,3] Finally, to determine the individual function, one needs both absolute GFR, as presented here, and a gamma-camera study.

Renal tracers

As stated in Chapter 2, renal plasma flow varies physiologically over many situations. Also, it can only be estimated – not measured – by tubular tracers. Therefore, only glomerular tracers will be addressed here.

To measure glomerular filtration, glomerular tracers are needed, i.e. tracers that are freely filtered, without protein binding, nor secretion, nor reabsorption. The gold standard for glomerular filtration is inulin, which is not radioactive (at least for human use). However, inulin is not widely available because it is no longer authorized for human use in any country; also, its dosage is hampered by strong interferences. Radiotracers have the advantage of both easy and reliable dosage and lack of toxicity.

The most common glomerular tracers are detailed in Table 3.1. Among radiotracers, ^{51}Cr-EDTA is considered the most reliable, with pure glomerular filtration, a high and stable (both in vitro and in vivo) labelling yield and only little protein binding. However, it is not available in any country. EDTA has a low and constant extrarenal clearance of ca. 4 ml/min; its urinary clearance underestimates inulin clearance by about 5% (probably because of its anionic charge). These two small biases compensate and, as a whole, EDTA plasma clearance matches inulin urinary clearance quite well.[4] Typical activity for a clearance is 7 MBq.

DTPA also has good characteristics but protein binding should be checked because contradictory studies were published, probably depending on the brand used.[5–8] It is suitable for imaging, so it makes it possible to assess both absolute (by clearance) and relative (by means of a gamma-camera) renal function with a single tracer. Typical activity is

Table 3.1 Glomerular radiotracers

		Labelling	MW	Filtration fraction	Secretion	Extraction coefficient	Protein binding
DTPA	Diethylene pentacetic acid	^{99m}Tc ^{169}Yb ^{113m}In ^{140}La	393 D	15–20%	–	15–20%	0–10%
EDTA	Ethylene-diamine-tetraacetic acid Iothalamate	^{51}Cr ^{125}I ^{131}I COLD	292 D 614 D	15–20% 15–20%	– 10–20%	15–20%	<5% 4–25%
	Diatrizoate	^{125}I	636 D	15–20%	–		

10 MBq for clearance but if imaging is performed, the activity should be much higher.

Diatrizoate is less commonly used but it is a valuable alternative. Conversely, iothalamate is not only filtered but also secreted. Its protein binding roughly cancels the effect of secretion so, even if it is only a second choice tracer, it is acceptable to determine GFR.

Methods

The clearance can be determined either by the plasma disappearance (then called plasma clearance), by the kidney uptake or by the elimination in the urine (then called urinary clearance).

Urinary clearance

Theory

Urinary clearance is sometimes called renal clearance. (Note that though urinary and renal clearances are the same for perfect glomerular tracers, it is not the case for all tracers, e.g. DMSA has a urinary clearance that is only about one quarter that of its whole renal clearance.) The clearance is defined as the imaginary plasma flow that is totally clear of tracer. The urinary clearance C can therefore be calculated as the urinary flow scaled to plasma by the urinary-to-plasma concentration ratio:

$$C = \frac{U}{P} \times V = \frac{U \times V}{P} \qquad (1)$$

where V is the urinary flow and U and P are the urinary and plasmatic concentrations of tracer, respectively. If the renal

blood flow is F, the amount of tracer extracted per unit of time is given by:

$$UV = F(P_A - P_V) \qquad (2)$$

where P_A and P_V are the arterial and venous concentrations of the tracer, respectively. The extraction coefficient, defined as the ratio of the arterio-venous difference to the arterial concentration:

$$E = \frac{P_A - P_V}{P_A} \qquad (3)$$

characterizes the ability of an organ to take up a substance. From (1), (2) and (3), it follows that the clearance is:

$$C = EF \qquad (4)$$

The clearance is therefore the product of the input function to the kidney (namely the plasma flow F) and the extraction rate E, which characterizes the kidney efficiency. This is why clearance is a good parameter for the function of perfused kidney. It works as if the role of the kidneys were to extract inulin (or any glomerular tracer) from the plasma. One should, however, keep in mind that it is only a means to quantify the function and that the real role of the kidneys is to regulate the body fluids'.

Plasma flow varies more than clearance and regulation processes ensure that over a wide range, variations of plasma flow F are compensated by opposite variations of the extraction coefficient E.

According to equation (1), for a reliable measurement of clearance, one must assume that both the clearance and the plasma concentration do not vary over the time of measurement. Though GFR has some variations over the nycthemeral cycle, they can be considered to be slight and slow enough compared to the sampling periods. So as not to induce additional variation, it is recommended that the subject does not eat meat nor undertake heavy exercise before or during the test. To keep variations on P as low as possible, two protocols can be used:

- either a single intravenous injection followed by plasma sampling and urine collection over short timed periods (P should then not vary much during this period);
- or a continuous infusion where P reaches a plateau.

A simplified alternative to the latter is to use a subcutaneous injection; most often using iothalamate. Variations on the urinary flow V and, as a consequence, on the urinary concentration U are not a problem because no bias is induced when considering the integrated urinary sample as a whole.

As urinary clearance techniques reflect only the kidneys, these techniques have an excellent accuracy. However, reliable urine sampling is not easy and it is important to be aware that the reference method should be to catheterize the bladder, rinse it with serum after voiding and chase the rest of urine by air insufflation. This is quite invasive and hardly ever done. As a consequence, urine clearance techniques are imprecise. To improve precision, the sampling should be repeated during the test and the calculated values averaged over every period.

For DTPA, it was also suggested to monitor voiding by the means of a gamma-camera and to make correction for residual activity in the bladder.[9] All these techniques also neglect the transit time (intrarenal and ureteral). In practice, this assumption is valid except during the first minutes of the test.

Bolus-injection, urinary clearance

For this technique, GFR is determined over several periods by formula (1) while sampling both plasma and urine. The final result is given by the average of GFR values calculated for each period. The following recommendations apply:

- the patient should be at relative rest, not undertaking heavy exercise;
- the patient should not eat meat just before or during the test;
- the patient should be well hydrated to ensure a good urinary flow (i.e. 7–10 ml/kg body weight initially then compensating urinary flow);
- urinary flow should be checked aiming for at least 3 ml/min; periods with a urinary flow under 1 ml/min should be discarded;
- the injection is usually performed intravenously, as a bolus; no calibration is required; in fact, any injection scheme can be used, so extravasation, if any, is not a problem for the reliability of the determination;
- urine should be collected over several (at least three) timed periods (typically 30–60 minutes); voiding should be complete;
- plasma sampling should be obtained around the middle of each period (see Figure 3.1).

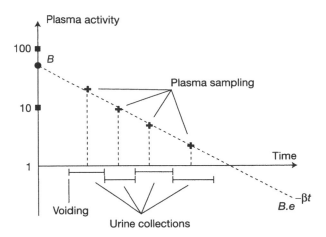

Figure 3.1 While activity is decreasing, plasma samples are taken around the middle of the urine collections.

The reproducibility of GFR between periods gives an idea of the final precision.

Continuous-infusion, urinary clearance

For this technique, the plasma concentration is made more stable. The principle is in fact exactly the same as for bolus injection, but for the injection scheme tracer is infused intravenously at a constant rate by means of a pump. It is more cumbersome but it has an advantage over the single-shot technique: the assumption that P is constant during the sampling periods is more realistic; this improves precision and also baseline and test condition studies (q.v.) are made easier. The details of this technique are described hereafter.

Plasma clearance

To avoid urine sampling, which is time-consuming and imprecise, one can make the assumption that the plasma disappearance perfectly matches urinary appearance. To gain precision, one then loses accuracy because extrarenal clearance may make this assumption invalid. However, in practice, the glomerular tracers used have only a very small extrarenal clearance so plasma clearances perform very well, except for very low GFR or in cases of oedema or ascites where the extrarenal clearance can no longer be neglected in comparison with GFR.

Continuous-infusion, plasma clearance

The principle of this technique is the same as for urinary clearance, except that the output urinary flow $U \times V$ is estimated from the pump flow, hereafter referred to as R. This assumption is reasonable when the tracer is at a steady-state, i.e. when the plasma concentration has reached a plateau. At this time, the input R is perfectly compensated by the output UV. The clearance is then simply given by:

$$C = \frac{R}{P} \qquad (5)$$

The general principle is therefore to sample plasma until a plateau is reached and then to determine the plateau level P. The pump should be calibrated in flow and, most importantly, have a constant flow. The specific activity of the infused solution should be determined. To save time in reaching the plateau, a priming activity is injected as a bolus before infusion. The following recommendations apply:

- no special hydration (avoid dehydration);
- prepare a solution of tracer diluted in glucose solution (5%), typically 500 ml;
- determine the product of the specific activity of the solution and the pump flow by 'infusing' several (typically four) counting tubes with a typical volume of 3 ml given by the pump;
- priming activity (suggested 22 kBq/kg BW);
- infusion with a precision pump (suggested at 7 kBq/ (ml/min GFR) as predicted by creatinine);
- start plasma sampling after 90 minutes, continue at least 4 h, typically with a plasma sample every hour; note that no special care on time is required because only the value of the plateau is sought.

As an example, if the standard counting tubes (3 ml) give 300 000 cpm, the specific activity of the solution is 100 000 cpm/ml. If the infusion rate is 30 ml/h (0.5 ml/min), the activity is infused at a rate R = 50 000 cpm/min. If the plateau is measured at 500 cpm/ml in plasma, the final clearance is:

$$C = \frac{R}{P} = \frac{50\ 000\ \text{cpm/min}}{500\ \text{cpm/ml}} = 100\ \text{ml/min} \qquad (6)$$

This technique has several advantages, the first of which is that nearly no methodological error is possible. It is therefore very robust. It also provides good precision and makes baseline and test condition studies possible. For this, the baseline clearance is determined, then a new plateau is sought after the stimulation.

The drawbacks are that the patient must stay at least 4 h with the infusion line and that potential impurities may accumulate over time in the plasma and bias the method. Also, due to less-permeable compartments, plasma clearance may overestimate urinary clearance.[10] It is frequently considered to be cumbersome; however, it requires no precise time determination and the calibration of the injected activity is made much easier and more reliable than for single-shot plasma clearance. Finally, in our institution, trained nurses consider it no more demanding than single-shot techniques.

Bolus-injection, plasma clearance

This technique, the most widely used, comes last because its theory is more complex. Reordering equation (1) and making it time-dependent results in:

$$C \times P(t) = U(t) \times V(t) \qquad (7)$$

After integration:

$$C \int_0^\infty P = \int_0^\infty UV \qquad (8)$$

Considering that there is no extrarenal clearance, the total activity found in urine corresponds to the injected activity Q:

$$\int_0^\infty UV = Q \qquad (9)$$

Therefore:

$$C = \frac{Q}{\int_0^\infty P} \qquad (10)$$

The plasma clearance is therefore the ratio of the injected activity to the integral of the plasmatic concentration over time, i.e. the area under the plasma–time activity curve. Both these values must be determined.

Determining the area under the plasma–time activity curve

The continuous plasma–time activity curve needs to be sampled. To interpolate between the sampling points and to extrapolate to the infinite, a mathematical model is required. Compartmental theory indicates that in many cases, the sum of two exponentials is a good model:

$$P(t) = A \times e^{-\alpha t} + B \times e^{-\beta t} \qquad (11)$$

The clearance is then:[11]

$$C = \frac{Q}{\dfrac{A}{\alpha} + \dfrac{B}{\beta}} \qquad (12)$$

The function described in equation (11) has four parameters. A theoretical minimum of four blood samples is therefore necessary to assess it. In practice, because of statistical errors, at least six to eight samples should be taken between 5 and 10 minutes and several hours after injection.

To alleviate the burden of many samples, many simplified techniques were proposed. Instead of using a model with two exponentials, one possibility is to consider only the late exponential (the first one corresponds to the time to nearly reach a steady-state between plasma and interstitial fluid). For this, sampling must start after 90 min and only two samples are necessary (more can be done). The model for the plasma time–activity curve becomes:

$$P(t) = B \times e^{-\beta t} \tag{13}$$

The clearance is then:

$$C = \frac{Q\beta}{B} \tag{14}$$

Neglecting the first exponential induces an underestimation of the area under $P(t)$ and, therefore, an overestimation of the clearance. To compensate for it, Chantler[4,12] proposed using a linear correction (note that Chantler's and Brochner–Mortensen coefficients are different for children):

$$C = \frac{Q\beta}{B} \times 0.93 \tag{15}$$

However, the area due to the first exponential is fairly constant, whatever the GFR, so the relative error is more important for high GFR (when the area is small). To take this into account, Brochner–Mortensen[13] introduced a parabolic correction, which has to be applied after scaling by BSA:

$$C_{corrected} = 0.99 \times C - 0.0012 \times C^2 \tag{16}$$

$$\text{where } C - \frac{Q\beta}{B} \times \frac{1.73 \ m^2}{BSA}$$

However, this parabolic correction is not suitable for determining very high clearances in hyperfiltration. Indeed, this formula intrinsically precludes finding any value over 204 ml/min. Even if such values are clearly outside usual ones, this strongly suggests that extrapolation with this formula deviates from true GFR for high values.

A variant of this method was proposed by Russell using two samples:[14]

$$C = \left[\frac{Q \ln \left(P(t_1)/P(t_2) \right)}{t_2 - t_1} \right.$$

$$\left. \times \exp \left(\frac{t_1 \ln P(t_2) - t_2 \ln P(t_1)}{t_2 - t_1} \right) \right]^{0.979} \tag{17}$$

This formula, which seems complex, can be simplified if one considers a single-exponential model, as in eqn (13). It is easily shown that:

$$\frac{\ln(P(t_1)/P(t_2))}{t_2 - t_1} = \beta \tag{18}$$

$$\exp \left(\frac{t_1 \ln P(t_2) - t_2 \ln P(t_1)}{t_2 - t_1} \right) = B^{-1} \tag{19}$$

So eqn (17) can be simplified:

$$C = \left(\frac{Q\beta}{B} \right)^{0.979} \tag{20}$$

and it becomes very similar to eqn (15). Russell's two-sample method can therefore be considered as another compensa-

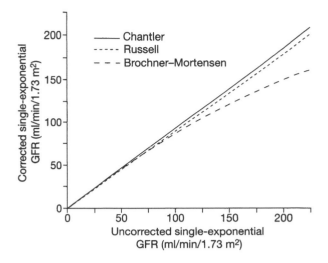

Figure 3.2 Effects of corrections for single-exponential techniques.

tion for neglecting the first exponential. Thus it is applicable to single-exponential techniques with more than two points. In fact, Chantler's and Russell's methods are very similar whereas Brochner–Mortensen gives significantly lower values at high GFR (see Figure 3.2).

Most of the other methods are single-sample methods where the area under the curve is estimated from a single point. The technique proposed by Christensen and Groth,[15] which was chosen by international consensus, is based upon an assumption on extracellular volume. It was published as an iterative calculation. However, Watson demonstrated that the same result could be reached from the solution of a second-degree equation.[16] For this, the first step is to estimate ECV from BSA:

$$ECV \cong 8116.6 \ ml/m^2 \times BSA - 28.2 \ ml \tag{21}$$

Then, one must calculate the parameters of the second-degree equation:

$$a = 1.7 10^{-6} \ min^{-2} \times t^2 - 0.0012 \ min^{-1} \times t$$
$$b = -7.75 10^{-4} \ min^{-2} \times t^2 + 1.31 \ min^{-1} \times t \tag{22}$$

$$c = ECV \times \ln \left(\frac{ECV}{V_D(t)} \right)$$

and solve the equation with:

$$C = \frac{b + \sqrt{b^2 - 4ac}}{2a} \ ml/min \tag{23}$$

This technique can be used for any sampling time.

Other methods are empirical and formulae for the most common ones are detailed in Table 3.2.

Table 3.2 Most commonly used empirical methods with a single sample (distribution volumes are expressed in litres, GFR is expressed in ml/min). Time t is given in minutes

Author	Sampling time	Formula*
Russell[14] (one sample)	Variable	$GFR = \left(-0.278 \times t + 119.1 + \dfrac{2405}{t}\right) \times \ln[V_D(t)] + \left(0.946 \times t - 400.2 - \dfrac{206.8}{t}\right)$
Morgan[17]	3 h	$GFR = -23.92 + 2.78 \times V_D(180\ \text{min}) - 0.0111 \times V_D(180\ \text{min})^2$
Constable[18]	3 h	$GFR = 24.5 \times \sqrt{V_D(180\ \text{min}) - 6.2} - 67$
Fawdry[19]	3 h	$GFR = 31.94 \times \sqrt{V_D(180\ \text{min}) + 16.92} - 161.7$

*Here, for Russell's formula, the coefficients were adapted to match distribution volume expressed in litres (instead of millilitres as in the original publication).

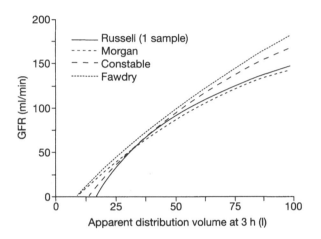

Figure 3.3 GFR values given by various formulae for a single sample taken at 3 h postinjection. The Christensen and Groth formula cannot be easily depicted here because it depends on BSA.

Table 3.3 Normal values for extracellular volume (ECV) in l/kg, W being body weight (kg) and A age (yr)

Author	Tracer	Value
Pierson[21]	Sulphate	$ECV = (0.47 - 0.0014 \times A) \times W$ for males $ECV = (0.451 - 0.0021 \times A) \times W$ for females
Froissart[22]	EDTA	$ECV = 0.149 \times W + 5.15$ for males $ECV = 0.140 \times W + 4.77$ for females
Ernest[22]	Sulphate Bromide	$ECV = (0.186 \pm 0.039) \times W$ $ECV = (0.16 \pm 0.30) \times W$

Figure 3.3 shows that, for a large range of values, the different formulae give similar results. Major differences can be seen only for very high values and very low values (where single-sample techniques are not recommended). Here again, the lower the expected GFR, the later should be the plasma sampling, ideally ranging from about 2 hours for normal function up to about 24 hours for severe renal failure.[20] However, among single-sample methods, only Christensen and Groth's and Russell's make it possible to choose time sampling.

Single-sample methods are simple and they have proven accuracy. However, they rely on the exact determination of the injected dose and any error in this determination will induce a similar error in GFR. An advantage of a mono-exponential method over single-sample methods is therefore that determining the distribution volume (which is of the order of the extracellular volume) may help to detect errors in the determination of the injected activity. Normal values

for ECV, found in Table 3.3, vary greatly between individuals and within the published data. Comparing the apparent distribution volume to these normal values can help to detect gross errors (Table 3.3).

Whatever the technique, time sampling depends on renal function: the higher the function, the faster the tracer disappears from the plasma and the earlier must the plasma samples be taken.[24] In practice, it is recommended that the function first roughly estimated by a formula using plasma creatinine (Cockcroft and Gault[25] or MDRD[26]; see Chapter 2); then for an estimated normal function, the last sample taken at 3 h postinjection is sufficient. For mildly impaired function, one should wait for 4–6 h; for severely impaired function, the last sample should be taken the following day.

In practice:

- the patient should be at relative rest, not undertaking heavy exercise;
- the patient should not eat meat just before or during the test;
- no special hydration is needed (avoid dehydration);
- the injected activity must be determined in comparison to a standard (see below);

- the injection must be performed strictly intravenously, as a bolus; time must be recorded with precision;
- plasma sampling should be performed on the arm contralateral to the injection site; time should be recorded with precision;
- sampling time(s) depend(s) on the chosen method (see Table 3.2).

Determining the injected activity

Determining the injected activity is a key point for plasmatic methods because any error induces the same error in the determined value of clearance. In all cases, the injected activity is compared to a standard. For this, two volumes are prepared from the same stock solution of radiotracer: one is injected into the patient and the other is diluted into a vial of precisely known volume (typically 250 ml), which can be considered as a reference patient (of known distribution volume and null clearance). Samples are then taken from this vial and counted in a well, just as plasma samples are counted. To compare the amount injected into the patient and the amount put into the standard, three techniques can be used: mass, volume or activity.

The mass method consists of weighing both the patient and standard syringes before and after injection to determine the injected weight. Care must be taken not to change the needle and cap on each syringe, or to rinse or aspirate blood into the syringe lest gross errors be induced.

The activity method consists of externally counting the syringes before and after injection. Care must be taken to keep strictly the same geometry of counting. For high activities of ^{99m}Tc, an activimeter may be enough. In other cases, a sufficiently sensitive device must be used.

For the volume methods, a sterile graduated pipette is used to insert a known volume of solution into a syringe. Another pipette is used for the standard. After injection, the syringe and needle, as well as all the injective devices (such as catheters) are rinsed into a known volume of solution. An aliquot of this solution is counted and the determined activity is subtracted from the activity initially inserted into the syringe. Finally, the difference is compared to the volume in the standard.

For these methods, recommendations and prepared charts can be found in the international consensus.[1]

Baseline and test condition studies

To perform baseline and test condition studies, only urinary techniques or plasmatic continuous infusion can be used. This is useful to assess the glomerular filtration reserve during an infusion of neoglucogenic amino acids or dopamine or both.[27] The maximum effect is usually obtained after 1–2 hours of infusion. The effect of conversion enzyme inhibitors can be assessed in the same way.

External detection

To avoid plasma or urine sampling and injected activity calibration, several techniques were proposed to measure the absolute function directly by camera only, among which the most widely known is the method of Schlegel[28,29] adapted by Gates.[30] The principle of all these methods is to assess the kidney uptake as a fraction of the injected activity. Authors claimed that these techniques were able to measure relative and absolute function at the same time. Though attractive, camera-based methods are not precise and the best known among them, the Gates technique, is even less precise than creatinine-based formulæ.[31–37] Other methods with better accuracy[38–40] have been published but none of them has proven reliable enough to replace clearances. Using transmission maps[41,43] may improve these methods, especially for high GFR values. However, it is not recommended that these techniques are used, at least until serious validation is published (most of the evaluations of the publications claimed only correlation – not agreement – with a reference, which is not sufficient[43]).

Another published approach was to use the absolute uptake of ^{99m}Tc-DMSA to assess renal function.[44] This approach is flawed and can lead to erroneous conclusions (see Figure 3.4).[45]

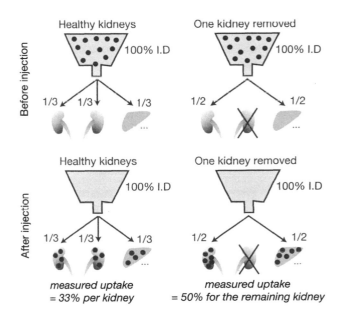

Figure 3.4 Illustration of the error made when considering that absolute DMSA uptake can determine renal function (the values are simplified for clarity; a more precise model can be found elsewhere[45]): at the plateau, the injected activity is either taken by one or othe of the kidneysr or by another organ. When removing one kidney, the same amount of tracer is divided into two parts instead of three so, even without any functional compensation, the uptake of the remaining kidney increases just because more tracer is available.

To monitor relative and rapid changes of GFR over time, the use of an external probe can, however, be recommended.[46] No value of GFR is provided but this method shows variations in GFR (given by the variations of the slope of recorded activity over time). This may be especially useful in intensive care units.

Patient scaling

In adults, GFR is usually scaled to body surface area (BSA). In 1916, Dubois and Dubois published a formula to calculate the surface of skin based on morphological data.[47] This formula was derived from morphological parameters determined on a few individuals. Since then, other papers were published improving this formula. BSA has become a standard to assess body dimension, mixing weight and height to scale physiological parameters and to adapt drug doses.

Several formulae are available to estimate BSA. The classic formula by Dubois and Dubois was devised nearly a century ago on eight adults and two children.[47] Other formulae were published with more numerous samples (see Table 3.4).

Scaling is especially important for children (see Chapter 4) and overweight subjects. It is carried out using the following formula:

$$GFR_{norm.} = GFR_{raw} \times \frac{1.73 \text{ m}^2}{BSA} \qquad (24)$$

Body surface area has been used for many years both to normalize physiological parameters and to calculate doses of drugs (e.g. in chemotherapy). It may seem surprising that the surface of the skin is commonly used for such purposes. Indeed, to our knowledge, no strong physiological evidence for this use has been shown and using BSA for this purpose is questioned.[53–55] Because of this, it was suggested that

normalizing GFR to extracellular volume (ECV) would be more physiologic.[55,56] It was therefore claimed that, in a single-exponential model, ECV is given by Q/A, GFR is given by $Q\alpha/A$ and therefore GFR can be expressed in terms of ECV as α, which is the inverse of a time constant. This approach would solve the normalization problem and make it easy to resolve the difficulties in determining the injected dose. However, such an approach does not take into consideration that the single-exponential model is not realistic, so Q/A and $Q\alpha/A$ are only rough approximations for ECV and GFR. The errors do not compensate for each other and, in a two-exponential model (see equation (11)), the ratio is not merely given by α but by:

$$\frac{GFR}{ECV} = \alpha\beta \frac{\alpha B + \beta A}{\alpha^2 B + \beta^2 A} \qquad (25)$$

A second argument against this approach is that a small error in one of two samples would be compensated for when calculating GFR but not when calculating GFR/ECV.[56] Moreover, ECV may not be such a good parameter to scale GFR because: (1) GFR does not physiologically adapt to ECV changes; (2) GFR does not regulate ECV; and (3) ECV may vary rapidly in some circumstances, with no similar variation in GFR. (For instance, a patient in heart failure receiving diuretics will have a major decrease in ECV, but no change in GFR in the absence of functional renal failure. Using GFR/ECV would give the false impression that renal function is improving with diuretics. This effect would be much less visible with BSA because the change in weight does not affect BSA as much as it affects ECV (in an average adult, a loss of 4 l of fluid would result in a −25% change in ECV but only a −2% change in BSA).) A similar approach was proposed for use with external detection ('FUR' or 'fractional uptake rate').[57] Another publication suggested using only the slope to determine GFR.[58] To our knowledge, no evaluation of this method was published afterwards but, at least in our experience, it does not perform well and we do not recommend this approach. Finally, though it is probably imperfect, we suggest keeping the classical normalization by BSA.

Table 3.4 Formulae for body surface area (BSA) expressed in m². Here, H refers to height in cm and W to body weight in kg

Authors	Formula
Dubois and Dubois[47]	$BSA = 0.007184 \times H^{0.725} \times W^{0.425}$
Gehan and George[48]	$BSA = 0.02350 \times H^{0.42246} \times W^{0.51456}$
Haycock[49]	$BSA = 0.024265 \times H^{0.3964} \times W^{0.5378}$
Boyd[50]	$BSA = 0.0003207 \times H^{0.3} \times (1000 \times W)^{0.7285 - 0.0564 \times \log_{10} W}$
Mosteller[51]	$BSA = \frac{\sqrt{H \times W}}{60}$
Livingston[52]	$BSA = 0.1173 \times W^{0.6466}$ if $W > 10$ kg $BSA = 0.1037 \times W^{0.6724}$ if $W \leq 10$ kg

Which method

Among external techniques, dynamic gamma-camera methods (such as Gates') are even less precise than creatinine-based methods; static methods (DMSA) are both imprecise and inaccurate; external probe techniques (Rabito) are efficient for monitoring changes but cannot assess absolute function. We do not recommend their use to determine absolute renal function. We do reiterate, however, that gamma-camera techniques are the technique of choice to determine the relative renal function.

Urinary techniques are cumbersome, very accurate, but they lack precision. Plasma clearances are precise and have a decent accuracy. Among plasmatic techniques, the multi-sample technique is cumbersome and should now be reserved for validation studies. The simplest technique, namely the plasma clearance after bolus injection with a single sample, is applicable in many cases with both good precision and accuracy (about 5 ml/min).[31,36,37,59]

In the determination of the optimal method to assess GFR, a few questions arise:

- does the patient have oedema, ascites or third space?
- what is the expected renal function (as roughly estimated by Cockcroft and Gault or MDRD formulae) (see Chapter 2)?
- is robustness critical?
- is it for research purposes?
- is a comparison between baseline and test conditions (such as ACE test or assessment of the functional glomerular reserve) considered?
- is hyperfiltration considered?

If the patient has oedema, ascites or third space, urinary clearances are mandatory (by bolus injection or continuous infusion or even after subcutaneous injection).

If the expected GFR is below 30 ml/min, a mono-exponential technique with late sampling (up to 24 h) should be considered. Between 15 and 30 ml/min, Christensen and Groth may still be acceptable.[60]

If a baseline period followed by a test period must be performed, the only way is to use a continuous infusion technique.

If robustness is critical (for example for a kidney donor), it is advisable either to use the continuous infusion technique or to combine plasma and urinary clearance.

For research purposes, it is advisable to use multisample methods or continuous infusion.

In any other cases, a single-shot, simplified, plasma clearance performs well. Among the multiple variants, the international consensus[1] selected the Christensen and Groth[15] technique with only one sample. It is simple and accurate. The drawback of this technique is that any error in the injected activity induces a similar error in GFR, with no possibility of detecting it.

To avoid this problem, a single exponential can be used. This is the choice of the British Nuclear Medicine Society. Claiming that the international recommendation is 'inade-quate'[61,62] seems, however, overstated. When using the single-exponential approach, the Bröchner–Mortensen correction is recommended, except when there may be

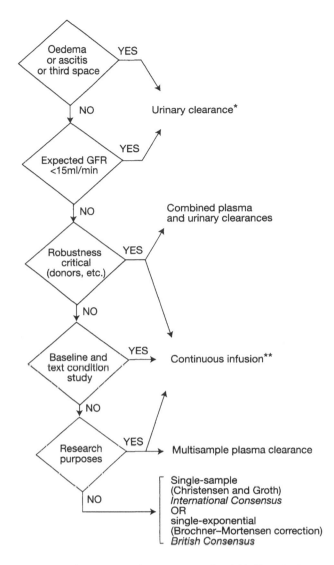

Figure 3.5 Strategy for choosing a method '(*either single-shot or continuous; **plasma and/or urinary clearances).

hyperfiltration (in this case, use Chantler's correction). If a single exponential is to be chosen, the question of the number of samples arises: it was recently shown that using more than two samples does not greatly improve the precision;[63] however, it does improve robustness.

To summarize, the choice of the method can be taken from Figure 3.5. Choice is left to the reader to follow either the international consensus,[1] preferring simplicity with good precision, or the British consensus,[61] preferring robustness.

References

1. Blaufox MD, Aurell M, Bubeck B, et al. Report of the Radionuclides in Nephrourology Committee on renal clearance. J Nucl Med 1996; 37: 1883–90.

2. Durand E, Prigent A. The basics of renal imaging and function studies. Q J Nucl Med 2002; 46: 249–67.

3. Prigent A, Cosgriff P, Gates GF et al. Consensus report on

quality control of quantitative measurements of renal function obtained from the renogram: International Consensus Committee from the Scientific Committee of Radionuclides in Nephrourology. Semin Nucl Med 1999; 29: 146–59.

4. Chantler C, Garnett ES, Parsons V, Veall N. Glomerular filtration rate measurement in man by the single injection methods using 51Cr-EDTA. Clin Sci 1969; 37: 169–80.

5. Carlsen JE, Moller ML, Lund JO, Trap-Jensen J. Comparison of four commercial Tc-99m(Sn)DTPA preparations used for the measurement of glomerular filtration rate: concise communication. J Nucl Med 1980; 21: 126–9.

6. Rehling M, Nielsen SL, Marqversen J. Protein binding of 99mTc-DTPA, 51Cr-EDTA and 125I-iothalamate. Nucl Med Commun 1997; 18: 324.

7. Rehling M. Stability, protein binding and clearance studies of [99mTc]DTPA. Evaluation of a commercially available dry-kit. Scand J Clin Lab Invest 1988; 48: 603–9.

8. Brochner-Mortensen J. Current status on assessment and measurement of glomerular filtration rate. Clin Physiol 1985; 5: 1–17.

9. Bianchi C, Coli A, Gallucci L et al. The measurement of glomerular filtration rate in children by 131-I-hypaque and external counting. J Nucl Biol Med 1967; 11: 143–51.

10. Hellerstein S, Berenbom M, Alon U, Warady BA. The renal clearance and infusion clearance of inulin are similar, but not identical. Kidney Int 1993; 44: 1058–61.

11. Sapirstein L, Vidt D, Mandel M, Hanusek G. Volumes of distribution and clearances of intravenously injected creatinine in the dog. Am J Physiol 1955; 181: 330–6.

12. Chantler C, Barratt TM. Estimation of glomerular filtration rate from plasma clearance of 51-chromium edetic acid. Arch Dis Child 1972; 47: 613–7.

13. Brochner-Mortensen J. A simple method for the determination of glomerular filtration rate. Scand J Clin Lab Invest 1972; 30: 271–4.

14. Russell CD, Bischoff PG, Kontzen FN et al. Measurement of glomerular filtration rate: single injection plasma clearance method without urine collection. J Nucl Med 1985; 26: 1243–7.

15. Christensen AB, Groth S. Determination of 99mTc-DTPA clearance by a single plasma sample method. Clin Physiol 1986; 6: 579–88.

16. Watson WS. A simple method of estimating glomerular filtration rate. Eur J Nucl Med 1992; 19: 827.

17. Morgan WD, Birks JL, Sivyer A, Ghose RR. An efficient technique for the simultaneous estimation of GFR and ERPF, involving a single injection and two blood samples. Int J Nucl Med Biol 1977; 4: 79–83.

18. Constable AR, Hussein MM, Albrecht MP et al. Single sample estimates of renal clearances. Br J Urol 1979; 51: 84–7.

19. Fawdry RM, Gruenewald SM. Three-hour volume of distribution method: an accurate simplified method of glomerular filtration rate measurement. J Nucl Med 1987; 28: 510–3.

20. Brochner-Mortensen J, Rodbro P. Selection of routine method for determination of glomerular filtration rate in adult patients. Scand J Clin Lab Invest 1976; 36: 35–43.

21. Pierson RN Jr, Wang J, Colt EW, Neumann P. Body composition measurements in normal man: the potassium, sodium, sulfate and tritium spaces in 58 adults. J Chronic Dis 1982; 35: 419–28.

22. Froissart M, Houillier P, Leviel F, Paillard M. Mesures simul-

tanées du débit de filtration glomérulaire (DFG) et du volume extra-cellulaire (VEC) par le 51Cr-EDTA en perfusion continue: valeurs normales. [Simultaneous measurements of GFR and ECV by continuous infusion of 51Cr-EDTA: normal values]. Médecine Nucléaire: imagerie fonctionnelle et métabolique 1998; 22: 148.

23. Ernest D, Hartman NG, Deane CP et al. Reproducibility of plasma and extracellular fluid volume measurements in critically ill patients. J Nucl Med 1992; 33: 1468–71.

24. Russell CD. Optimum sample times for single-injection, multi-sample renal clearance methods. J Nucl Med 1993; 34: 1761–5.

25. Cockcroft DW, Gault MH. Prediction of creatinine clearance from serum creatinine. Nephron 1976; 16: 31–41.

26. Levey AS, Bosch JP, Lewis JB et al. A more accurate method to estimate glomerular filtration rate from serum creatinine: a new prediction equation. Modification of Diet in Renal Disease Study Group. Ann Intern Med 1999; 130: 461–70.

27. ter Wee PM, Tegzess AM, Donker AJ. Renal reserve filtration capacity before and after kidney donation. J Intern Med 1990; 228: 393–9.

28. Schlegel JU, Halikiopoulos HL, Prima R. Determination of filtration fraction using the gamma scintillation camera. J Urol 1979; 122: 447–50.

29. Schlegel JU, Hamway SA. Individual renal plasma flow determination in 2 minutes. J Urol 1976; 116: 282–5.

30. Gates GF. Glomerular filtration rate: estimation from fractional renal accumulation of 99mTc-DTPA (stannous). AJR Am J Roentgenol 1982; 138: 565–70.

31. Itoh K. Comparison of methods for determination of glomerular filtration rate: Tc-99m-DTPA renography, predicted creatinine clearance method and plasma sample method. Ann Nucl Med 2003; 17: 561–5.

32. Russell CD, Dubovsky EV. Gates method for GFR measurement. J Nucl Med 1986; 27: 1373–4.

33. Mulligan JS, Blue PW, Hasbargen JA. Methods for measuring GFR with technetium-99m-DTPA: an analysis of several common methods. J Nucl Med 1990; 31: 1211–9.

34. Goates JJ, Morton KA, Whooten WW et al. Comparison of methods for calculating glomerular filtration rate: technetium-99m-DTPA scintigraphic analysis, protein-free and whole-plasma clearance of technetium-99m-DTPA and iodine-125-iothalamate clearance. J Nucl Med 1990; 31: 424–9.

35. Durand E, Prigent A, Gaillard J. Comparison between 9 methods for estimation of glomerular filtration rate (G.F.R.) with simultaneous injections of 51Cr-EDTA and 99mTc-DTPA. In: Taylor A, Jr., Nally J, Thomsen H, eds. Radionuclides in Nephrology. Reston: Society of Nuclear Medicine; 1997: 112–20.

36. Fawdry RM, Gruenewald SM, Collins LT, Roberts AJ. Comparative assessment of techniques for estimation of glomerular filtration rate with 99mTc-DTPA. Eur J Nucl Med 1985; 11: 7–12.

37. Galli G, Rufini V, Vellante C, D'Errico G, Piraccini R. Estimation of glomerular filtration rate with 99Tc(m)-DTPA: a comparative assessment of simplified methods. Nucl Med Commun 1997; 18: 634–41.

38. Piepsz A, Dobbeleir A, Erbsmann F. Measurement of separate kidney clearance by means of 99mTc-DTPA complex and a scintillation camera. Eur J Nucl Med 1977; 2: 173–7.

39. Rehling M, Moller ML, Lund JO et al. 99mTc-DTPA gamma-

camera renography: normal values and rapid determination of single-kidney glomerular filtration rate. Eur J Nucl Med 1985; 11: 1–6.

40. Moonen M, Jacobsson L, Granerus G et al. Determination of split renal function from gamma camera renography: a study of three methods. Nucl Med Commun 1994; 15: 704–11.

41. Carlsen O. The gamma camera as an absolute measurement device: determination of glomerular filtration rate in 99mTc-DTPA renography using a dual head gamma camera. Nucl Med Commun 2004; 25: 1021–9.

42. Inoue Y, Ohtake T, Homma Y et al. Evaluation of glomerular filtration rate by camera-based method in both children and adults. J Nucl Med 1998; 39: 1784–8.

43. Bland JM, Altman DG. Statistical methods for assessing agreement between two methods of clinical measurement. Lancet 1986; 1: 307–10.

44. Groshar D, Embon OM, Frenkel A, Front D. Renal function and technetium-99m-dimercaptosuccinic acid uptake in single kidneys: the value of in vivo SPECT quantitation. J Nucl Med 1991; 32: 766–8.

45. Durand E, Prigent A. Can dimercaptosuccinic acid renal scintigraphy be used to assess global renal function? Eur J Nucl Med 2000; 27: 727–30.

46. Rabito CA, Moore RH, Bougas C, Dragotakes SC. Noninvasive, real-time monitoring of renal function: the ambulatory renal monitor. J Nucl Med 1993; 34: 199–207.

47. DuBois D, DuBois E. A formula to estimate the approximate surface area if height and weight are known. Arch Int Med 1916; 17: 863–71.

48. Gehan EA, George SL. Estimation of human body surface area from height and weight. Cancer Chemother Rep 1970; 54: 225–35.

49. Haycock GB, Schwartz GJ, Wisotsky DH. Geometric method for measuring body surface area: a height-weight formula validated in infants, children, and adults. J Pediatr 1978; 93: 62–6.

50. Boyd E. The growth of the surface area of the human body. Minneapolis: University of Minnesota Press, 1935.

51. Mosteller RD. Simplified calculation of body-surface area. N Engl J Med 1987; 317: 1098.

52. Livingston EH, Lee S. Body surface area prediction in normal-weight and obese patients. Am J Physiol Endocrinol Metab 2001; 281: E586–91.

53. Gurney H. How to calculate the dose of chemotherapy. Br J Cancer 2002; 86: 1297–302.

54. Peters AM. Expressing glomerular filtration rate in terms of extra-cellular fluid volume. Nephrol Dial Transplant 1992; 7: 205–10.

55. Peters AM, Gordon I, Sixt R. Normalization of glomerular filtration rate in children: body surface area, body weight or extracellular fluid volume? J Nucl Med 1994; 35: 438–44.

56. Piepsz A, Ham HR. How good is the slope of the second exponential for estimating 51Cr- EDTA renal clearance? Nucl Med Commun 1997; 18: 139–41.

57. Rutland M, Que L, Hassan IM. 'FUR' – one size suits all. Eur J Nucl Med 2000; 27: 1708–13.

58. Galli G, Rufini V, Meduri G. A simplified determination of glomerular filtration rate with 99Tcm-DTPA. Nucl Med Commun 1994; 15: 831–5.

59. Picciotto G, Cacace G, Cesana P et al. Estimation of chromium-51 ethylene diamine tetra-acetic acid plasma clearance: a comparative assessment of simplified techniques. Eur J Nucl Med 1992; 19: 30–5.

60. Rehling M, Rabol A. Measurement of glomerular filtration rate in adults: accuracy of five single-sample plasma clearance methods. Clin Physiol 1989; 9: 171–82.

61. Fleming JS, Nunan TO. The new BNMS guidelines for measurement of glomerular filtration rate. Nucl Med Commun 2004; 25: 755–7.

62. Fleming JS, Zivanovic MA, Blake GM et al. Guidelines for the measurement of glomerular filtration rate using plasma sampling. Nucl Med Commun 2004; 25: 759–69.

63. De Sadeleer C, Van Laere K, Georges B et al. Influence of time interval and number of blood samples on the error in renal clearance determination using a mono-exponential model: a Monte Carlo simulation. Nucl Med Commun 2000; 21: 741–5.

4 Measurement of GFR in children by means of radionuclide techniques

Amy Piepsz, Hamphrey Ham

Introduction

The question arises whether radionuclide techniques can be useful in children for the determination of overall renal function. The answer is dependent on several factors:

- Does the radionuclide technique offer an accurate measurement of renal function for the whole range of clearance values?
- Does it represent a noninvasive approach, friendly to the child, delivering a rather negligible amount of radiation and resulting in an acceptable cost for the society?
- Does it provide information which cannot be given by the nonradioactive measurements, and is it significantly more accurate than these traditional methods?

This chapter will consider these different points and will try to demonstrate that radionuclide plasma clearances, specifically tailored to the child, may offer to the clinician an interesting tool in the daily practice of nephro-urology.

Gamma camera or plasma samples

There is no doubt – and this has been extensively developed in several chapters of this book – that gamma cameras can provide accurate estimation of relative function and renal drainage, for each kidney individually. Beside relative function, camera methods allowing estimation of absolute single kidney clearance are also available. They are based on the amount of tracer taken up by the kidney and expressed in percentage of what has been injected or what has reached the plasma. However, factors such as background correction, inaccuracy of plasma curves derived from heart structures, estimation of kidney depth and correction for attenuation, all contribute to some degree of inaccuracy. Plasma sample clearances are definitely more accurate.[1] It is therefore not surprising that until now no guidelines have been produced related to gamma camera clearances. This chapter will be devoted exclusively to plasma sample methods.

Glomerular or tubular tracers

Several complex as well as simplified algorithms have been produced for both glomerular and tubular tracers and are extensively used in clinical practice. It has been shown however (see Chapter 1) that parenchymal function is better represented by the glomerular filtration rate than by tubular clearance, the latter being heavily influenced by some extrarenal factors such as salt load, level of hydration, pH of urine, level of stress, etc. These factors may be responsible for a lesser degree of day-to-day reproducibility when dealing with tubular tracers.[2]

We will therefore, in this chapter, focus essentially on the determination of glomerular filtration rate.

Tc-99m DTPA or Cr-51 EDTA

Both tracers can be used for the determination of GFR and the correlation between EDTA and DTPA clearance is excellent.[3] However, the binding between chromium 51 and EDTA is better than the chelation of Tc-99m on DTPA, while the protein binding of DTPA seems higher than to EDTA, although this point remains controversial.[4] It has been shown that filtered and unfiltered DTPA blood samples result in quite different clearances.[5] We have personally experienced during DTPA renography in children some accumulation of tracer in the stomach, as well as late diffusion of the tracer into the joints.

Radiation burden

For Cr-51 EDTA, the effective dose is approximately 0.011 mSv/examination regardless of the age of the child, providing that the dose is adapted according to body weight. This is at least one hundred times less than the radiation burden related to an intravenous urography, which, in favourable conditions, results in an effective dose of 1 mSv. In cases of poor renal function (10 ml/min/1.73 m^2), the radiation dose is twice as high.

For 99mTc-DTPA, the effective dose is approximately 0.1 mSv/examination.[6]

Methods

We will successively consider, for paediatric applications, the different modalities of plasma clearance estimation using glomerular tracers and single shot techniques: the multiple blood sample technique, the slope-intercept method, the single sample method and the slope method.

Multiple blood sample technique

This methodology has been extensively described in Chapter 3.

The technique is nowadays considered as a reference technique for the determination of GFR, comparable to inulin clearance, despite some well-known methodological limitations and assumptions. Considering the paediatric point of view, the main limitation is related to the number of blood samples needed to define accurately the entire plasma curve. Placing a permanent venous catheter during the test might solve this difficult constraint, although such a procedure is dependent on sufficient calibre of the vein. Moreover, those using this technique have experienced difficulties in getting blood through the catheter rapidly enough, thus introducing uncertainties related to the plasma concentration as well as to the exact time of sampling. In a recent multicentric study in children,[7] several patients' data had to be deleted, because of inaccuracies in the timing of blood sampling particularly for the initial values, when the plasma disappearance slope is very steep.

Slope-intercept method

It is based (see Chapter 3) on the fact that the early exponential may be neglected, insofar as a correction factor is introduced. As a matter of fact, the clearance is overestimated if no correction is introduced and the overestimation, expressed in percentage of the clearance, increases when clearance increases.

The technique is the same as the one applied to adults. After intravenous injection of the tracer, blood is taken at approximately 2 and 4 h, allowing the determination of the late slope of the plasma disappearance curve. The distribution volume is obtained by dividing the injected dose by the intercept of the slope on the y-axis. Clearance is equal to the distribution volume multiplied by the slope.

It is mandatory that the exact time of blood sampling should be noted. If the counting and dilution are performed by an experienced technologist, no additional blood sample is needed between 2 and 4 h. It has been demonstrated[8] that, in order to improve significantly the accuracy of the slope, one should add at least 13 blood samples between 2 and 4 h. There is therefore no real advantage to adding one or even two blood samples.

Two correction factors, adapted to the child, are available and allow to correct for having neglected the early exponential. One has been calculated by Chantler[9] in a series of children having undergone a clearance measurement by means of a reference method (amount excreted in the urine divided by plasma concentration). It is a constant factor, by which the obtained clearance should be multiplied.

$Cl_1 = 0.87 \times Cl_2$

Cl_1 = clearance corrected for the first exponential

Cl_2 = noncorrected clearance

The other one has been developed by Bröchner–Mortensen[10] and takes into account the fact that the factor is theoretically increasing when clearance increases. The equation of correction is therefore quadratic.

$Cl_1 = (1.01 \times Cl_2) - (0.0012 \times Cl_2^2)$

Cl_1 = clearance corrected for the first exponential

Cl_2 = noncorrected clearance

The possible drawback of the latter correction factor is the fact that the equation has been established on the basis of reference clearance values not higher than 130 ml/min. For higher clearance values, the correction factor results in an underestimation of the true renal clearance.

Single blood sample clearance

It is a significant simplification, for those who are dealing with children, to use one blood sample instead of two. This type of clearance is however derived from an empirical formula, and is different for adults and children. Since only one single blood sample is available, one can only calculate a 'distribution volume', in other words a ratio between injected dose and plasma concentration at a given time. The only way to transform such a ratio into a clearance value is to construct an abacus, in which a reference clearance is plotted against this 'distribution volume'. If a sufficiently large number of patients is selected, covering the whole range of ages and clearance values, then it is possible to derive an equation relating both parameters. However, the relation between slope intercept clearance and 'distribution volume' is a complex one and it is obvious, from the equations describing the two methods, that the single blood sample clearance cannot, by definition, be valid for the whole range of clearance values[11] and is not applicable to low clearance values.

Several algorithms have been developed for the child. Groth and Aasted[12] based their method on an empirically estimated distribution volume of Cr EDTA. Others have published algorithms applicable to both adults and children.[13,14] Although theoretically comfortable, this last approach represents a compromise resulting in less accurate results then with an algorithm adapted to the child.

Ham and Piepsz[15] have directly compared the plasma concentration at 2 hours with the clearance calculated using the slope-intercept method. From this comparison, they derived an equation which can be applied whatever the age of the patient, the coefficient of correlation between both parameters being close to 1.0 for all age groups.

$$GFR = 2.602\ V_{120} - 0.273$$

where

$$V_{120} = \frac{Dose}{A_{120}}$$

A_{120} being the plasma concentration at 120 min.

The blood sampling can be performed anywhere between 110 and 130 min, providing that the exact time (t) of sampling has been precisely indicated and that the following correction has been introduced:

$$A_{120} = A_{(t)} \cdot e\ (0.08)(t - 120)$$

The final result has to be corrected for body surface.

The validity of the method has been established by applying the method to a second large group of children. In this control group, the correlation between both methods was close to the identity line, allowing to use the concentration at 2 h to predict the clearance with the slope-intercept method (Figure 4.1). The method has been tested from 0 to 15 years. Recently, it has been shown that one can use the same algorithm for patients between 15 and 30 years. It should be underlined again that the method is not valid for clearance values below 30–35 ml/min/1.73 m^2. Therefore, any patient referred for a clearance measurement, and having a history of chronic renal failure or a clearly abnormal plasma creatinine value cannot benefit from the single sample clearance method.

Slope method

It has been proposed, instead of using the slope-intercept method or the single-sample method, to limit the test to the determination of the slope by means of three blood samples.[16]

The advantage of this method is that one gets rid of the measurements of the injected dose and the measurement of

the standard of the dose. Moreover, no body surface correction is needed since the clearance, using this method, is automatically calibrated by means of the distribution volume of the tracer:

Clearance = slope × distribution volume

Slope = clearance/distribution volume

The slope is therefore the rate by which the tracer is eliminated from the distribution volume of the tracer.

In our opinion however, the disadvantages are obvious.

When using the slope-intercept method, an error on the slope is more or less compensated by an inverse error on the distribution volume. On the contrary, using the slope only, the error on the slope constitutes the error on the final result. This explains why the slope method is less reproducible than any method of clearance measurement.[17]

The second disadvantage of the method is the number of blood samples to be taken: for those in favour of the method, fitting a slope on three blood samples is sufficient, providing that the correlation coefficient on the fit is at least 0.99. However, five blood samples at least are needed in order to reach the same accuracy as for the slope-intercept method. This constraint limits the use of the method when applied to children.

The advantage of correcting the clearance for age by means of the distribution volume of the tracer instead of the body surface is strongly debated. Indeed, the distribution volume used, when considering the slope method, is not a true physiological one, close to the extracellular volume, but simply a mathematical interpolation of the slope. There is no true evidence that one correction is superior to the other.

Finally, one has to take into account the fact that the clinician is familiar with the concept of clearance, expressed in ml/min. It is hard to believe that he would be prepared to abandon this parameter and to adopt instead the concept of a simple rate.

Quality control

No special difficulties are related to the determination of radionuclide clearance by means of blood samples, providing that some minimal precautions are taken. The measurement of dose, standard of dose, dilution of the standard and measurements in a well counter of both the patient's plasma and the dilution of the standard, are simple and accurate measurements, which, in the hands of an experienced technologist, should not result in significant errors.[6] On the other hand, one should be sure that the exact time of sampling has been noted and not some approximation of the time, which could significantly affect the final result.[8] When using the slope-intercept method, the distribution volume, obtained by interpolating the slope, is usually between

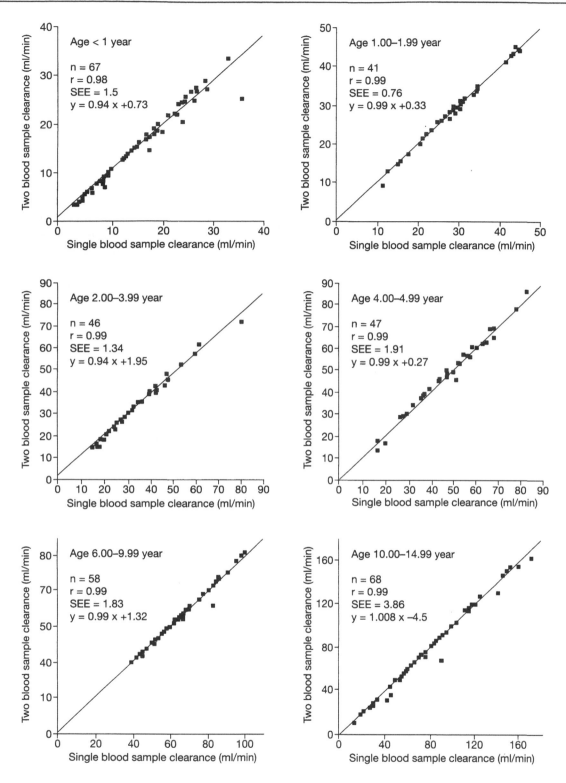

Figure 4.1 Using the linear converting equation obtained from the whole basic group (GFR = 2.602 V_{120} – 0.273), the V_{120} in the test group was converted into an estimate of GFR. Figure 4.1 shows the correlation between this estimate and the corresponding two-blood sample GFR. For all age groups, the linear correlation function relating this parameter and the two-blood sample clearance was close to the identity line with high coefficient of correlation and low s.e.e. (With permission from reference 15.)

20–35% of body weight. Any value below 15% or higher than 40% should raise a suspicion of error.

One argument against the single sample method is the fact that no such quality control is possible, since only a plasma concentration and a dose are available. Recently however, a method has been proposed and validated in children, allowing to circumscribe this difficulty.[18] One can artificially reconstruct three different slopes, by considering, on the y-axis, three different distribution volumes corresponding respectively to 20, 25 and 30% of body weight and by joining these values to the plasma concentration at 2 h. Three artificial slope-intercept clearances can then be calculated and compared to the single sample clearance. It has been demonstrated that, when the maximal difference between each of these artificial clearances and the single sample clearance is higher than 10 ml/min/1.73 m^2, one can suspect an error either on the injected dose or on the plasma concentration at 2 h.

Day-to-day reproducibility of renal clearance

The day-to-day reproducibility of GFR measurement by means of plasma sample method has been tested in both adults and children[2,19,20] and has shown a mean reproducibility around 6% (SD of the individual differences).

A difference of 10 ml/min/1.73 m^2 or more between two successive examinations can therefore be considered as a significant change.

Normal values

Getting normal values in children, while these values are changing in function of age, represents a major challenge, since nothing such as real normal values can be obtained, because of evident ethical reasons.

Some 'normal' values have been published.[21] They were selected retrospectively, on the basis of a simultaneous Tc-99m DMSA acquisition, showing a normal left-to-right ratio (between 45–55%) and normal parenchymal imaging. The reason for performing the examinations was the detection of scars 6 months after acute urinary tract infection. In some patients, the tests were performed during the acute phase of infection, because at that time the authors were not aware of the fact that significant hyperfiltration can be transitorily associated with acute infection.[22] Some of these estimated normal values might therefore be overestimated and, because we were dealing with patients and not with normal children, some others might be underestimated.

From the published data, it appears that normal values, corrected for body surface, are increasing with age during the first 2 years and remain stable afterwards until the adult period. Since body surface correction is an imprecise method, subjected to individual fluctuations of weight, one reasonable option for the future could be to present the normal values without correction for body surface and to determine, like for the children's growth charts, the normal percentiles in function of age.

Clinical advantages compared to traditional nonradioactive methods

Compared to creatinine clearance, the main advantage of radionuclide methods is that there is no need for urine collection, which, in routine situations, represents a main source of precision errors.

Compared to plasma creatinine and derived algorithms, they are (as shown in Chapter 5) much more accurate, the creatinine-derived algorithms giving rise to extreme errors in about one out of four determinations. It is for instance obvious, from the nonlinear relation between plasma concentration and clearance, that up to half of the renal function can be lost before any significant increase in plasma creatinine occurs.

One important tool for a nephrologist is to be able to detect the first signs of renal function impairment, particularly in the monitoring of nephrotoxic drugs. This is a major role of radionuclide methods, as demonstrated by those clinical centres who are using them extensively. Hyperfiltration, as can be observed for instance in juvenile diabetes, can best be quantified and monitored by these methods.

Conclusion

In paediatric patients, two simplified radionuclide methods are nowadays available, the single 2-h blood sample method and, in cases of clearance below 30–35 ml/min/1.73 m^2, the slope-intercept method using two blood samples, with the specific paediatric correction for having neglected the first exponential.

These methods allow an accurate estimation of GFR for all levels of clearance. They provide extremely reproducible results. They are noninvasive and easy to perform for both the young patient and the physician in charge of the test.

References

1. Fleming JS, Keast CM, Waller DG, Ackery D. Measurement of glomerular filtration rate with 99mTc-DTPA: a comparison of gamma camera methods. Eur J Nucl Med 1987; 13: 250–3.

2. Piepsz A, Tondeur M, Kinthaert J, Ham HR. Reproducibility of technetium-99m mercaptoacetyltriglycine clearance. Eur J Nucl Med 1996; 23: 195–8.

3. Hilson AJW, Mistry RD, Maisey MN. Tc-99m-DTPA for the

measurement of glomerular filtration rate. Br J Radiol 1976; 49: 794–6.

4. Rehling M, Nielsen LE, Marqversen J. Protein binding of 99Tcm-DTPA compared with other GFR tracers. Nucl Med Commun 2001; 22: 617–23.

5. Mulligan JS, Blue PW, Hasbargen JA. Methods for measuring GFR with technetium-99m DTPA: An analysis of several common methods. J Nucl Med 1990; 31: 1211–19

6. Piepsz A, Colarinha P, Gordon I et al. Guidelines for glomerular filtration rate determination in children. Eur J Nucl Med 2001; 28: BP31–6.

7. Piepsz A, Gordon I, Hahn K et al. Determination of the technetium-99m mercaptoacetyltriglycine plasma clearance in children by means of a single blood sample: a multicentre study. The Paediatric Task Group of the EANM. Eur J Nucl Med 1993; 20: 244–8.

8. De Sadeleer C, Van Laere K, Georges B et al. Influence of the time interval and the number of blood samples on the error in the clearance determination using a monoexponential model: a Monte Carlo simulation. Nucl Med Commun 2000; 21: 741–5.

9. Chantler C, Barratt TM. Estimation of glomerular filtration rate from plasma clearance of 51 Chromium Edetic Acid. Arch Dis Child 1972; 47: 613–17.

10. Bröchner-Mortensen J, Haahr J, Christoffersen J. A simple method for accurate assessment of the glomerular filtration rate in children. Scand J Clin Lab Invest 1974; 33: 139–43.

11. Waller DG, Keast CM, Fleming JS, Ackery DM. Measurement of glomerular filtration rate with Technetium-99m DTPA: Comparison of plasma clearance techniques. J Nucl Med 1987; 28: 372–7.

12. Groth S, Aasted M. 51-Cr EDTA clearance determined by one plasma sample in children. Clin Physiol 1984; 4: 75–83.

13. Bubeck B, Piepenburg R, Grethe U et al. A new principle to normalize plasma concentration allowing single sample clearance determinations in both children and adults. Eur J Nucl Med 1992; 19: 511–16.

14. Russell CD, Dubovsky EV, Scott JW. Simplified methods for renal clearance in children. Scaling for patient size. J Nucl Med 1991; 32: 1821–5.

15. Ham HR, Piepsz A. Estimation of glomerular filtration rate in infants and children using a simple plasma sample method. J Nucl Med 1991; 32: 1294–7.

16. Peters AM, Henderson BL, Lui D. Comparison between terminal slope rate constant and 'slope/intercept' as measures of glomerular filtration rate using the single-compartment simplification. Eur J Nucl Med 2001; 28: 320–6.

17 Piepsz A, Ham H. How good is the slope of the second exponential for estimating 51 Cr EDTA renal clearance. Nucl Med Commun 1997; 18: 139–41.

18. De Sadeleer C, Piepsz A, Ham H. Post-test quality control for single blood sample technique in glomerular filtration rate measurement. Eur J Nucl Med 2004; 31: S412 (abstr).

19. Brochner-Mortensen J, Rohbrandt K, Lauritzen RB. Precision of single injection (51Cr)EDTA plasma clearance and endogenous creatinine clearance determinations in children. Scand J Clin Lab Invest 1977; 37: 625–9.

20. Donath A. The simultaneous determination in children of glomerular filtration rate and effective renal plasma flow by the single injection clearance technique. Acta Paediatr Scand. 1971; 60: 512–20.

21. Piepsz A, Pintelon H, Ham HR. Estimation of normal 51Cr EDTA clearance in children. Eur J Nucl Med 1994; 21: 12–16.

22. Arnello F, Ham HR, Tondeur M, Piepsz A. Evolution of single kidney glomerular filtration rate in urinary tract infection. Pediatr Nephrol 1999; 13: 121–4.

5 Assessment of GFR in adults: the point of view of the nephrologist

Laurent Juillard, Maurice Laville

Glomerular filtration rate is only one of the several markers that describe renal performance. Renal blood flow, tubular functions involved in protein and electrolyte reabsorption and secretion of xenobiotics, are critical and relevant parameters when considering kidney exocrine function. Moreover, kidneys are endocrine organs involved in the long-term regulation of blood pressure by the secretion of renin and other components of the renin–angiotensin system, such as control of erythropoiesis by erythropoietin, and of phosphate and calcium metabolism by vitamin D hydroxylation.

Nevertheless, glomerular filtration rate estimated by serum creatinine remains the standard marker for renal function in a clinical routine, although the relation between the two parameters is complex.[1-3] First, the relationship between serum creatinine and glomerular filtration rate is exponentially inverse (Figure 5.1). Therefore in most patients, about 50% of glomerular filtration rate may be lost before serum creatinine reaches an abnormal value. Second, as creatinine is a degradation product of muscles, its serum level depends on age, sex (Figure 5.2),[4] and weight, with all these parameters integrated into the formulae of creatinine clearance estimation.[5-7] Plasma creatinine is also influenced by protein diet,[8] calibration of measurement[9] and tubular reabsorption.[10] As a consequences there is no normal value of serum creatinine for all individuals, and hence a given creatinine value must be always interpreted, and also serum creatinine is an insensitive marker for beginning renal failure (i.e. chronic renal disease stage 2). Nevertheless, when glomerular filtration rate decreases below 60 ml/min, plasma creatinine becomes an operational marker for the longitudinal follow-up of chronic renal disease in an individual patient, even if glomerular filtration rate measurement remains highly recommended.[11] Different methods for measurement(s) and estimation of glomerular filtration rate are summarized in Tables 5.1 and 5.2. It must be pointed out that measurement(s) of glomerular filtration rate by reference methods is not easy to perform, when using urine and blood samples drawn at precise time intervals, especially in a 'single shot' method that estimates renal function by the disappearance of a substance after an intravenous bolus injection. Another limitation of the use of plasma creatinine and formulae for estimation is for asymmetric renal diseases such as renal artery stenosis, unilateral ureteral obstruction and

Figure 5.1 The inverse exponential relationship between glomerular filtration rate measured with inulin clearance and serum creatinine level in adults (personal data).

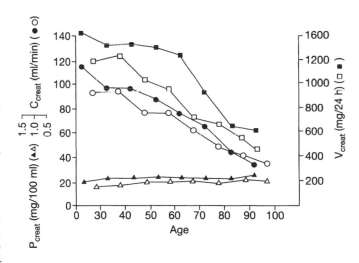

Figure 5.2 Age-related decrease in creatinine clearance (C_{Creat}) and urinary creatinine excretion (V_{Creat}) with no change in plasma creatinine (P_{Creat}) in normal individuals (black symbols: men; open symbols: women).[4]

Table 5.1 Methods for clinical use

- Measurement of GFR: clearances
  Substances
  - Endogenous: urea, creatinine, cystatin C
  - Chemicals: inulin, polyfructosan (with caution for allergy)
  - Radiopharmaceuticals: ^{51}Cr-EDTA, ^{99m}Tc-DTPA, ^{125}I-iothalamate
  - Contrast media: Iohexol,

  Models (exogenous substances)
  - Infusion with timed urine collections and plasma samples
  - Bolus with plasma samples with/without timed urine collections

- Estimation of GFR: formulas
  Cockcroft and Gault
  MDRD
  Mean of urea and creatinine clearances

Table 5.2 GFR estimation formulae

- Cockcroft and Gault (Ref. 5)
  Ccr* = [(140 − age) × weight]/72 × Pcr (mg/dl)
  Ccr* = [(140 − age) × weight]/0.814 × Pcr (μmol/l)
  *ml/min, correct by 0.85 for women.

- Complete MDRD (Ref. 6)
  GFR* = 170 × $Scr^{-0.999}$ × $age^{-0.176}$ × $SUN^{-0.170}$ × $Alb^{+0.318}$
  *ml/min/1.73 m^2, correct by 0.762 for women and 1.18 for blacks.

- Simplified MDRD (Ref. 11)
  GFR* = 186 × $Scr^{-1.154}$ × $age^{-0.203}$
  *ml/min/1.73 m^2, correct by 0.742 for women and 1.21 for blacks.

Table 5.3 Pitfalls of global assessment of renal function

- Contralateral compebsation results in
  Late diagnosis
  Silent aggrevation
- Unilateral/assymetrical renal disease
  Disease of upper urinary tract
    Hypoplasia
    Obstruction: hydronephrosis, stones
    Pyelonephritis and vesico-ureteral reflux
  Renal vascular disease
    Progressive renal artery stenosis and thrombosis

Table 5.4 Indications of renal function evaluation: estimation (E) and measurement (M)

- Screen for renal damage:
  General population (E)
  High-risk patients: diabetes, hypertension, elderly, medical or surgical history including genetics and professional exposures (M)
  Special settings: living kidney donors (M)
- Follow patients with chronic renal disease:
  Rate of progression, events (M)
  Treatment adjustments (M)
- Clinical research:
  Intervention studies (M)

pyelonephritis. The loss of unilateral function will not necessarily affect plasma creatinine, especially in cases of contralateral compensation. Functional imaging of the single kidney split function (e.g. renal scintigraphy) is mandatory to evaluate the performance of a damaged kidney (Table 5.3).

The growing use of formulae for creatinine clearance estimation as a marker of renal function leads to a better recognition of chronic renal failure in the general population. As a result, patients and general practitioners question the possibility of an increased risk for health associated with a decline in creatinine clearance, and the need of interventions performed to avoid progression of chronic renal failure.[12] These questions are pertinent as chronic renal failure represents an increased risk for end-stage renal disease and also a very significant and independent risk factor for cardiovascular morbidity and mortality.[13,14]

For the nephrologist, an abnormal renal function is a strong indicator of renal disease, especially if either prior serum creatinine or estimated creatinine clearance values are unaltered, or if seen together with clinical signs of hypertension or oedemas, or biological abnormalities (especially urinary abnormalities, such as proteinuria and haematuria) (Table 5.4). Therefore, after finding an abnormal creatinine or estimated creatinine clearance value during a routine test for renal function, it is critically important to recover prior results and to run serum creatinine measurements that will establish the progression or stability of renal disease. If plasma creatinine is stable with no change in lean body mass, interventions will be limited to a conservative treatment for renal protection, correcting any metabolic abnormalities, and reducing increased cardiovascular risk, depending on the stage of the chronic renal disease (Table 5.5). However, the decreased rate of GFR from the normal range to a value as low as 60 ml/min cannot be retrospectively estimated from the previous plasma creatinine data. In the case of a significant increase in plasma creatinine, specific evaluations should be performed and further investigations such as renal biopsy will need to be discussed.

Renal function measurements are also used to grade the severity of renal diseases found by clinical or biological abnormalities. For example, after the finding of a micro-

Table 5.5 Stages of chronic renal disease

Stage	Description	GFR (ml/min/1.73 m²)*
1	Kidney damage** with normal GFR	≥90
2	Kidney damage with mild ↓ GFR	60–89*
3	Moderate ↓ GFR	30–59
4	Severe ↓ GFR	15–29
5	Kidney failure	<15 or dialysis

*For at least 3 months. **Abnormalities of BP, urine, morphology, pathology.
K/DOQI clinical practice guidelines (Ref. 11)

scopic haematuria isolated or associated with a proteinuria <0.5 g/24 h, a renal biopsy could be carried out to confirm IgA nephropathy only if the results trigger a decision for therapeutic intervention;[15] also finding an abnormal renal function will be a pertinent indicator for a decision to carry out a biopsy. Consequently, it is critical to perform an initial accurate renal function measurement to keep as a reference during evaluation, especially at the early stage of most nephropathies. Thereafter, this initial evaluation will help the diagnosis of progressive renal disease and use of therapeutics. Moreover, the initial evaluation will be critical to test the efficiency of the therapeutics and to help decide whether to stop or pursue the use of toxic drugs, such as immuno-suppressive drugs or high-dose steroids.

When the diagnosis of chronic renal disease is established, renal function evaluation is mandatory at all stages to initiate therapeutics aimed at correcting or preventing the complications of renal function loss, mainly anaemia and calcium-phosphate metabolism disorders. Finally, renal function evaluation should be used at the late stage of renal failure in conjunction with the assessment of metabolic abnormalities and clinical tolerance in order to decide when to start dialysis treatment. After starting dialysis, renal function evaluation remains mandatory to measure residual glomerular filtration rate. Especially in peritoneal dialysis, renal function estimated by the mean of creatinine and urea clearances is critical; the clearance could reach a value between 60 and 70 l/week with 1 ml/min of residual renal function corresponding to up to 10 l/week of the total clearance in peritoneal dialysis.[16,17]

Another field of renal function evaluation is organ transplantation, especially kidney transplantation. Systematic glomerular filtration rate measurements are mandatory in the follow-up of kidney transplantation to screen for acute rejection and chronic graft rejection, in both cases to adjust immunosuppressive therapy.[18] Indeed, some drugs given after transplantation will have an impact on renal function of the graft, and also on the native kidneys after heart and liver transplantation.[19] Calcineurin inhibitors are efficient drugs but at high risk of nephrotoxicity.[20–22] In the case of worsening of the renal function not related to an immunologic process, another immunosuppressive drug can be used.[18] Renal function must be systematically measured with reference methods before carrying out heart and liver transplantations to indicate a concomitant kidney transplantation. This situation is particularly challenging as a significant part of renal function loss may be a consequence of relative hypovolaemia or decreased cardiac output and therefore potentially reversible.[23,24]

Renal function measurement is the cornerstone test before kidney nephrectomy in the living donor.[25] Concomitantly with cardiovascular risk assessment, renal function must be measured by reference methods. Measurements of renal functional reserve could be recommended to predict the adaptation capacities of a single kidney after nephrectomy. Glomerular filtration rate is measured in basal condition and repeated after a rich protein meal or amino acid perfusion: these interventions could lead to a 20% increase in basal value in normal renal subjects. The preservation of functional reserve would allow the acceptance of older living donors with a glomerular filtration rate below the normal range, corrected for the physiological decrease of 1 ml/min/year, for donors over 40 years of age.[26]

For general practitioners, the estimation of creatinine clearance by formulae should be systematic before any prescription of drugs in order to detect unrecognized kidney function impairment, especially in lean elderly women; that is, the major population at risk for undiagnosed chronic renal disease. However, renal function must be measured before the induction of the nephrotoxic treatment and monitored systematically during chronic treatment and after a temporary treatment with nephrotoxic drugs, keeping in mind that plasma creatinine changes allow only the detection of significant renal loss (decline greater than 25–50%) with poor sensitivity.[11] As most drugs have predominant renal elimination, dosages should be adjusted when creatinine clearance is under 30 ml/min, which is common in elderly patients.[27,28]

Currently, the major challenge for optimal treatment in chronic renal failure is the late nephrology referral,[29] denying access to early and efficient conservative treatment, a situation that could be prevented by systematic screening of creatinine clearance. In this regard, the wide diffusion of formulae to estimate glomerular filtration rate will be a significant advance, if proven interventions for reducing progression of chronic renal failure and protecting against cardiovascular complications are applied to patients. Health systems organizing screening to prevent chronic renal disease will be the price to pay for stopping the chronic renal failure epidemic in developed countries.

References

1. Levey AS, Perrone RD, Madias NE. Serum creatinine and renal function. Annu Rev Med 1988; 39: 465–90.
2. Perrone RD, Madias NE, Levey AS. Serum creatinine as an index of renal function: new insights into old concepts. Clin Chem 1992; 38: 1933–53.
3. Levey AS, Coresh J, Balk E et al. National Kidney Foundation practice guidelines for chronic kidney disease: evaluation, classification, and stratification. Ann Intern Med 2003; 139: 137–47.
4. Kampmann J, Siersbaek-Nielsen K, Kristensen M, Hansen JM. Rapid evaluation of creatinine clearance. Acta Med Scand 1974; 196: 517–20.
5. Cockcroft DW, Gault MH. Prediction of creatinine clearance from serum creatinine. Nephron 1976; 16: 31–41.
6. Levey AS, Bosch JP, Lewis JB et al. A more accurate method to estimate glomerular filtration rate from serum creatinine: a new prediction equation. Modification of Diet in Renal Disease Study Group. Ann Intern Med 1999; 130: 461–70.
7. Manjunath G, Sarnak MJ, Levey AS. Prediction equations to estimate glomerular filtration rate: an update. Curr Opin Nephrol Hypertens 2001; 10: 785–92.
8. Lew SW, Bosch JP. Effect of diet on creatinine clearance and excretion in young and elderly healthy subjects and in patients with renal disease. J Am Soc Nephrol 1991; 2: 856–65.
9. Coresh J, Eknoyan G, Levey AS. Estimating the prevalence of low glomerular filtration rate requires attention to the creatinine assay calibration. J Am Soc Nephrol 2002; 13: 2811–2; author reply 2812–6.
10. Sjostrom PA, Odlind BG, Wolgast M. Extensive tubular secretion and reabsorption of creatinine in humans. Scand J Urol Nephrol 1988; 22: 129–31.
11. National Kidney Foundation. K/DOQI clinical practice guidelines for chronic kidney disease: evaluation, classification, and stratification. Am J Kidney Dis 2002; 39 (Suppl 1): S1–266.
12. Stevens LA, Levey AS. Clinical implications of estimating equations for glomerular filtration rate. Ann Intern Med 2004; 141: 959–61.
13. Go AS, Chertow GM, Fan D et al. Chronic kidney disease and the risks of death, cardiovascular events, and hospitalization. N Engl J Med 2004; 351: 1296–305.
14. Weiner DE, Tighiouart H, Amin MG et al. Chronic kidney disease as a risk factor for cardiovascular disease and all-cause mortality: a pooled analysis of community-based studies. J Am Soc Nephrol 2004; 15: 1307–15.
15. Laville M, Alamartine E. Treatment options for IgA nephropathy in adults: a proposal for evidence-based strategy. Nephrol Dial Transplant 2004; 19: 1947–51.
16. Bargman JM, Golper TA. The importance of residual renal function for patients on dialysis. Nephrol Dial Transplant 2005; 20: 671–3.
17. Kuno T, Matsumoto K. Clinical benefit of preserving residual renal function in patients after initiation of dialysis. Blood Purif 2004; 22 (Suppl 2): 67–71.
18. Pascual M, Theruvath T, Kawai T et al. Strategies to improve long-term outcomes after renal transplantation. N Engl J Med 2002; 346: 580–90.
19. Ojo AO, Held PJ, Port FK et al. Chronic renal failure after transplantation of a nonrenal organ. N Engl J Med 2003; 349: 931–40.
20. Keogh A. Calcineurin inhibitors in heart transplantation. J Heart Lung Transplant 2004; 23(Suppl): S202–6.
21. Cattaneo D, Perico N, Gaspari F, Remuzzi G. Nephrotoxic aspects of cyclosporine. Transplant Proc 2004; 36 (Suppl): 234S–9S.
22. Ziolkowski J, Paczek L, Senatorski G et al. Renal function after liver transplantation: calcineurin inhibitor nephrotoxicity. Transplant Proc 2003; 35: 2307–9.
23. Cipullo R, Finger MA, Ponce F et al. Renal failure as a determinant of mortality after cardiac transplantation. Transplant Proc 2004; 36: 989–90.
24. Skluzacek PA, Szewc RG, Nolan CR 3rd et al. Prediction of GFR in liver transplant candidates. Am J Kidney Dis 2003; 42: 1169–76.
25. Rule AD, Larson TS, Bergstrahl EJ et al. Measured and estimated GFR in healthy potential kidney donors. Am J Kidney Dis 2004; 43: 112–9.
26. Laville M, Hadj-Aissa A, Pozet N et al. Restrictions on use of creatinine clearance for measurement of renal functional reserve. Nephron 1989; 51: 233–6.
27. Rowe JW, Andres R, Tobin JD et al. The effect of age on creatinine clearance in men: a cross-sectional and longitudinal study. J Gerontol 1976; 31: 155–63.
28. Fuller NJ, Elia M. Factors influencing the production of creatinine: implications for the determination and interpretation of urinary creatinine and creatine in man. Clin Chim Acta 1988; 175: 199–210.
29. Lameire N, Wauters JP, Teruel JL et al. An update on the referral pattern of patients with end-stage renal disease. Kidney Int Suppl 2002; 80: 27–34.

6 Assessment of GFR in children: the point of view of the paediatric nephrologist

Jean-Pierre Guignard

Glomerular filtration rate (GFR)

Glomerular filtration rate is the best estimate of the functional renal mass. It is the most widely used indicator of kidney function in patients with renal disease. The assessment of GFR is of great value in a variety of clinical conditions, since an estimate of GFR may be required to rationally prescribe fluids, electrolytes or drugs excreted by the kidney.

Physiology of glomerular filtration

Ultrafiltration occurs through the permselective capillary wall. Ultrafiltration is driven by Starling forces across the glomerular capillaries. The glomerular barrier filters molecules on the basis of size and electric charges. The molecular weight cut-off for the filter is approximately 70 kDa. With a molecular weight (MW) of 69 kDa, albumin passes through the filter in minute quantities. The glomerular filter is freely permeable to those molecules with a MW less than 7 kDa. Filtration of proteins, with consequent proteinuria, is increased in a number of glomerular diseases associated with the loss of negative charges on the glomerular filtration barrier.

Concept of clearance

The most common measurement of GFR is based on the concept of clearance, which relates the quantitative urinary excretion of a substance per unit time to the volume of plasma that, if 'cleared' completely of the same substance, would yield a quantity equivalent to that excreted in the urine. The clearance of substance (x) is expressed by the formula:

$$C_x = U_x \cdot V/P_x$$

where V represents the urine flow rate, U_x and P_x the urine and plasma concentration of the substance x, respectively.

Markers of GFR

For its plasma clearance to be equal to the rate of glomerular filtration, a marker must have the following properties: (a) it must be freely filterable through the glomerular capillary membranes; and (b) it must be biologically inert and neither reabsorbed nor secreted by the renal tubules. Several substances, endogenous or exogenous, have been claimed to have the above properties: creatinine, inulin, iohexol, and three compounds labelled with radioisotopes: diethylenetri-aminepenta-acetic acid (DTPA); ethylenediaminetetra-acetic acid (EDTA) and sodium iothalamate (Table 6.1). The experimental evidence that this is true has only been produced for inulin. While inulin is the most accurate marker, creatinine is the most commonly used in children.

Methods available for assessing GFR

A variety of glomerular markers (Table 6.1) can be used to assess GFR, using different methods, the principles of which are described below.

Table 6.1 Characteristics of the glomerular markers

	Inulin	Creatinine	Iohexol	DTPA	EDTA	Iothalamate
Molecular weight	5200	113	811	393	292	637
Elimination half-life (min)	70	200	90	110	120	120
Plasma protein binding (%)	0	0	<2	5	0	<5
Space of distribution	EC	TBW	EC	EC	EC	EC

DTPA, diethylenediaminepenta-acetic acid; EDTA, ethylenediaminetetra-acetic acid; EC, extracellular space; TBW, total body water.

The standard urinary clearance UV/P

Endogenous markers

The urinary excretion of the marker is measured over a few hours, and its excretion rate is divided by the plasma concentration present during the urine collection period. When urine flow rate is expressed in ml/min per 1.73 m^2, the UV/P formula also expresses GFR in ml/min per 1.73 m^2. Duration of the collection may last from 3 to 24 h. Short periods are most suitable in children in order to avoid inaccuracies in urine collection. Creatinine is the endogenous marker that is used for assessing GFR.

Exogenous markers

The exogenous marker is infused at a constant rate over 3 to 4 hours, in order to achieve constant plasma concentrations. To shorten the time of equilibration, a priming dose of the marker is administered at the onset of the clearance study. When stable plasma concentrations are attained, urine and blood samples are collected at regular intervals, and the UV/P ratio is calculated. Inulin is the most accurate marker of GFR.

The constant infusion technique without urine collection

The constant infusion technique[1,2] assumes that the rate of infusion of a marker (x) needed to maintain constant its plasma concentration is equal to the rate of its excretion. After equilibration of the marker in its distribution space, the excretion rate must thus be equal to the rate of infusion (IR), hence the formula:

$$C_x = U_x \cdot V/P_x = IR_x/P_x$$

When the flow rate of the test solution containing the marker is expressed in ml/min per 1.73 m^2, so the clearance is C_x.

To accelerate the achievement of a steady concentration of the marker, a loading dose precedes the constant iv infusion. The constant infusion method may overestimate GFR if steady concentrations of the marker are not achieved when the plasma concentration is measured. Depending on the conditions, the equilibration of the marker within its distribution space may only be achieved after several hours of constant infusion. In newborn infants, the proportionally greater extracellular space and the low GFR require a much longer period for steady plasma concentrations to be attained. Inulin is the marker of choice for this technique, which is usually used when urine collection is not possible (see below).

Plasma disappearance curve (single injection technique)

The plasma disappearance curve is most often used when assessing GFR with radionuclides. Infusion of radionuclides for several hours is indeed undesirable, and they are best reserved for single injection studies in which the radioisotope is more rapidly eliminated from the kidney. Commonly used markers include ^{99m}Tc-DTPA, ^{51}Cr-EDTA and ^{125}I-iothalamate. Clearance values derived from the plasma disappearance curve should be analysed critically, the more so in patients with reduced GFR, and those with oedema and circulatory disturbances.

Plasma concentration

The concentration of endogenous markers such as creatinine increases when GFR decreases. Several attempts have been made to develop reliable methods that will allow a correct estimate of creatinine clearance from its plasma concentration (P_{creat}) alone, without urine collection. A formula has thus been developed to estimate GFR from the child's creatinine plasma concentration and height:

$$GFR = k \times height/P_{creat},$$

where k is a constant, height represents the body height and P_{creat} the plasma creatinine concentration. This formula is based on the assumption that creatinine excretion is proportional to body height and inversely proportional to plasma creatinine.[3] The value of factor k can be obtained from the formula $k = GFR \times height/P_{creat}$. Under steady-state conditions, k should be directly proportional to the muscle component of body weight, which corresponds reasonably well to the daily urinary creatinine excretion rate.

Cystatin C

The serum concentration of cystatin C has been proposed to assess GFR.[4] There is as yet no convincing evidence that the serum concentration of this marker will prove superior to that of creatinine in estimating the level of renal function.

Estimation of GFR in clinical practice with different markers

Inulin

The marker

Inulin, a fructose polysaccharide derived from dahlia roots and Jerusalem artichokes, has a MW of approximately 5.2 kDa. It is inert and not metabolized. Evidence that inulin in neither reabsorbed nor secreted by the renal tubules has been well demonstrated in experimental micropuncture studies.[5,6]

The clearance (UV/P) of inulin is independent of its plasma concentration. The renal excretion of inulin occurs exclusively by glomerular filtration, its clearance is the most accurate index of GFR. Estimates of inulin clearance provide

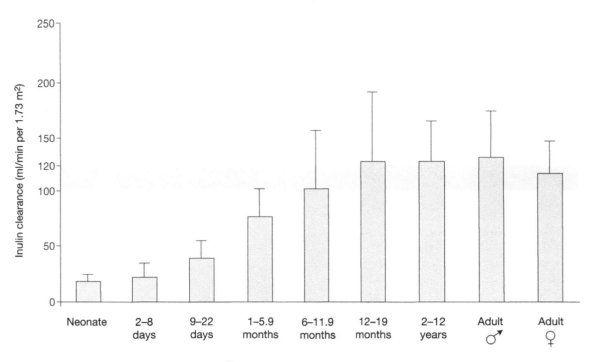

Figure 6.1 Inulin clearance as a function of age $\overline{X} \pm SD$.

the basis for a standard reference against which the route or mechanism of excretion of other substances can be ascertained.

Sinistrin is a readily soluble preparation of polyfructosan with side-branching (extracted from the bulb of *Urginea maritima*), more suitable for clinical use and readily available in Europe. This compound is identical to inulin.

Inulin urinary clearance

Inulin or sinistrin urinary clearance (UV/P) is the gold standard for the assessment of GFR. In the classical method, inulin is administered as a priming dose to achieve plasma concentrations close to 200–400 mg/l. It is then constantly infused to maintain constant levels over the 3-hour clearance study.

The rise in GFR from birth to adulthood is illustrated in Figure 6.1. Mature values of GFR range from 100–120 ml/min per 1.73 m². In a study by Koopman in adult volunteers, GFR, as assessed by inulin clearance, had a circadian rhythm.[7] It started to decrease during late afternoon or evening, and rose again at the end of the night. The mean amplitude of the rhythm was 36 ml/min.

The constant infusion technique of inulin without urine collection

The constant infusion technique of inulin without urine collection yields reproducible results,[1,2] as long as sufficient time is given for steady concentrations to be reached.[8] This may take as long as 12 h in adults[8] and even longer in infants.[9] During the equilibration period, inulin is excreted by filtration, while at the same time diffusing into the extracellular space. Calculations of the infusion (IR/P) clearance before equilibra-

tion occurs thus falsely increase the estimation, yielding values of clearance up to 30% above the urinary clearance. The shorter the time of infusion, the larger is the overestimation. The constant infusion method is useful when timed urine collections are difficult or unreliable, such as in small babies, children with hydronephrosis, or those with neurogenic bladder.

The result of the study comparing the '3-hour constant infusion' with the urinary clearance of inulin in 60 children older than 1 year showed a significant correlation, but the calculated regression line differed significantly from the line of identity and the scatter of points was considerable.[10] These results did not confirm an earlier report by Cole et al[2] demonstrating virtual superposition of inulin clearances values generated with and without urine collection.

Creatinine

The marker

Creatinine is the anhydre of creatine, a compound present in skeletal muscle as creatine phosphate. It has a MW of 113. The serum creatinine levels reflect total body supplies of creatinine and correlate with muscle mass. After an initial decrease during the first month of life it increases steadily with age (Figures 6.2 and 6.3). The excretion rate varies according to body weight and age, both reflecting muscle mass (Table 6.2). The renal excretion pattern of endogenous creatinine is very similar to that of inulin in humans and several animal species. However, in addition to being filtered through the glomerulus, creatinine is secreted in part by the renal tubular cells.

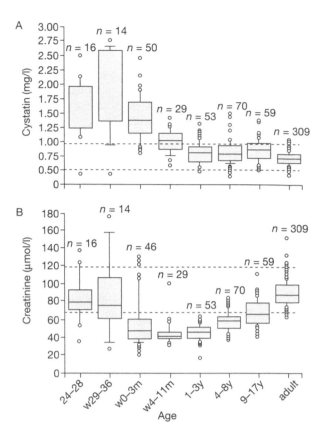

Figure 6.2 Changes in plasma creatinine (A) and urea (B) concentrations during the first 100 hours of life of premature neonates of variable gestational age. The shaded area represents 95% CIs for the mean plasma creatinine or urea of all infants. Adapted from reference 56.

Figure 6.3 Box plot distributions showing (A) cystatin C and (B) creatinine values (10th, 25th, 50th and 90th centiles) across the age groups. The categories of 24–36 and 29–36 weeks refer to gestational ages of preterm babies. Dotted lines indicate 95% confidence interval of adult range. Preterm babies born between 24–36 weeks gestation were one day old. Adapted from reference 30.

Table 6.2 Plasma creatinine in children

Age	Plasma creatinine		Creatininuria	
	µmol/l	mg/dl	µmol/kg per day	mg/kg per day
<2 years	35–40	0.4–0.5	62–88	7.1–9.9
2–8 years	40–60	0.5–0.7	108–188	12.2–21.2
9–18 years	50–80	0.6–0.9	132–212	14.9–23.9

Adapted from Garcia Nieto V, Santos F. Pruebas funcionales renales. In: Garcia Nieto V, Santos F (eds), Nefrologia Pediatrica. Grupo Aula Medica, Madrid, pp. 15–26, 2000.

The validity of creatinine as a marker of GFR has been questioned because creatinine is not only secreted by the renal tubular cells, but could also be reabsorbed under certain conditions. Such reabsorption has been shown to occur in rats[11] and dogs at low urine flow rates.[12] Substantial tubular secretion and reabsorption of creatinine has been suggested in humans in relation to the degree of hydration,[13,14] as well as in very premature infants.

Overestimation of GFR by creatinine clearance is usually more evident at low GFR. Indeed, as GFR falls progressively during the course of renal diseases, the renal tubular secretion of creatinine represents an increasing fraction to urinary excretion, so that creatinine clearance may substantially exceed the actual GFR. Diffusion of creatinine into the gut may also decrease the accuracy of its clearance in uraemic patients. At normal plasma concentrations, the amount of creatinine entering the gut is negligible. It may become significant during renal failure when the plasma creatinine concentration increases.[15] This phenomenon explains in part why creatinine clearance overestimates true GFR in patients with renal failure.

Measurement of creatinine

Creatinine concentration in plasma and urine is usually based on the Jaffe reaction, characterized by the production of an orange-red colour when creatinine reacts with alkaline sodium picrate. The method is not very specific, noncreatinine chromogens generating sufficient colour to account for 0.2–0.3 mg/dl (~30 µmol/l) of 'false creatinine'. The interference of noncreatinine chromogen obviously is highest at the lowest values of creatinine, as present in newborn infants.[16] Negative interference by conjugated and unconjugated bilirubin makes the use of the Jaffe reaction questionable in neonates. Other interference substances include aceto-acetate, pyruvate, uric acid, the cephalosporins and cotrimoxazole.[16] Enzymatic methods have been developed that are more specific than the Jaffe reaction.

Determination of serum creatinine by isotope dilution mass spectrometry has been described as the potentially 'definitive' method.[17] High performance liquid chromatography will undoubtedly become the reference method for creatinine determination,[18] even if its routine use is still not possible in most clinical laboratories.

Creatinine urinary clearance (UV/P)

The urinary clearance of creatinine is the most commonly used method for assessing GFR in children. The urine is collected over 4–24 h, and the plasma sample collected at the mid urine collection period. The plasma creatinine concentration can be significantly increased by eating cooked-meat.[19] Drugs such as trimethroprim[20] and cimetidine[21] increase the plasma creatinine by interfering with the renal tubular secretion, presumably by competition for the organic cation secretory pathway.[20]

The estimation of GFR by measuring the urinary clearance of creatinine yields values that have been shown to correlate variably with inulin clearance. The best correlation is seen when GFR is normal. This agreement usually results from the balance of two artifacts: (1) the excretion rate of creatinine is higher than the filtered rate because of the tubular secretion of creatinine and (2) the measured plasma creatinine is higher than the true creatinine because of the presence of noncreatinine chromogens that interfere with a standard colorimetric analysis of creatinine in the Jaffe reaction. Overestimation of GFR by the urinary clearance of creatinine is usually maximal at low levels of GFR.[22,23] The ratio of the urinary clearance of creatinine to urinary inulin clearance has been shown to vary from 1.14 to 2.27 in adult subjects. It was suggested long ago that the clearance of creatinine should be discarded as a precise estimate of GFR as this clearance varies as a consequence of tubular secretion of creatinine in mature individuals. In Kim et al's study, 42% of patients with definitely diminished renal function would have been diagnosed as normal if only creatinine had been checked.[24] Like those of Rosenbaum,[25] data obtained by Guignard et al[10] in 72 children older than one year showed a substantial overestimation of GFR by creatinine clearance at all levels of GFR.

Assessment of GFR by the formula $(2C_{creat} + C_{urea})/3$

In children undergoing simultaneous inulin and creatinine urinary clearance studies[10] the overestimation of GFR by creatinine clearance was 'corrected' when the clearance of urea was also taken into account. When using the formula '$(2C_{creat} + C_{urea})/3$', the regression line correlating this formula to inulin clearance was indistinguishable from the line of identity (Figure 6.4). The scatter of points around the regression line was, however, not negligible.

Figure 6.4 Relationship between standard urinary clearance of inulin and the $(2C_{creat} + C_{urea})/3$ formula. Adapted from reference 10.

Clearly, creatinine clearance alone is not a good alternative to inulin clearance when a precise measurement of GFR is needed. The use of the formula '$(2C_{creat} + C_{urea})/3$', calculated over 3–4 h in well-hydrated children, is recommended when the clinical situation does not warrant the cumbersome measurement of inulin clearance or when the technique is not available.

The GFR = k . height/P_{creat} formula

Numerous studies have used this index first described in 1976,[26,27] providing conflicting results. A critical review of the use of this formula has been published by Haycock.[28] The formula provides useful data when used cautiously. It cannot be used in obese or malnourished children in whom body height does not accurately reflect muscle mass. Ideally, the exact value of k should be derived from the laboratory where the plasma creatinine is measured, and from inulin clearance as the reference method for estimating GFR. The values of k, as derived from creatinine clearance in different age groups by Schwarz and colleagues[3] are given in Table 6.3. In a study involving 200 patients aged 1 month to 23 years, Haenggi et al[14] compared the values of k derived from the urinary clearance of inulin to that derived from simultaneous creatinine urinary clearance. The value of k derived from creatinine or inulin clearance differed significantly in children undergoing water diuresis (urine flow rate 8.5 ml/min per 1.73 m²), being lower when calculated from C_{inulin}. In hydropenic children the values of k were identical whether derived from C_{inulin} or C_{creat} (49 ± 2 and 50 ± 3, respectively). Increased secretory rates of creatinine at high urine flow rates probably account for the elevated value of k calculated from C_{creat} in well-hydrated children. Extensive tubular secretion and reabsorption of creatinine in relation to the degree of hydration has been well described in humans.[11] Whatever the limitation in the accuracy of the estimate of GFR by the k . height/P_{creat} formula, the use of the formula has proved valuable as a rapid estimate of GFR in clinical practice.

Table 6.3 Values of k for various age groups

	k values when P_{creat} expressed in	
	μmol/l	mg/dl
Low birth-weight infants <2.5 kg	29	0.33
Normal infants 0–18 months	40	0.45
Girls 2–16 years	49	0.55
Boys 2–13 years	49	0.55
Boys 13–16 years	62	0.70

Adapted from references 3 and 14.

Cystatin C

Cystatin C, a nonglycosated 13-Da basic protein, is a proteinase inhibitor involved in the intracellular catabolism of proteins.[29] It is produced by all nucleated cells at a constant rate apparently independent of inflammatory conditions, muscle mass and gender.[30] It is freely filtered across the glomerular capillaries, almost completely reabsorbed and catabolized in the proximal tubular cells.[31] Being reabsorbed, cystatin is not a classical glomerular marker, as strictly defined.[32] Fully automated assays using particle-enhanced turbidimetry[33] or particle-enhanced nephelometry[34] are available for the measurement of cystatin in plasma and serum.

Cystatin C does not appear to cross the placenta and there is no correlation between maternal and neonatal serum cystatin C levels.[35] Cystatin C concentrations are highest at birth, and then decrease to stabilize after 12 months of age (Figure 6.3).[30] Whether cystatin C is significantly higher in premature infants as compared to term infants is not yet clear.[30,36] The reference interval for serum cystatin C has been estimated as ranging from 0.70 to 1.38 mg/l in children older than 1 year.[37]

Serum cystatin C increases when GFR decreases. The reciprocal values of cystatin C correlate linearly with GFR and cystatin C has been claimed to be at least as good a measure of GFR as serum creatinine in adults.[38] In children aged 1.8–18.8 years with various levels of GFR, serum cystatin C has been found to be broadly equivalent to serum creatinine as an estimate of GFR.[4] The fact that cystatin C is independent of age, gender, height and body composition[36] has been considered an advantage.

The major drawbacks in using cystatin C are that it is not a classical glomerular marker, and that its clearance can consequently not be calculated. Numerical estimates of GFR can also not be rationally derived from its plasma clearance. A recent study by Martini et al[39] compared the reliability of different estimates of GFR to distinguish impaired from normal GFR, with a cut-off at 100 ml/min per 1.73 m². While plasma cystatin was slightly superior to the plasma creatinine concentration to diagnose renal insufficiency, it was significantly less sensitive than both the urinary clearance of creatinine and the estimate k × height/P_{creat}. The authors

concluded that simply measuring the child's height in addition to its plasma creatinine was a simpler, cheaper and better means of rapidly assessing GFR in children than measuring the plasma cystatin C. The recent observation by Knight et al[40] that cystatin C is influenced by factors other than renal function alone casts doubt on the real value of cystatin C as the best estimate of GFR. In this very large study involving 8058 inhabitants of the city of Groningen, multivariate serum cystatin C-based estimates were indeed not superior to equivalent serum creatinine-based estimates.[40]

Assessment of GFR in neonates

Inulin as a marker of GFR in the neonate

Studies comparing the clearance of inulin with that of other glomerular markers have led to the hypothesis that glomerular pore size could be related to body size, and that inulin may not be freely filtered by the immature glomerulus.[41] This hypothesis has not been confirmed by studies of inulin handling in rats[42] or fetal lambs,[43] both failing to demonstrate any restriction to the filtration of inulin. The same conclusion was reached from clinical studies in preterm infants showing that high-molecular-weight inulin or polysaccharides did not accumulate in the plasma of very immature babies infused with these glomerular markers for several days, thus excluding any retention of the larger molecules.[44,45]

Standard urinary inulin clearance studies performed during the first two days of life of preterm and term neonates have shown that GFR at birth is approximately 20 ml/min per 1.73 m² in term neonates and 10 ml/min per 1.73 m² in preterms of 28 weeks of gestation.[46] The GFR matures rapidly in the early postnatal period, doubling during the first two weeks of life (Figure 6.5).[46] The speed of the maturation is somewhat slower in the most premature infants.

Conflicting results have been produced in neonates studied by the inulin constant infusion technique over a few hours. While Cole and Leake and their colleagues[2,47] found an excellent correlation between the constant infusion clearance and the urinary clearance of inulin (R = 0.999), Guignard and coworkers[48] found the constant infusion technique to greatly overestimate (~30%) the urinary clearance of inulin in infants. The overestimation declined with time but remained substantial after 3 h of infusion. The same conclusion was reached by Coulthard[9] who also observed an overestimation of GFR by the constant infusion technique, in spite of the fact that the plasma inulin concentration was apparently stable. Reliable estimates of GFR could however be obtained when inulin was constantly infused for 24 h. The main disadvantage of the method is that it requires a constant infusion of long duration. Results comparing data obtained by the plasma disappearance curve technique with those obtained by the urinary clearance of inulin are conflicting. Early optimistic results[49] have not been

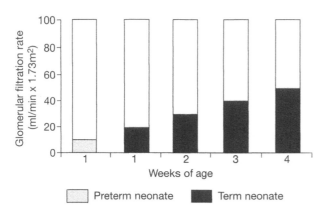

Figure 6.5 Postnatal increase in glomerular filtration rate in term and preterm infants. Adapted from reference 46.

confirmed. A 30% overestimation of the true GFR was described by Fawer and colleagues in neonates 1–3 days old.[50]

Creatinine as a marker of GFR in the neonate

In tiny premature neonates, the clearance of creatinine underestimates inulin clearance.[51,52] Animal studies suggest that endogenous creatinine is significantly reabsorbed by the immature tubule.[53,54] Creatinine reabsorption by the immature kidney probably occurs by passive back-diffusion of filtered creatinine across leaky tubules. Significant reabsorption of filtered creatinine supposedly accounts for the transient increase in plasma creatinine in the first three days of life of very low birth-weight infants (Figure 6.2).[55–57] After the neonatal period P_{creat} rises steadily throughout infancy and childhood towards adult levels (Table 6.2).

In spite of its drawbacks creatinine clearance has been used commonly to assess GFR in neonates. Studying very low birth-weight (VLBW) infants, Stonestreet et al[52] have reported a correlation coefficient of 0.78 when values of creatinine clearance were compared to those of inulin clearance. In recent studies in premature and term neonates[57,58] creatinine clearance has been shown to be low at birth and to rise rapidly after birth. The slope of maturation was steeper in the most mature infants.[58] The increase in creatinine clearance correlated with the postnatal increase in systemic blood pressure,[58,59] as well as with gestational and postnatal age.[57,58] Creatinine clearance close to 42 ml/min per 1.73 m² in term neonates, and 27 ml/min per 1.73 m² in preterms less than 27 weeks of gestation were recorded on the 52nd day of life.[57] Mature levels close to 100 ml/min per 1.73 m² are reached at the end of the first year of life.

References

1. Earle DP, Berliner RW. A simplified clinical procedure for measurement of glomerular filtration rate and renal blood flow. Proc Soc Exp Biol Med 1946; 62: 262–264.

2. Cole BR, Giangiacomo J, Ingelfinger JR et al. Measurement of renal function without urine collection. A critical evaluation of the constant-infusion technic for determination of inulin and para-aminohippurate. N Engl J Med 1972; 287: 1109–14.

3. Schwartz GJ, Brion LP, Spitzer A. The use of plasma creatinine concentration for estimating glomerular filtration rate in infants, children, and adolescents. Pediatr Clin North Am 1987; 34: 571–90.

4. Stickle D, Cole B, Hock K et al. Correlation of plasma concentration of cystatin C and creatinine to inulin clearance in a pediatric population. Clin Chem 1998; 44: 1334–8.

5. Marsh D, Frasier C. Reliability of inulin for determining volume flow in rat renal cortical tubules. Am J Physiol 1965; 209: 283–6.

6. Tanner GA, Klose RM. Micropuncture study of inulin reabsorption in Necturus kidney. Am J Physiol 1966; 211: 1036–8.

7. Koopman MG, Koomen GCM, Krediet RT et al. Circadian rhythm of glomerular filtration rate in normal individuals. Clin Sci 1989; 77: 105–11.

8. Hellerstein S, Barenbom M, Alon U et al. The renal clearance and infusion clearance of inulin are similar, but not identical. Kidney Int 1993; 44: 1058–61.

9. Coulthard MG. Comparison of methods of measuring renal function in preterm babies using inulin. J Pediatr 1983; 102: 923–30.

10. Guignard JP, Torrado A, Feldmann H, et al. Assessment of glomerular filtration rate in children. Helv Pediatr Acta 1980; 35: 437–47.

11. Namnum P, Insogna K, Baggish D, et al. Evidence for bidirectional net movement of creatinine in the rat kidney. Am J Physiol 1983; 244: F719–23.

12. Lee KE, Behrendt U, Kaczmarczyk G, et al. Estimation of glomerular filtration rate in conscious dogs following a bolus of creatinine. Pflügers Arch 1983; 396: 176–8.

13. Sjöstrom PA, Odlind BG, Wolgast M. Extensive tubular secretion and reabsorption of creatinine in humans. Scand J Urol Nephrol 1988; 22: 129–31.

14. Haenggi MH, Pelet J, Guignard JP. Estimation of glomerular filtration rate by the formula GFR = K × T/Pc. Arch Pediatr 1999; 6: 165–72.

15. Jones JD, Burnett PC. Implication of creatinine and gut flora in the uremic syndrome: induction of 'creatininase' in colon contents of the rat by dietary creatinine. Clin Chem 1972; 18: 280–4.

16. Rossano TG, Ambrose RT, Wu AHB, et al. Candidate reference method for determining creatinine in serum: method development and interlaboratory validation. Clin Chem 1990; 36: 1951–5.

17. Welch MJ, Cohen A, Hertz HS, et al. Determination of serum creatinine by isotope dilution mass spectrometry as a candidate definitive method. Anal Chem 1986; 58: 1681–5.

18. Ambrose RT, Ketchum DF, Smith JW. Creatinine determined

by 'high-performance' liquid chromatography. Clin Chem 1983; 29: 256–9.

19. Meyersohn M, Conrad KA, Achari R. The influence of a cooked meat meal on creatinine plasma concentration and creatinine clearance. Br J Clin Pharmacol 1983; 15: 227–30.

20. Guignard JP, Tabin R, Vienny H, et al. Effect of trimethoprim-sulfamethoxazole on renal function. Curr Ther Res 1983; 34: 801–6.

21. Dubb JW, Stole RM, Familiar RG. Effect of cimetidine on renal function in normal man. Clin Pharmacol Ther 1978; 24: 76–83.

22. Arant BS, Edelmann CM, Spitzer A. The congruence of creatinine and inulin clearance in children: use of the Technicon Auto-Analyser. J Pediatr 1972; 81: 559–61.

23. Dodge WF, Travis LB, Daeschner CW. Comparison of endogenous creatinine clearance with inulin clearance. Am J Dis Child 1967; 113: 683–92.

24. Kim KE, Onesti G, Ramirez O, et al. Creatinine clearance in renal disease: A reappraisal. Br Med J 1969; 4: 11–14.

25. Rosenbaum JL. Evaluation of clearance studies in chronic kidney disease. J Chronic Dis 1970; 22: 507–14.

26. Counahan R, Chantler C, Ghazali S, et al. Estimation of glomerular filtration rate from plasma creatinine concentration in children. Arch Dis Child 1976; 51: 875–8.

27. Schwartz GJ, Haycock GB, Edelmann CM Jr, et al. A simple estimate of glomerular filtration rate in children derived from body length and plasma creatinine. Pediatrics 1976; 58: 259–63.

28. Haycock GB. Creatinine, body size and renal function. Pediatr Nephrol 1989; 3: 22–4.

29. Olafsson I. The human cystatin C gene promoter: functional analysis and identification of heterogenous mRNA. Scand J Clin Lab Invest 1995; 55: 597–607.

30. Finney H, Newman DJ, Thakkar H, et al. Reference ranges for plasma cystatin C and creatinine measurements in premature infants, neonates and older children. Arch Dis Child 2000; 82: 71–5.

31. Tenstad O, Roald AB, Grubb A, et al. Renal handling of radio-labelled human cystatin C in the rat. Scand J Clin Lab Invest 1996; 56: 409–14.

32. Pitts RF, ed. Physiology of the Kidney and Body Fluids. 2nd edn. Chicago: Yearbook Medical Publishers Inc, 1988.

33. Kyhse-Andersen J, Schmidt C, Nordin G, et al. Serum cystatin C, determined by a rapid automated particle-enhanced turbimetric method, is a better marker than serum creatinine for glomerular filtration rate. Clin Chem 1994; 40: 1921–6.

34. Finney H, Newman DJ, Grubb W, et al. Initial evaluation of cystatin C measurement by particle-enhanced immuno-nephelometry on the Behring nephelometer systems (BNA, BNII). Clin Chem 1997; 4: 1016–22.

35. Cataldi L, Mussap M, Bertelli L, et al. Cystatin C in healthy women at term pregnancy and in their infant newborns: relationship between maternal and neonatal serum levels and reference values. Am J Perinatol 1999; 16: 287–95.

36. Harmoinen A, Ylinen E, Ala-Houhala M, et al. Reference intervals for cystatin C in pre- and full-term infants and children. Pediatr Nephrol 2000; 15: 105–8.

37. Bökenkamp A, Domanetzki M, Zinck R, et al. Reference values for cystatin C serum concentration in children. Pediatr Nephrol 1998; 12: 125–9.

38. Randers E, Erlandsen EJ. Serum cystatin C as an endogenous

marker of the renal function – a review. Clin Chem Lab Med 1999; 37: 389–95.

39. Martini SS, Prévot AY, Werner D, et al. Diagnostic value of cystatin C as a marker of glomerular filtration rate indication. J Am Nephrol 2001; 12: 226A.

40. Knight EL, Verhave JC, Spiegelman D, et al. Factors influencing serum cystatin levels other than renal function and the impact on renal function measurement. Kidney Int 2004; 65: 1416–21.

41. Arturson G, Groth T, Grotte G. Human glomerular membrane porosity and filtration pressure: dextran clearance data analysed by theoretical models. Clin Sci 1971; 40: 137–58.

42. Harris CA, Baer PG, Chirito E, et al. Composition of mammalian glomerular filtrate. Am J Physiol 1974; 227: 972–6.

43. Rankin JH, Gresham EL, Battaglia FC, et al. Measurement of fetal renal inulin clearance in a chronic sheep preparation. J Appl Physiol 1972; 32: 129–33.

44. Coulthard MG, Ruddock V. Validation of inulin as a marker for glomerular filtration in preterm babies. Kidney Int 1983; 23: 407–9.

45. Wilkins BH. The glomerular filterability of polyfructosan-S in immature infants. Pediatr Nephrol 1992; 6: 319–22.

46. Guignard JP, Torrado A, Da Cunha O, et al. Glomerular filtration rate in the first three weeks of life. J Pediatr 1975; 87: 268–72.

47. Leake RD, Trygstad CW, Oh W. Inulin clearance in the newborn infant: relationship to gestational and postnatal age. Pediatr Res 1976; 10: 759–62.

48. Alinei P, Guignard JP. Assessment of glomerular filtration rate in infants. Helv Pediatr Acta 1987; 42: 253–62.

49. Svenningsen NW. Single injection polyfructosan clearance in normal and asphyxiated neonates. Acta Paediatr Scand 1975; 64: 87–95

50. Fawer CL, Torrado A, Guignard JP. Single injection clearance in the neonate. Biol Neonat 1979; 35: 321–4.

51. Coulthard MG, Hey EN, Ruddock V. Creatinine and urea clearances compared to inulin clearance in preterm and mature babies. Early Hum Dev 1985; 11: 11–19.

52. Stonestreet BS, Bell EF, Oh W. Validity of endogenous creatinine clearance in low birthweight infants. Pediatr Res 1979; 13: 1012–14.

53. Alt JM, Colenbrander B, Forsling ML, et al. Perinatal development of tubular function in the pig. Q J Exp Physiol 1984; 69: 693–702.

54. Matos P, Duarte-Silva M, Drukker A, et al. Creatinine reabsorption by the newborn rabbit kidney. Pediatr Res 1998; 44: 639.

55. Guignard JP, Drukker A. Why do newborn infants have a high plasma creatinine? Pediatrics 1999; 103: e49.

56. Miall LS, Henderson MJ, Turner AJ, et al. Plasma creatinine rises dramatically in the first 48 hours of life in preterm infants. Pediatrics 1999; 104: e76.

57. Gallini F, Maggio L, Romagnoli C, et al. Progression of renal function in preterm neonates with gestational age 32 weeks. Pediatr Nephrol 2000; 15: 119–24.

58. Bueva A, Guignard JP. Renal function in preterm neonates. Pediatr Res 1994; 36: 572–7.

59. Fawer CL, Torrado A, Guignard JP. Maturation of renal function in full-term and premature neonates. Helv Paediat Acta 1979; 34: 11–21.

Obstruction in adults

7 Introduction and the role of nuclear medicine

Patrick H O'Reilly

Introduction

Obstructive uropathy in adults can be of upper tract origin (e.g. ureteric stone), or lower tract origin (e.g. prostatic hypertrophy).

Upper tract obstruction may be acute or chronic. Chronic obstruction can be subdivided into three types – unequivocal where the cause and effect are established beyond doubt; equivocal where the upper tract is dilated but not necessarily obstructed, and end-stage, where there is a postobstructive, non-functioning kidney.

Lower tract obstruction may interact with the upper tract, for example in high-pressure chronic retention where the obstructed high-pressure bladder causes slow but steady upper tract dilatation and hydronephroisis.

This classification is demonstrated in Figure 7.1.

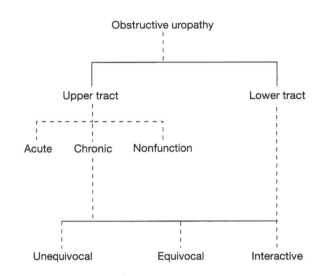

Figure 7.1 Obstructive uropathy.

Acute obstruction

Acute obstruction to the upper urinary tract is usually caused by a ureteric stone which has passed from the renal pelvis to become arrested at the pelviureteric junction (PUJ), the ureter or at the vesicoureteric junction (VUJ). Occasionally an injudicious gynaecological suture during hysterectomy or colposuspension can cause the same thing. Acute ureteric colic is usually extremely painful, often the worst pain the patient has ever experienced (including females who have been through childbirth!). Traditionally, the diagnostic tool has been the intravenous urogram (IVU) where a series of radiographs are taken following the injection of contrast medium. In acute obstruction there will be a dense nephrogram and delayed films will demonstrate a dilated ureter down to the level of the stone. In recent years, uroradiologists have been recommending computed tomography (CT) scanning as a preferable diagnostic test;[1] indeed, there have been energetic debates around the statement that 'the IVU should be relegated to history'. The reasons for this are several but include the fact that virtually all stones are visible on a CT scan whereas only 70–80% of stones are seen on a plain radiograph. Furthermore, if the patient's loin pain is not

due to a stone, the CT may well show up an alternative cause, which an IVU rarely does. Opposition to this development has included the fact that the IVU is cheap and easy and does not require the presence of a radiologist, that CT scanning carries a greater radiation dose for the patient. The latter argument has disappeared somewhat with the recent development of rapid multiplanar CT scanners, and there is no doubt that a quick (a matter of seconds or minutes) unenhanced CT scan can settle once and for all any doubts about the presence of a urinary calculus. Nonetheless, there remains a role for the IVU where the radiologist or CT scanner is not available, and the single-shot IVU (full-length postmicturition prone film 20 minutes after contrast injection) is very valuable for follow up of a known calculus.

There is a limited role in acute obstruction for nuclear medicine studies.[2,3] A standard ^{99m}Tc-MAG3 renogram can be helpful to demonstrate preserved split renal function and an absence of complete obstruction in patients with small calculi prior to discharge from hospital for conservative management at home in the hope that the stone will pass spontaneously.

Unequivocal chronic obstruction

Unequivocal chronic obstruction refers to the finding of a dilated upper urinary tract with a demonstrable nonacute cause for that dilatation, indicating genuine obstruction. There are many examples of this – a pelvic carcinoma (e.g. colon, ovary), retroperitoneal fibrosis, transitional cell cancer of the bladder (in the region of the ureteric orifice) or ureter, etc.

Such a diagnosis is usually the result of imaging studies, especially CT scanning or magnetic resonance (MR) scanning, where the anatomical problem and its effect on the upper urinary tract become obvious.

Nuclear medicine has an important role in this situation. ^{99m}Tc-MAG3 scanning will determine the degree of obstruction, but also the effect the obstructing lesion has had on underlying renal function. This is important since it will guide the clinician towards the vital decision regarding renal conservation after removal of the obstructing lesion, or nephrectomy if the residual renal function is seriously and irreversibly reduced. If the split renal function suggests that the kidney would be incapable of sustaining dialysis-free life should anything destroy the contralateral kidney, then nephrectomy is the usual course of action. As a rule of thumb, split function of less than 10% is indicative of such a situation. However, in current urological practice, there are other considerations. For example, if one is talking of split function, it begs the question *split function of what?* In many cases, if time allows it, a GFR should be obtained to get a proper estimate of single kidney GFR before making the decision regarding nephrectomy. Furthermore, that decision should not be made on one split function estimate alone, and at least two should be available. There is also a need to address the role of intra-ureteric stents or percutaneous nephrostomy drainage of the obstructed kidney for a period of time to assess recoverability of function before deciding between nephrectomy or conservation. Thus, a two stage approach to the situation is often the best course of action, first to deal with the primary pathology, and thereafter to assess the renal status. Naturally, if the primary pathology has destroyed the outflow tract in the presence of poor function, then the decision for nephrectomy becomes clearer.

Equivocal chronic obstruction

Dilatation does not necessarily mean obstruction. This adage was increasingly appreciated by urologists during the 1970s as it became clear that several conditions mimicked obstruction on scans and IVUs, and yet the dilated upper tract was, in fact, just that – dilated but working perfectly well and completely unobstructed. Dilated renal pelves mimicking pelviureteric

junction obstruction, dilated ureters from primary non-obstructive megaureter, or previous vesicoureteric reflux, and other conditions were clarified mainly by the development of diuresis renography.

Diuresis renography

This test was developed to distinguish between the dilated nonobstructed and the dilated obstructed upper urinary tract.[4,5] Standard renography produces a rising curve in both these conditions, the first from stasis of urine allowing the tracer to accumulate rather than leave the upper tract, and the other from genuine impedance to outflow. If a diuretic is administered at 20 minutes, usually 40 mg frusemide, it has been shown that within 3–6 minutes, the flow rate of urine through the upper tract increases from about 1–2 ml/min to 10–12 ml/min. In the obstructed upper tract, this exacerbates the obstruction and no elimination occurs. In the nonobstructed tract, stasis is eliminated, and excretion occurs secondary to the sudden increase in flow. Thus, the rising obstructed renogram curve continues to rise, while the rising stasis curve falls suddenly, in the same way as a normal renogram curve, distinguishing between the two conditions and guiding the urologist towards surgery or conservative management. This development was a major step forward in urological management of the dilated upper urinary tract and is widely used in current practice. For the best and most reliable results, certain guidelines are required.

Guidelines for the performance of diuresis renography

Patient preparation

The patient should be well hydrated for the test. Dehydration results in falsely rising curves due to slow urine flow through the kidneys, and thus mimicks obstruction. It is standard practice to give the patient 500 ml of fluid to drink on arrival in the department before the test.

Choice of radiopharmaceutical

While ^{99m}Tc-DTPA and ^{123}I-hippuran were both widely used in the 1970s and 1980s, ^{99m}Tc-MAG3 is now regarded as the agent of choice.

Dose of diuretic

Forty mg of intravenous frusemide is the normal dose. In children under 16, 0.5 mg/kg is recommended.

Timing of diuretic

The classic renogram involved injection of the diuretic 20 minutes after the radiopharmaceutical. It was subsequently found that the maximum flow rate of urine following frusemide injection occurred at 15 minutes. Thus, a second type of renogram – the F-15 study – was developed, where the radiopharmaceutical was administered 15 minutes after the diuretic. This was found to reduce the equivocal rate of 17% in the F+20 study to around 3–5%. More recently, a study giving the frusemide and radiopharmaceutical at the same time – the F0 diuresis renogram – showed that this is an acceptable method also. Most workers believe, however, that the F-15 technique is the preferred method.

Injection technique

It is important to flush through the intravenous cannula after injection of radiopharmaceutical. If this is not done, some radiopharmaceutical may linger in the syringe or vein, and subsequent movement will cause a small secondary injection of the agent which may mimic obstruction or render the test equivocal.

The effect of posture

In some dilated upper tracts, particularly where the dilatation is sufficient to render normal peristaltic transport inefficient, urine flow from upper to lower urinary tract may depend to a large extent on posture. Thus, when the patient is supine, urine flow may be slow, and the renogram curve will show a rising pattern, mimicking obstruction. When the patient is erect, however, excretion will be normal. It is standard practice to perform diuresis renography with the patient sitting. If the test is done supine for any reason, then further images should be obtained erect at the end of the study.

A further postural consideration is the possibility of nephroptosis. This refers to a hypermobile kidney, a rare condition, usually found in slim females under the age of 40, where the right kidney is in normal position supine, but moves downwards and forwards when the individual is erect. This means the gamma camera will be looking at the right kidney end-on, presenting a small image and resulting in an artificially reduced split function estimate. The excretion curve will be normal, but reduced in size due to the artificially reduced functional estimate. In this situation, a ^{99m}Tc-DMSA scan erect and supine will confirm the condition, and interpretation of the diuresis renogram will be more reliable.

The effect of the bladder on the upper tract

Bladder dysfunction can affect upper tract urodynamics. This is particularly so in the condition of high pressure chronic retention where prostatic hypertrophy causes chronic retention of urine, which is held under high pressure in the bladder. This impairs intraureteric transport of urine leading to dilatation of the ureters and slow, insidious renal failure. Such patients depend on two factors to slow this process – the passage of small amounts of urine from the bladder every 2–3 hours, and the erect position to allow gravitational transport of urine as discussed above. Renogram studies in such cases demonstrate an obstructed pattern supine, but elimination in response to the passage of urine (which takes some of the pressure off the bladder), or a change from the supine to the erect position.

Where these guidelines are observed, the results of diuresis renography should be reliable and the equivocal rate very low. Thus, the dilated obstructed upper urinary tract requiring correction, will accurately be distinguished from the dilated nonobstructed tract, which is harmless and requires no intervention. This topic is covered in detail in Chapter 9.

Value of radionuclide studies in evaluation of the treatment of PUJ obstruction

Open procedures for the treatment of pelviureteric junction (PUJ) obstruction include the Anderson Hynes dismembered pyeloplasty, the Culp deWeerd spiral flap procedure and the Foley Y–V technique, of which the former is the most widely used. Newer methods to treat the condition include antegrade endopyelotomy, retrograde endopyelotomy (Acusize), balloon dilatation and laparoscopic pyeloplasty. It has hitherto been assumed that open pyeloplasty gives a lasting beneficial result in terms of preserved function and improved drainage, and to date, the results of the newer noninvasive techniques have been said to be not as good. However, little data exist in the literature on just how effective and durable open pyeloplasty really is, and its role as a gold standard has been questioned occasionally at endourology meetings. Our investigations into this subject suggest that open dismembered pyeloplasty is indeed the 'gold standard'.[6]

We examined the records of 56 patients having an Anderson Hynes pyeloplasty under the care of two surgeons between 1981 and 1994. Renographic data on preoperative split renal function and diuretic drainage characteristics were examined and charted according to the responses in the original description of the procedure. All patients had had preoperative ^{123}I-hippuran renograms using the standard F+20 or F-15 techniques and a dedicated Scintronix gamma camera system. Patients were then contacted and invited to return to the hospital for a consultation and an up-to-date diuresis renogram to compare with their original preoperative status.

Ultimately, 24 patients agreed and underwent F+20 technetium-labelled mercaptoacetyltriglycine (^{99m}Tc-MAG3) diuresis renograms. The renal function data were subjected to statistical analysis using the Wilcoxon signed ranks test to investigate the functional results of surgery. The drainage characteristics were analysed by a urologist and a radiologist by eyeballing the responses in the usual clinical manner. $T\frac{1}{2}$ times were not required. All patients were subsequently informed of their results.

The dismembered Anderson–Hynes pyeloplasties had been performed 6–19 years previously with a mean of 10.6 years. The mean age of the patients at the time of surgery was 39 years (range 12–72). Nineteen cases demonstrated an improvement in split renal function (79%). The median improvement was from 32–44% ($P = 0.005$). All 24 cases had demonstrated preoperative obstruction. Twenty-three of these (96%) showed improved drainage – normal in nine cases, dilated nonobstructed in ten cases, equivocal in four cases, and obstructed in one case. In the four equivocal responders, function had increased in three (by +3%, +10% and +17%) and the equivocal washout undoubtedly represented a volumetric phenomenon – slow washout through a nonobstructed but high-capacity system. All patients were asymptomatic.

These results would only be possible by the application of standardized, reproducible, diuresis renography technique. They set the standard for the newer techniques which challenge traditional open surgery. There is no doubt that proper assessment of the various treatments of upper urinary tract obstruction cannot be credible without assessment of results by the same standardized, reproducible radionuclide methods described above by all workers in the field. This was lacking in several of these presentations, reflecting a common pattern in urological practice. Many previous reports, especially from the USA, have failed to incorporate pre- and postoperative assessments of function and drainage, relying on eyeballing IVUs or CT, or relying on symptomatic status, two highly subjective and scientifically dubious means of assessment. As demonstrated above, guidelines on standardization of such evaluation already exist in the nuclear medicine literature.[7] They must be encouraged for all workers in the field to allow comparison of different techniques, and of the same techniques between different centres, and it behoves the nuclear medicine community to educate and encourage their urological colleagues to utilize these techniques to the advantage of everyone, especially the patient.

Recovery of function after relief of obstructive uropathy

The nature and extent of recovery following relief of obstructive uropathy will depend on whether the underlying obstruction involves both ureters (or the only ureter of a single functioning kidney) or whether the obstruction is unilateral with a normally functioning contralateral kidney. In the latter circumstances it would be expected that the normal kidney would maintain homeostasis whereas with bilateral ureteric obstruction, global renal function will be impaired.

Bilateral ureteric obstruction (BUO) or unilateral ureteric obstruction (UUO) in a single functioning kidney

This situation typically occurs in high-pressure chronic retention of urine (HPCR) secondary to benign prostatic hypertrophy (BPH) or pelvic malignant disease. Occasionally it develops due to a stone or pelvi-ureteric junction (PUJ) obstruction in a single kidney.

Changes occurring during the period of obstruction

The primary abnormality determining renal function in obstructive uropathy is a reduction in glomerular filtration rate. Salt and water retention are common accompaniments resulting in the clinical features of hypertension, peripheral oedema and, in more severe cases, signs of congestive cardiac failure, especially in patients with chronic bilateral ureteric obstruction.[8] Approximately 50% of patients with HPCR develop hypertension making it the commonest surgically reversible cause of this condition.

The fractional excretion of potassium is less than might be predicted from the glomerular filtration rate and hence potassium retention can also occur. Defective urinary concentrating and acidifying ability develop as a result of increased flooding of the distal nephron with solute from more proximal nephron segments as well as a defective response of the distal tubular mechanism to the normal hormonal influences.

Changes following the relief of obstruction

[99m]TcDTPA GFR studies in patients with HPCR during and after relief of obstruction by urethral catheterization have clarified the changes which occur after relief of obstruction.

Renal functional recovery appears to occur in two phases. There is an initial tubular phase during which sodium and water balance is restored (thus blood pressure normalizes and signs of congestive cardiac failure diminish) and plasma creatinine falls. There is then a secondary phase when glomerular filtration rate slowly recovers. Changes in the tubular phase of recovery are maximal during the first few days following relief of obstruction, but may continue for up to 2 weeks. The second glomerular phase takes place between 2 weeks and 3 months.[9]

The radiographic contrast medium, Iohexol, is handled by glomerular filtration with clearances very similar to those of inulin. In the above study, simultaneous iohexol clearance completely mimicked DTPA clearance, confirming the accuracy of radionuclide ^{99m}Tc-DTPA GFR measurements, and also the correctness of these conclusions regarding renal functional recovery.

Unilateral ureteric obstruction (UUO) with normal contralateral functioning kidney

In clinical practice this situation is most commonly represented by unilateral UPJ obstruction. There are a number of studies, including that described above, demonstrating that unilateral function can be improved, or at least deterioration prevented, by appropriate surgical intervention. Following the relief of obstruction, free water excretion, demonstrating a relative concentrating defect, can be demonstrated, but normal homeostasis is almost invariably maintained by the normally functioning contralateral kidney. There are, however, very rare reports of postobstructive diuresis due to defective urinary concentrating mechanisms following relief of obstruction in a unilateral UPJ patient.

Prediction of recovery of function after relief of unilateral obstruction

In clinical practice it is common to have to decide whether an obstructed kidney is worth salvaging. This can be very difficult. There are many case reports in the literature indicating worthwhile functional recovery following relief of obstruction in what was previously thought to be a radiologically non-functioning kidney. The duration of the obstruction can sometimes be measured, for instance after surgical trauma, and recovery has been documented following obstruction which is known to have been present for a number of years. Conversely, short periods of obstruction can also be associated with irrecoverable function. The completeness of obstruction and particularly the presence of infection are critical in determining ultimate outcome, the combination of obstruction and infection being particularly poor prognostic features.

The measurement of split renal function on standard renography together with assessment of renal cortical thickness on ultrasound are often used as a clinical guide as to whether to perform reconstructive surgery or nephrectomy. When the split function is less than 10% then the value of salvage is often questioned. Percutaneous nephrostomy is sometimes used in such circumstances to try to see what recovery can be obtained in the affected kidney. However, this presents a dilemma of how long to leave the nephrostomy, bearing in mind that recovery may be ongoing for up to 3 months. There is also some evidence from experimental studies that the presence of a normal contralateral kidney actually provides a disincentive for the unilaterally obstructed kidney to recover because normal homeostasis is maintained without it.

Recently, evidence in children has shown that ^{99m}Tc-DMSA scanning during the obstructed state may provide a better predictor of split renal function following relief of obstruction in an affected kidney.[10] This has yet to be confirmed in adults, but the evidence to date is convincing, once more establishing the vital role of radionuclide studies in obstructive uropathy.

Conclusion

There is no doubt that nuclear medicine has contributed a huge amount to current urological management. Imaging techniques such as urography, ultrasound, CT scanning and MR imaging are all vitally important diagnostic techniques, but none has yet been shown to give accurate reliable information on quantitative renal function and urodynamics, information which only nuclear medicine can provide and which is so crucial in the assessment of obstructive uropathy.

References

1. Lorbeboym M, Kapustin Z, Elias S et al. The role of renal scintigraphy and unenhanced helical computerized tomography in patients with ureterolithiasis. Eur J Nucl Med 2000; 27: 441–6.

2. Sfakianakis GN, Cohen DJ, Braunstein RH et al. MAG3-F0 scintigraphy in decisions making for emergency intervention in renal colic after helical CT positive for a urolith. J Nucl Med 2000; 41: 1813–22.

3. De Decker N, Elkholti M, Gouldouzian M et al. Value of renography in the work-up of patients with renal colic admitted in an emergency department. Eur J Nuc Med 2000; 27: 1096 (abstract).

4. O'Reilly PH, Testa HJ, Lawson RS et al. Diuresis renography in equivocal urinary tract obstruction. Br J Urol 1978; 50: 76–80.

5. O'Reilly PH. Diuresis renography 8 years later: An update. J Urol 1986; 136: 993–9.

6. O'Reilly PH, Brooman PJC, Mak S et al. The long term results of Anderson Hynes pyeloplasty. Brit J Urol Int 2001; 87: 1–4.

7. O'Reilly PH, Aurell M, Britton K et al. Consensus on diuresis renography for investigating the dilated upper urinary tract. J Nuc Med 1996; 37: 1872–6.

8. Jones DA, George NJR, O'Reilly PH. Reversible hypertension associated with unrecognised high pressure chronic retention of urine. Lancet 1987; 2: 1052–4.

9. Jones DA, George NJR, O'Reilly PH et al. The biphasic nature of renal functional recovery following relief of chronic obstructive uropathy. Br J Urol 1988; 61: 192–7.

10. Thompson A, Gough DCS. The use of renal scintigraphy in assessing the potential for recovery in the obstructed renal tract in children. BJU International 2001; 87: 853–6.

8 The contribution of radiology

Michel Claudon, Damien Mandry, Jean-Nicolas Dacher

Introduction

Definition

Urinary obstruction was defined by Whitaker in 1978[1] as 'a narrowing of the urinary tract such that the proximal pressure must be raised to transmit the usual flow through it'.

Dilatation of the urinary tract is a well-described consequence of obstruction. However, dilatation may be encountered without any significant increase in intrapelvic pressure; as is the case in patients with megacalicosis. Nonobstructive dilatation can also be found in patients who had their obstruction recently relieved.

Organic dilatation has to be differentiated from functional dilatation. For example in vesico-ureteral reflux, dilatation is the consequence of an abnormal urinary flow. The urinary tract is not narrowed.

Three types of obstruction have been described:

- *Acute obstruction* is characterized by an increase in intrapelvic pressure (10–50 mmHg). Ureteral peristalsis augments initially, then it diminishes or even disappears. At the same time, blood flow transiently increases. A few hours later, arteriolar vasoconstriction occurs, which leads to a decreased renal blood flow and glomerular filtration.
- *Chronic obstruction* may be complete or partial. Dilatation is present whereas the urinary tract pressure is usually normal. Parenchymal atrophy can occur. Renal damage can be reversible in the early stages.
- In *intermittent obstruction*, a moderate narrowing of the urinary tract leads to acute obstruction when the urinary flow increases above a given threshold. This situation is usually associated with uretero-pelviceal junction syndrome (UPJ).

Causes of obstruction

These are either congenital or acquired. Acquired disease can be classified as follows:

- Intraluminal: calculi, blood clot, sloughed papilla, fungus ball
- Wall disease: urothelial tumours, tuberculosis, malakoplakia, schistosomiasis, postoperative strictures
- Extraluminal: pelvic and retroperitoneal tumours, retroperitoneal fibrosis, gynaecological and gastrointestinal lesions, aneurysms.

Objectives of imaging techniques

The management of a patient presenting with a suspected acute or chronic urinary tract obstruction requires the following questions to be addressed:

- Is there an obstruction?
- Where is the level of the obstruction?
- What is the cause of the obstruction?
- What is the degree of the obstruction?

There are five imaging techniques used by radiologists for this purpose: plain radiograph (KUB for kidney, ureters and bladder), ultrasound and Doppler, CT scan, intravenous urography (IVU) and MRI. All of these can provide both anatomical and functional information, except KUB and nonenhanced CT scan.

KUB

KUB is mainly used to detect calcified urinary stones. Even though 90% of calculi contain calcium, not all of them are visible on a plain film. Some are small, others are superimposed on bones, or on dilated bowel loops. In addition, pelvic phleboliths, which are frequent in adults, can be confusing, and sometimes require additional evaluation by CT or IVU.

The sensitivity and specificity of KUB in the diagnosis of urolithiasis is low (respectively 45% and 77%) as compared with CT.[2] The CT scout view is comparable to plain film.[3]

Ultrasound

Anatomical evaluation

Ultrasound was used early in the evaluation of urinary tract obstruction. In 1978, Ellenbogen et al. studied 67 patients and found greyscale ultrasound to have a sensitivity of 98% in the detection of urinary tract obstruction.[4] The grading of the obstruction was based on the degree of dilatation of the excretory cavities by analogy with IVU. These authors had noticed a low rate of false negative cases (2%) contrasting with a high rate of false positive cases (26%).

The greater than 90% sensitivity of greyscale ultrasound in the diagnosis of chronic obstruction (dilatation) has since been confirmed. The scarcely reported false-negative cases were related to hypovolemia, dehydration, retroperitoneal fibrosis, metastases, intermittent and partial obstruction.[5] Specificity of US remains lower, as various conditions can be misdiagnosed as obstruction; large extrarenal pelvis, megacalicosis, peripelvic cyst, dilated vessels (i.e. in the case of arteriovenous fistula or renal varices). In addition, a full bladder with retained micturition and/or vesicoureteral reflux can induce dilatation without obstruction.

In the case of acute obstruction, the renal pelvis may be normal sized at a very early stage, after fornix rupture, or look normal when an echogenic contentm such as a clot, fills the cavities.[6-8]

There has been no recently published study evaluating the accuracy of ultrasound in the diagnosis of urinary tract obstruction. However, an improvement can be postulated with the introduction of harmonic and compound techniques, which decrease the level of noise and improve the contrast to noise ratio (Figure 8.1).[9]

The value of greyscale ultrasound in the diagnosis of the level and cause of the obstruction mainly depends on the patient's physical status (obesity, dilated bowel loops). Renal calyces, renal pelvis and the upper ureter can be evaluated in almost all patients using a transrenal view. The lower ureter and the bladder can also be observed via a transvesical or endocavitary approach. However, the lumbar and pelvic portions of the ureter often remain difficult to visualize due to the interposed bowel loops.

Stone detection is based on the depiction of a hyperechoic structure with acoustic shadowing. Twinkling artifact has been reported as a useful colour Doppler US sign; it is a posterior tail of various colours, which is the consequence of phase distortion at the surface of the stone when irregular.[10] The main locations of stones are the pelvicaliceal system, the level of the iliac vessels crossing and the uretero-vesical junction. In this latter location, a residual oedema can be the only sign of a recent migration of a stone through the lower ureter meatus. The accuracy of US for stone detection is increasing but remains limited. In the early 1990s, US was evaluated, and the reported sensitivity and specificity respectively ranged from 12 to 89% and 78–92%.[11,12] When associated with KUB, the sensitivity reaches 80–100%,[13-15] but still remains lower than that of nonenhanced CT (77% vs 92%).[16]

Physiological dilatation of the upper urinary tract can be observed in pregnant women, especially on the right side. This is due to compression of the ureter by the enlarged uterus and to a decreased ureteral peristalsis. This can lead to a difficult differential diagnosis with obstruction related to stone migration, which is not rare during pregnancy. The ability of colour Doppler to differentiate vessels (iliac vessels) from dilated ureter has been shown.[17] Colour Doppler may also detect a crossing vessel in the case of UPJ syndrome (Figure 8.2).

Figure 8.1 New greyscale ultrasound modes, such as harmonic imaging, allow a nice depiction of renal calyces and pelvis dilatation.

Figure 8.2 In this case of UPJ syndrome complicated by urinary infection, colour Doppler mode shows an arteriovenous pedicle crossing the uretero-pelvic junction.

Figure 8.3 High RI (0.95) in the case of acute obstruction in a patient presenting with an obstruction due to urolithiasis.

Functional evaluation

Increased resistive index

Platt et al[18–21] showed that an increased resistive index (RI > 0.70) recorded from the interlobar arteries Doppler waveforms could help in diagnosing acute obstruction (Figure 8.3). This author subsequently reported an improved sensitivity from a unilateral elevation of the RI as compared with the opposite kidney, with a significant threshold of ΔRI − 0.1. Overall accuracy ranged from 0.77 to 0.96. The increased resistive index was considered independently from dilatation of the collecting system. Haemodynamic change was shown to be able to develop prior to dilatation. It was thought to be related to the early renal blood flow changes that have previously been described in animal models.[22]

However, this theory gave rise to controversy; Tublin[23] and Lee[24] reported much lower sensitivity (19–44%). Partial obstruction, intermittent obstruction due to stone migration, and nonsteroidal anti-inflammatory drugs have been reported as potential causes of false-negative cases. In addition, elevated RI is common in infants. Moreover, it has been shown that RI correlated poorly with renal blood flow changes. Conversely, RI index modification correlated with the urinary tract pressure.[22,25]

Diuretic sonography has been proposed to increase the sensitivity of the RI. A greater than 15% increase in RI over baseline after diuretic administration has been shown in obstructive kidney.[26,27] Preliminary injection of saline and Lasix has also been suggested in order to sensitize RI measurement.[28,29]

Asymmetric ureteral jets

Ureteral jets within the bladder can be shown via transabdominal approach at the level of the trigone by colour Doppler. Hence, obstruction could be suspected in a patient with absent or weak jet as compared to the normal side.[30] Optimal hydration of the patient is required. False-negative cases of ureteric jet may be encountered in patients with partial relief of their obstruction after medical treatment.

Unenhanced CT scan

Unenhanced CT scan is now widely accepted as the reference method for the detection of stone.[31] It is not expected to provide any functional information, but can show morphological signs of obstruction.

The acquisition protocol associates low kVs and a high pitch index for dose reduction. A very short acquisition time is allowed by multidetector technology. Native images have to be individually studied. Multiplanar reconstructions and attenuation measurements can then be performed.

Even if composed of uric acid, stones appear as dense structures (Figure 8.4A). The sensitivity and specificity of unenhanced CT scan in the detection of stone are close to 100%.[32,33] There is no correlation between the attenuation level and the chemical composition of the stone. Stones as small as 1 mm are usually demonstrated. Smaller-diameter calculi can be detected if they are very dense. In slim patients it might be difficult to distinguish ureters from adjacent intestinal loops or vessels. Differential diagnoses should be considered, including ureteral neoplasms and blood clots, which may have moderately elevated attenuation values. As previously mentioned in the KUB section, other calcified structures should also be discussed, including arterial calcifications and phleboliths. A tissue rim is highly suggestive of stone (92–100%),[34] whereas a radiolucent centre[35] and the presence of a comet sign are specific for phleboliths with a predictive positive value of 100%.[36]

Moderate to marked uretero-hydronephrosis can easily be recognized, especially on multiplanar reconstruction images. The dilated ureter can then be followed down to the level of the obstruction. A high-density intraluminal structure is suggestive of stone (Figure 8.4B,C).

The accuracy of perirenal oedema in the prediction of acute obstruction is high, with a reported PPV of 94%.[37] Perirenal oedema is not clearly understood. It could be related to water resorption through the capsule. This indirect sign seems reliable, with a low interobserver variability.[38]

The major limitations of unenhanced CT for lumbar pain diagnosis are extrarenal processes and vascular causes (including renal infarction and renal vein thrombosis). Contrast medium injection is required whenever nonenhanced CT does not clearly demonstrate the cause of an obstruction.

A

B   C

Figure 8.4 Evaluation by non-enhanced CT scan of a left ureterohydronephrosis due to the migration of a calculus. A: Axial sweep shows the stone obstructing a thickened wall ureter. B and C: Coronal and sagittal reformatted images demonstrate both the upper urinary tract dilatation and the obstructing stone.

Enhanced CT and intravenous urography

Iodinated contrast agent administration has been used for decades in the evaluation of urinary tract disease. As a result

of the dynamic enhancement of the kidneys and urinary tract, both anatomical and functional information are provided. The method of analysis has been extensively described for IVU. However, CT appears to be more accurate due to its higher spatial and contrast resolution, shorter acquisition time, multiplanar, 3D and MIP (maximum intensity projection) reconstruction capabilities. The diagnosis of the level and cause of obstruction is more straightforward with CT.[39] However, the higher image quality obtained on CT scan images should be balanced with its higher radiation dose.

Anatomical and functional evaluation in acute and chronic obstruction

The dilatation of the collecting system depends on the level and degree of obstruction (Figure 8.5). In cases of chronic obstruction, a negative pyelogram can be observed on CT as compared with the normal side. A fluid–fluid interface due to gravity can be observed when the contrast medium slowly fills the dilated cavities. A level is created by the overlying

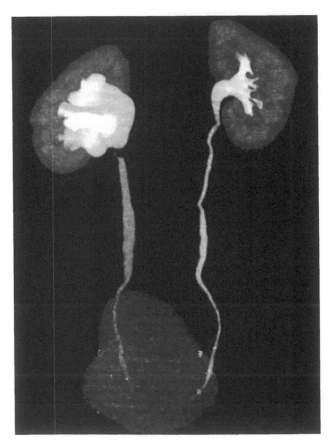

Figure 8.5 3D contrast enhanced CT scan of the urinary tract showing a moderate dilatation of the right renal cavities due to a compression of the ureteropelvic junction.

nonenhanced urine. This phenomenon is obvious on CT, and can be underestimated by IVU. At late stages, renal parenchyma atrophy occurs, scars and calyceal clubbing develop.

On the obstructed side, a delayed nephrogram as compared to the opposite kidney is a key functional sign for obstruction. Delayed enhancement can be seen at the level of the medulla with CT, in the cavities with both IVU and CT. Persistent nephrogram is suggestive of acute obstruction. Pelvicalyceal wall enhancement, which may be noticed on slightly delayed CT, is a nonspecific abnormality.

Functional protocol in intermittent obstruction

Diagnosis of intermittent obstruction may be challenging, as imaging is usually performed after an episode of unexplained lumbar pain. Examinations are normal when the obstruction is no longer present.

In order to reveal the obstruction, the urinary flow should be increased above the upper threshold allowed by the narrowing. Adapted from the Whitaker test principle,[1] a diuresis test has been proposed in order to sensitize IVU.[40] The protocol associates the administration of a high osmolarity contrast medium, optimal hydration of the patient (either by oral water or IV saline) and the injection of 40 mg of Lasix when the cavities become opacified. Films are obtained 5, 10, 30 and 60 minutes after contrast medium injection. An equivalent protocol can be applied with CT. Interpretation is based on clinical symptoms (pain), functional and morphological data (asymmetry of enhancement, dilatation of cavities). Patient position changes, which are expected to reproduce pain, may be indicated during IVU and CT.

Quantification using CT

The excellent spatial resolution and the linearity between the attenuation coefficient and iodine concentration have suggested that CT could be a valuable tool in evaluating the physiology of renal contrast media excretion.[41–43] A significant limitation is the dose delivered to the patient, even when using low kVs.

A simple method was initially described, using repeated scans at a single level through the kidney and aorta after contrast medium injection. Perfusion could be quantified from the comparison of the renal vs aortic attenuation.[44,45]

A more complex method has been adapted from the Patlak plot graphic analysis initially used in nuclear medicine. It is based on a bi-compartmental model and assumes a two-way diffusion of the contrast agent between plasma and extracellular fluids, with a one-way filtration from the plasma to the urine.[46] This graphic analysis plots the ratio of renal to aortic attenuation values (R(t)/A(t)) on the y-axis, and a 'normalized time' on the x-axis. This 'normalized time' is the ratio of the integral of vascular attenuation value (in an aortic region of interest or ROI) from $t = 0$ to time t to the vascular attenuation value at t $\left(\int_0^t A(t)/A(t) \right)$. The y-axis intercept estimates fractional vascular volume, and the slope of the plot is the renal clearance per unit volume in the renal ROI. This technique has been applied to electron beam computed tomography (EBCT)[47] and multiphasic helical CT.[48,49]

Good reproducibility and correlation with renal functional tests have been demonstrated.[49–51] Clinical experience has been obtained in patients presenting with diabetes,[52] renal artery stenosis[53] and, more recently, with hydronephrosis or pyelonephritis.[48]

MR urography: the one stop shop?

Since the first description by Hennig,[51] MR diagnostic capabilities have improved with higher spatial resolution, shorter acquisition time and sophisticated imaging sequences providing either high-quality images or functional information. MR now appears to be a promising technique for the evaluation of the urinary tract, especially in the case of chronic intermittent obstruction.

The specific advantages of MR are the capability to obtain multiplanar views, the absence of ionizing radiation and the good tolerance of gadolinium chelates as compared to iodinated agents. Contraindications are claustrophobia and the presence of a pacemaker. Limitations include its high cost, limited availability, and the need for sedation in young children.

Because of the long T2 of fluid in the collecting system, the initial studies have been performed using heavily T2-weighted sequences, allowing visualization of the urine-filled urinary tract.[55–57]

Based on T1-weighted sequences performed after the IV administration of gadolinium chelate, excretory MR provides both morphological and quantitative information about the urinary tract. Therefore, MR urography has been proposed to replace IVU in both children and adults.[58–61] The addition of fast 3D MR angiography provides valuable information on renal vasculature in patients in whom abnormal vascular anatomy or vascular disease may affect the urinary tract.[62]

If the initial results of MR urography reported by many studies are exciting, functional MR still requires larger clinical studies to obtain validation and to become a widely accepted standard examination.[63]

Static fluid MR urography

Distension of a nondilated renal collecting system is an important condition for optimal MR evaluation using T2-weighted sequences. The patient is not recommended to restrict water drinking. Oral hydration prior to the examination is not indicated, as it results in superimposition of fluid-filled bowel loops. IV infusion of saline allows optimal distension of non-dilated ureters. The injection of frusemide (5–20 mg a few minutes before starting the examination) has been recommended,[55,58,64] but it could alter functional study results. The field of view must include the entire urinary tract, with both kidneys, ureters and bladder.

Long echo times (effective TEs close to 1000 ms) produce high contrast, heavily T2-weighted images, resulting in bright signal from stationary fluid, and demonstrating urine within dilated or non-dilated calyces, pelvis and ureters. Collecting tubules may be demonstrated within the renal medulla. Using short TEs (approximately 100 ms) results in moderately T2-weighted images but allows better analysis of the content of the dilated cavities, ureteric wall and surrounding soft tissue. This can be very helpful in determining the nature of an extrinsic urinary obstruction.[62] Multislice sequences could provide better diagnostic information than thick-slab sequences, particularly in evaluating the cause of obstruction.[65] In addition, T2-weighted images demonstrate perirenal or periureteral fluid, which has been shown to be sensitive in the diagnosis of acute urinary obstruction.[66]

Static fluid sequences are often used as the first step of MR urography. They are particularly useful in cases of chronic obstruction with a nonfunctioning kidney.[57,67] They are effective in demonstrating the degree and level of obstruction, unless the upper tract dilatation is not sufficient.[68] The diagnostic capability of these sequences in congenital anomalies such as UPJ syndrome in children is excellent (Figures 8.6A,B and 8.7A,B).[68] MR sensitivity in detecting stones has initially been reported as low.[68] However, recent studies contradicted these preliminary results.[69] MR urography turns out to be a valuable, well-tolerated investigation for evaluating painful hydronephrosis in pregnancy. This is especially true for the diagnosis of obstructive urinary stone.[70,71] Lastly, MR is highly sensitive in the detection of urological complications after renal transplantation.[72]

Excretory MR urography

Excretory MR urography is based on the glomerular filtration of gadolinium chelates, which are not toxic for the kidney (within the usual dose range) and can be eliminated by dialysis.[58–60] IV administration of a half dose of gadolinium chelate (0.1 mmol/kg) is sufficient to evaluate the urinary tract.

A fast T1-weighted gradient-recalled-echo sequence with very short repetition and echo times can visualize enhanced urine[58] and allows the evaluation of normal and abnormal renal cavities and ureters at different times and in multiple planes. Gadolinium-enhanced T1-weighted MR urography depends on the renal excretory function: a satisfactory urographic effect is usually obtained up to a serum creatinine

A   B

Figure 8.6 Left upper tract chronic obstruction due to a metastatic lymph node. A: Long TE T2-weighted image shows the dilated ureter and renal cavities as well as the level of the obstruction. B: Short TE T2-weighted image demonstrates the presence of a small lymph node squeezing the ureter.

concentration of 2 mg/dl.[58] Due to longer acquisition times as compared with T2-weighted sequences, image quality can be altered by patient motion, especially in children.[73]

In excretory MR urography, the main drawback is gadolinium-related. Paramagnetic contrast agents shorten both T1 and T2 relaxation times of fluids and tissues. A drop in the signal due to T2 and T2* effects can be seen in the pyramids and renal cavities, where water resorption increases the concentration of gadolinium. The most effective way to prevent this problem is to inject furosemide shortly before the injection of the contrast agent.[58]

The diagnosis of obstruction on excretory MR urography is based on morphology (a persistent narrowing of the ureter below a dilated urinary tract), and function (delayed excretion of contrast into the collecting system and ureter).[67,74] However, there is no correlation between the grade of hydronephrosis and the delay in calyceal and ureteric excretion.[67] As compared with T2-weighted sequences, T1-weighted images are usually more effective in assessing the cause of obstruction. Their contrast is higher and the enhancement of pathological lesions is helpful.[58] In addition, renal scarring and cortical thinning is easily identified.[75]

3D MR angiography can be obtained during the initial injection of contrast agent, or secondarily. The enhanced vessels can be superimposed on the dilated urinary tract in order to plan the surgical approach.[62] The detection of a crossing vessel in a patient with UPJ syndrome remains a challenge. This is especially true in children.[76]

A   B

C

D

Figure 8.7 Marked left upper tract dilatation related to an obstructive primary megaureter. A, B: Long TE T2-weighted images showing the marked dilatation of renal cavities and ureter and the hypertonic distal aspect of the left ureter. C: Dynamic enhanced MRI clearly demonstrates both hydronephrosis and increased transit time of the contrast medium. D: Time–intensity curves confirm the asymmetry between both kidneys. Curves 1 and 2 correspond respectively to right and left parenchyma; curves 3 and 4 to left and right cavities.

Dynamic functional MR urography

The functional parameters which can be noninvasively approached by MR are multiple: glomerular filtration, tubular concentration and transit, blood volume and perfusion, diffusion and oxygenation.[77]

In the last decade, clinical studies have been based on exogenous contrast agents, such as ultra-small particles of iron oxide (USPIO)[78] and gadolinium chelates.[60,67,79]

Dynamic sets of coronal images across both kidneys were obtained after IV administration of a bolus of gadolinium chelate. MR renograms were computed from the changes in signal intensity of the total parenchyma, cortex, medulla and cavities.[80] Paediatric uropathies have been particularly studied, with the expectation that MRI might replace renal scintigraphy as a nonradiating method (Figure 8.7C).[59,60,67,79,81]

Currently, there is no consensus about the acquisition protocol, which requires multiple optimizations prior to performing clinical studies.

As previously described, a normal patient hydration before the examination is required. Saline infusion is recommended. The administration of furosemide remains debatable. In the first MR studies, Lasix injection was performed 20 minutes after injection of Gd chelate, as is routinee in renal scintigraphy.[59,60] However, this resulted in a long acquisition time (approximately one hour). Recently, an F-15 technique (Lasix 15 minutes before Gd) was introduced with good results.[67]

The acquisition plane is oblique coronal after determination of the long axis of the kidneys on sagittal views. Acquisition is based on single or multiple slice 2D or 3D technique, using fast, heavily T1-weighted acquisition, repeated every 3–5 seconds during the 10–20 minutes after injection.

Correction for body motion (mainly breathing) may be obtained after spatial registration. ROIs are usually drawn over a large area of parenchyma (including cortex and medulla), the entire kidney and the cavities.[79] When an obstruction is found in a duplex kidney, a separate analysis for both poles can be performed. Time–intensity curves obtained are similar to those of renal scintigraphy, which allow assessment of urinary excretion. Three segments can be described in this renogram: a short vascular phase, a second phase of slow signal increase until a maximum which can be used to assess split renal function, and a third phase of signal decrease due to contrast excretion (Figure 8.7D).[60]

Comparative analysis may reveal asymmetry in the kinetics of enhancement of the kidneys. Quantitative analysis is based on the determination of split renal function. Several methods have been described. Rohrschneider proposed quantifying the area under the curve of the second phase weighted by the volume of the parenchyma. This volume was inferred from a mid 1 cm thick slice obtained in the best coronal plane of the kidneys. This approach is well correlated with the quantification obtained from ^{99m}Tc-MAG3 scintigraphy.[79]

A simple estimation of parenchymal volume of each kidney by MR is also well-correlated with the split function assessment from renal scintigraphy in children ($r = 0.98$).[67] More recently, the estimation of the renal transit time from the qualitative analysis of dynamic images has been demonstrated as a good indicator of obstruction.[82] With dynamic contrast-enhanced methods, precise quantification remains limited as there is a nonlinear relationship between the signal intensity and the concentration of contrast medium. A signal drop at high concentration due to T2 and T2* effects can even be found, as previously mentioned.[81,83] Potential solutions to decrease this phenomenon include the optimization of the T1-weighted sequence parameters, the increase of urine flow rate by the injection of diuretics and the administration of low doses of gadolinium.[84] Macrovascular agents have a very low interstitial diffusion and enable lower T2 effect.[85]

Conclusion

For acute obstruction, nonenhanced CT is the first method performed in adults in many institutions, although the association of KUB and US remains an effective alternative. Doppler is only useful as an adjunct technique. CT scan is effective in demonstrating the level and cause of the obstruction in many cases. Contrast-enhanced CT should be performed when no abnormality has been detected by nonenhanced study and should be preferred to IVU.

The diagnosis of chronic obstruction is mainly based on the US or CT demonstration of a dilated excretory system. The level and the cause of obstruction are optimally determined by CT and MRI.

The demonstration of an intermittent obstruction may be challenging and requires an appropriate hydration, to reach a sufficient diuresis to overwhelm the capacity of drainage of the stenosed UP junction or ureter. This might represent one of the remaining indications for IVU. However, CT, US and MRI may be helpful in confirming the obstruction and its cause, such as a crossing vessel. Indication for surgery can be oriented by functional evaluation of the renal function, which can now be obtained with MRI in a similar way to scintigraphy.

References

1. Whitaker RH. Clinical assessment of pelvic and ureteral function. Urology 1978; 12: 146–50.
2. Levine JA, Neitlich J, Verga M et al. Ureteral calculi in patients with flank pain: correlation of plain radiography with unenhanced helical CT. Radiology 1997; 204: 27–31.
3. Chu G, Rosenfield AT, Anderson K et al. Sensitivity and value of digital CT scout radiography for detecting ureteral stones in patients with ureterolithiasis diagnosed on unenhanced CT. AJR Am J Roentgenol 1999; 173: 417–23.
4. Ellenbogen PH, Scheible FW, Talner LB, Leopold GR. Sensitivity of gray scale ultrasound in detecting urinary tract obstruction. AJR Am J Roentgenol 1978; 130: 731–3.
5. Talner LB. Does hydration prevent contrast material renal injury? AJR Am J Roentgenol 1981; 136: 1021–2.
6. Bryan PJ, Azimi F. Ultrasound in diagnosis of congenital hydronephrosis due to obstruction of pelviureteric junction. Urology 1975; 5: 17–20.
7. Hately W, Whitaker RH. How accurate is diagnostic ultrasound in renal disease? Br J Urol 1973; 45: 468–73.
8. Taylor KJ, Kraus V. Grey-scale ultrasound imaging: assessment of acute hydronephrosis. Br J Urol 1975; 47: 593–7.
9. Claudon M, Tranquart F, Evans DH et al. Advances in ultrasound. Eur Radiol 2002; 12: 7–18.
10. Chelfouh N, Grenier N, Higueret D et al. Characterization of urinary calculi: in vitro study of 'twinkling artifact' revealed by color-flow sonography. AJR Am J Roentgenol 1998; 171: 1055–60.
11. Haddad MC, Sharif HS, Shahed MS et al. Renal colic: diagnosis and outcome. Radiology 1992; 184: 83–8.
12. Soyer P, Levesque M, Lecloirec A et al. Evaluation of the role of echography in the positive diagnosis of renal colic secondary to kidney stone. J Radiol 1990; 71: 445–50.
13. al-Hassan HK, Sabha MN, Taleb HH, Leven HO. Value of ultrasound in persistent flank pain. Int Surg 1991; 76: 264–5.
14. Dalla Palma L, Stacul F, Bazzocchi M et al. Ultrasonography and plain film versus intravenous urography in ureteric colic. Clin Radiol 1993; 47: 333–6.
15. Hill MC, Rich JI, Mardiat JG, Finder CA. Sonography vs. excretory urography in acute flank pain. AJR Am J Roentgenol 1985; 144: 1235–8.
16. Catalano O, Nunziata A, Sandomenico F, Siani A. Acute flank pain: comparison of unenhanced helical CT and ultrasonography in detecting causes other than ureterolithiasis. Emerg Radiol 2002; 9: 146–54.
17. Grenier N, Pariente JL, Trillaud H et al. Dilatation of the collecting system during pregnancy: physiologic vs obstructive dilatation. Eur Radiol 2000; 10: 271–9.
18. Platt JF, Ellis JH, Rubin JM. Assessment of internal ureteral stent patency in patients with pyelocaliectasis: value of renal duplex sonography. AJR Am J Roentgenol 1993; 161: 87–90.
19. Platt JF, Rubin JM, Ellis JH. Distinction between obstructive and nonobstructive pyelocaliectasis with duplex Doppler sonography. AJR Am J Roentgenol 1989; 153: 997–1000.
20. Platt JF, Rubin JM, Ellis JH. Acute renal obstruction: evaluation with intrarenal duplex Doppler and conventional US. Radiology 1993; 186: 685–8.
21. Platt JF, Rubin JM, Ellis JH, DiPietro MA. Duplex Doppler US of the kidney: differentiation of obstructive from nonobstructive dilatation. Radiology 1989; 171: 515–7.
22. Claudon M, Barnewolt CE, Taylor GA et al. Renal blood flow in pigs: changes depicted with contrast-enhanced harmonic US imaging during acute urinary obstruction. Radiology 1999; 212: 725–31.
23. Tublin ME, Dodd GD 3rd, Verdile VP. Acute renal colic: diagnosis with duplex Doppler US. Radiology 1994; 193: 697–701.
24. Lee HJ, Kim SH, Jeong YK, Yeun KM. Doppler sonographic resistive index in obstructed kidneys. J Ultrasound Med 1996; 15: 613–8; quiz 9–20.

25. Cronan JJ, Tublin ME. Role of the resistive index in the evaluation of acute renal obstruction. AJR Am J Roentgenol 1995; 164: 377–8.

26. Mallek R, Bankier AA, Etele-Hainz A et al. Distinction between obstructive and nonobstructive hydronephrosis: value of diuresis duplex Doppler sonography. AJR Am J Roentgenol 1996; 166: 113–7.

27. Palmer JM, Lindfors KK, Ordorica RC, Marder DM. Diuretic Doppler sonography in postnatal hydronephrosis. J Urol 1991; 146: 605–8.

28. Bude RO, Platt JF, Wahl RL et al. Suspected obstructive pyelocaliectasis: Doppler ultrasonography compared with diuretic renal scintigraphy in proven cases. Can Assoc Radiol J 1996; 47: 101–6.

29. Bude RO, Rubin JM. Power Doppler sonography. Radiology 1996; 200: 21–3.

30. Burge HJ, Middleton WD, McClennan BL, Hildebolt CF. Ureteral jets in healthy subjects and in patients with unilateral ureteral calculi: comparison with color Doppler US. Radiology 1991; 180: 437–42.

31. Smith RC, Levine J, Dalrymple NC et al. Acute flank pain: a modern approach to diagnosis and management. Semin Ultrasound CT MR 1999; 20: 108–35.

32. Sheley RC, Semonsen KG, Quinn SF. Helical CT in the evaluation of renal colic. Am J Emerg Med 1999; 17: 279–82.

33. Yilmaz S, Sindel T, Arslan G et al. Renal colic: comparison of spiral CT, US and IVU in the detection of ureteral calculi. Eur Radiol 1998; 8: 212–7.

34. Heneghan JP, Dalrymple NC, Verga M et al. Soft-tissue 'rim' sign in the diagnosis of ureteral calculi with use of unenhanced helical CT. Radiology 1997; 202: 709–11.

35. Boridy IC, Nikolaidis P, Kawashima A et al. Ureterolithiasis: value of the tail sign in differentiating phleboliths from ureteral calculi at nonenhanced helical CT. Radiology 1999; 211: 619–21.

36. Traubici J, Neitlich JD, Smith RC. Distinguishing pelvic phleboliths from distal ureteral stones on routine unenhanced helical CT: is there a radiolucent center? AJR Am J Roentgenol 1999; 172: 13–7.

37. Takahashi N, Kawashima A, Ernst RD et al. Ureterolithiasis: can clinical outcome be predicted with unenhanced helical CT? Radiology 1998; 208: 97–102.

38. Guest AR, Cohan RH, Korobkin M et al. Assessment of the clinical utility of the rim and comet-tail signs in differentiating ureteral stones from phleboliths. AJR Am J Roentgenol 2001; 177: 1285–91.

39. Bosniak MA, Megibow AJ, Ambos MA et al. Computed tomography of ureteral obstruction. AJR Am J Roentgenol 1982; 138: 1107–13.

40. Delomez J, Claudon M, Darmaillacq C et al. Imagerie des tumeurs de la voie excrétrice supérieure. J Radiol 2002; 83: 825–38.

41. Brennan RE, Curtis JA, Pollack HM, Weinberg I. Sequential changes in the CT numbers of the normal canine kidney following intravenous contrast administration. II: The renal medulla. Invest Radiol 1979; 14: 239–45.

42. Jaschke W, Cogan MG, Sievers R et al. Measurement of renal blood flow by cine computed tomography. Kidney Int 1987; 31: 1038–42.

43. Jaschke W, Lipton MJ, Boyd DP et al. Attenuation changes of the normal and ischemic canine kidney. Dynamic CT scanning after intravenous contrast medium bolus. Acta Radiol Diagn (Stockh) 1985; 26: 321–30.

44. Miles KA. Measurement of tissue perfusion by dynamic computed tomography. Br J Radiol 1991; 64: 409–12.

45. Miles KA, Hayball MP, Dixon AK. Functional imaging of changes in human intrarenal perfusion using quantitative dynamic computed tomography. Invest Radiol 1994; 29: 911–4.

46. Blomley MJ, Dawson P. Review article: the quantification of renal function with enhanced computed tomography. Br J Radiol 1996; 69: 989–95.

47. Romero JC, Lerman LO. Novel noninvasive techniques for studying renal function in man. Semin Nephrol 2000; 20: 456–62.

48. Hackstein N, Bauer J, Hauck EW et al. Measuring single-kidney glomerular filtration rate on single-detector helical CT using a two-point Patlak plot technique in patients with increased interstitial space. AJR Am J Roentgenol 2003; 181: 147–56.

49. Hackstein N, Puille MF, Bak BH et al. Measurement of single kidney contrast media clearance by multiphasic spiral computed tomography: preliminary results. Eur J Radiol 2001; 39: 201–8.

50. Lerman LO, Flickinger AL, Sheedy PF 2nd, Turner ST. Reproducibility of human kidney perfusion and volume determinations with electron beam computed tomography. Invest Radiol 1996; 31: 204–10.

51. Miles KA, Leggett DA, Bennett GA. CT derived Patlak images of the human kidney. Br J Radiol 1999; 72(854): 153–8.

52. Tsushima Y, Blomley MJ, Kusano S, Endo K. Use of contrast-enhanced computed tomography to measure clearance per unit renal volume: a novel measurement of renal function and fractional vascular volume. Am J Kidney Dis 1999; 33: 754–60.

53. Lerman LO, Taler SJ, Textor SC et al. Computed tomography-derived intrarenal blood flow in renovascular and essential hypertension. Kidney Int 1996; 49: 846–54.

54. Hennig J, Nauerth A, Friedburg H. RARE imaging: a fast imaging method for clinical MR. Magn Reson Med 1986; 3: 823–33.

55. Rothpearl A, Frager D, Subramanian A et al. MR urography: technique and application. Radiology 1995; 194: 125–30.

56. Roy C, Saussine C, Jahn C et al. Fast imaging MR assessment of ureterohydronephrosis during pregnancy. Magn Reson Imaging 1995; 13: 767–72.

57. Roy C, Saussine C, Jahn C et al. Evaluation of RARE-MR urography in the assessment of ureterohydronephrosis. J Comput Assist Tomogr 1994; 18: 601–8.

58. Nolte-Ernsting CC, Bucker A, Adam GB et al. Gadolinium-enhanced excretory MR urography after low-dose diuretic injection: comparison with conventional excretory urography. Radiology 1998; 209: 147–57.

59. Rohrschneider WK, Becker K, Hoffend J et al. Combined static-dynamic MR urography for the simultaneous evaluation of morphology and function in urinary tract obstruction. II. Findings in experimentally induced ureteric stenosis. Pediatr Radiol 2000; 30: 523–32.

60. Rohrschneider WK, Hoffend J, Becker K et al. Combined static-dynamic MR urography for the simultaneous evaluation of morphology and function in urinary tract obstruction. I. Evaluation of the normal status in an animal model. Pediatr Radiol 2000; 30: 511–22.

61. Leppert A, Nadalin S, Schirg E et al. Impact of magnetic resonance urography on preoperative diagnostic workup in children affected by hydronephrosis: should IVU be replaced? J Pediatr Surg 2002; 37: 1441–5.

62. Roy C, Lefèvre F, Lemaitre L et al. IRM du haut appareil urinaire. J Radiol 2000; 81: 1085–95.

63. Huang AJ, Lee VS, Rusinek H. MR imaging of renal function. Radiol Clin North Am 2003; 41: 1001–17.

64. Hattery RR, King BF. Technique and application of MR urography. Radiology 1995; 194: 25–7.

65. Blandino A, Minutoli F, Gaeta M et al. MR pyelography in the assessment of hydroureteronephrosis: single-shot thick-slab RARE versus multislice HASTE sequences. Abdom Imaging 2003; 28: 433–9.

66. Regan F, Petronis J, Bohlman M et al. Perirenal MR high signal – a new and sensitive indicator of acute ureteric obstruction. Clin Radiol 1997; 52: 445–50.

67. Grattan-Smith JD, Perez-Bayfield MR, Jones RA et al. MR imaging of kidneys: functional evaluation using F-15 perfusion imaging. Pediatr Radiol 2003; 33: 293–304.

68. Blandino A, Gaeta M, Minutoli F et al. MR pyelography in 115 patients with a dilated renal collecting system. Acta Radiol 2001; 42: 532–6.

69. Magno C, Blandino A, Anastasi G et al. Lithiasic obstructive uropathy. Hydronephrosis characterization by magnetic resonance pyelography. Urol Int 2004; 72 Suppl 1: 40–2.

70. Roy C, Saussine C, LeBras Y et al. Assessment of painful ureterohydronephrosis during pregnancy by MR urography. Eur Radiol 1996; 6: 334–8.

71. Spencer JA, Chahal R, Kelly A et al. Evaluation of painful hydronephrosis in pregnancy: magnetic resonance urographic patterns in physiological dilatation versus calculous obstruction. J Urol 2004; 171: 256–60.

72. Cohnen M, Brause M, May P et al. Contrast-enhanced MR urography in the evaluation of renal transplants with urological complications. Clin Nephrol 2002; 58: 111–7.

73. Borthne A, Pierre-Jerome C, Nordshus T, Reiseter T. MR urography in children: current status and future development. Eur Radiol 2000; 10: 503–11.

74. Chu WC, Lam WW, Chan KW et al. Dynamic gadolinium-enhanced magnetic resonance urography for assessing drainage in dilated pelvicalyceal systems with moderate renal function: preliminary results and comparison with diuresis renography. BJU Int 2004; 93: 830–4.

75. Rodriguez LV, Spielman D, Herfkens RJ, Shortliffe LD. Magnetic resonance imaging for the evaluation of hydronephrosis, reflux and renal scarring in children. J Urol 2001; 166: 1023–7.

76. Zamparelli M, Cobellis G, Rossi L et al. Detection of crossing vessels at the ureteropelvic junction with fast MRI. Pediatr Med Chir 2003; 25: 50–2.

77. Grenier N, Basseau F, Ries M et al. Functional MRI of the kidney. Abdom Imaging 2003; 28: 164–75.

78. Schoenberg SO, Aumann S, Just A et al. Quantification of renal perfusion abnormalities using an intravascular contrast agent (part 2): results in animals and humans with renal artery stenosis. Magn Reson Med 2003; 49: 288–98.

79. Rohrschneider WK, Haufe S, Clorius JH, Troger J. MR to assess renal function in children. Eur Radiol 2003; 13: 1033–45.

80. Katzberg RW, Buonocore MH, Ivanovic M et al. Functional, dynamic, and anatomic MR urography: feasibility and preliminary findings. Acad Radiol 2001; 8: 1083–99.

81. Borthne A, Nordshus T, Reiseter T et al. MR urography: the future gold standard in paediatric urogenital imaging? Pediatr Radiol 1999; 29: 694–701.

82. Jones RA, Perez-Brayfield MR, Kirsch AJ, Grattan-Smith JD. Renal transit time with MR urography in children. Radiology 2004; 233: 41–50.

83. Carvlin MJ, Arger PH, Kundel HL et al. Use of Gd-DTPA and fast gradient-echo and spin-echo MR imaging to demonstrate renal function in the rabbit. Radiology 1989; 170: 705–11.

84. Lee VS, Rusinek H, Johnson G et al. MR renography with low-dose gadopentetate dimeglumine: feasibility. Radiology 2001; 221: 371–9.

85. Mandry D, Pedersen M, Odille F et al. Renal functional contrast-enhanced magnetic resonance imaging: evaluation of a new rapid-clearance blood pool agent (p 792) in Sprague-Dawley rats. Invest Radiol 2005; 40: 295–305.

9   The urologist's view

Stephen CW Brown

Introduction

The definition of urinary tract obstruction is a restriction to the flow of urine that gives rise to symptoms or threatens renal function. It may occur at any point from the minor calyces of the kidney to the external meatus of the urethra. It may be acute or chronic, complete or incomplete, upper or lower urinary tract depending on its origin in relation to the vesico-ureteric junction. Upper and lower urinary tract obstruction present different clinical issues and are therefore best considered separately. It is important, however, not to overlook the interaction between the upper and lower urinary tract, which is central to understanding the dynamics of the system as a whole.

Obstructive uropathy is a functional disturbance and therefore static imaging alone is inadequate for clinical evaluation. A dilated renal pelvis on intravenous urography or a large bladder residual volume on ultrasound may suggest obstruction, but does not equate with it. In order to evaluate the lower urinary tract, the urologist is able to perform direct pressure–flow studies in the form of conventional filling and voiding cystometry. In the upper tract such studies are invasive and more difficult to relate to physiological conditions. Nuclear medicine has provided the clinically acceptable investigative techniques that have become the mainstay of functional upper tract assessment. Nuclear medicine plays no part in the management of lower urinary tract obstruction and is not considered further.

Upper tract obstruction

Acute obstruction of the upper urinary tract typically presents with pain and sometimes with complicating factors such as infection and haematuria. The diagnosis is usually identifiable on static imaging alone. Chronic obstruction can present with or without pain and may come to light as a manifestation of resulting infection or even uraemia. There may be the palpable mass of a massively dilated renal pelvis. Commonly the first suggestion of obstruction is the finding of upper tract dilatation on X-ray or ultrasound.

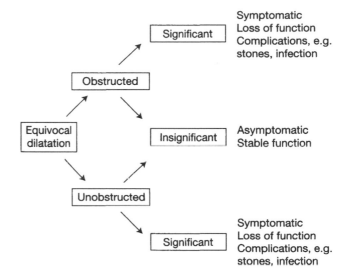

Figure 9.1   Diagnostic steps in the treatment of equivocal dilatation.

If a cause for the obstruction is evident, it is referred to as 'unequivocal'. Examples include ureteric calculi or urothelial tumours. Management is directed to relief of the obstruction and eradication of the cause. If no cause for the dilatation is evident, it is defined as 'equivocal'. It is necessary firstly to determine whether obstruction is present, and secondly whether it is clinically significant, warranting intervention (Figure 9.1). Ideally the diagnosis of obstruction made should equate with clinical significance and therefore dictate the intervention required and the predicted outcome. This is not always the case, but careful application of renography with close attention to all physiological factors involved gives the best clinical guidance in these challenging cases.

Investigation

Renography

The excretory role of the kidney lends itself to radionuclide scanning. The attachment of a gamma-emitting nuclide to a molecule that is excreted and concentrated in the urine provides an ideal radiopharmaceutical for the purpose. Standardized protocols are well documented and should be adopted to optimize the value of the investigation and enable comparison between centres.[1]

Protocol

Patients should be well hydrated and the bladder emptied immediately prior to the start of the test. ^{99m}Tc-MAG3 is the radiopharmaceutical of choice as it is predominantly secreted giving a rapid clearance but readily available. The dose is injected intravenously, taking care to avoid extravasation or contamination. Scanning proceeds for 20–40 min into the study and at least 15 min after the injection of diuretic in the case of diuresis renography. Digital images of the kidneys and bladder are stored for processing and interpretation. At the end of the procedure, the patient again empties the bladder. This reduces the radiation dose to the bladder and enables a check on the rate of urine production, which helps with interpretation.

Regions of interest (ROI) are drawn over both kidneys and the bladder and a C-shaped elliptical area around the kidneys for blood background estimation. The number of counts occurring in each ROI is computed for each time frame and the counts plotted against time. The background count is subtracted from the other three. The resulting time–activity curves constitute the renogram.

Interpretation

The normal kidney curves have three classic phases shown in curve (Figure 9.2A). The first reflects the speed of injection and the blood supply to the kidney. The second represents mainly the renal handling of the radiopharmaceutical and the third the efficiency of excretion of tracer in the urine. A normal pattern virtually excludes any degree of obstruction. If partial or complete obstruction is present, the depression of the slope of the second phase is representative of uptake decrease, an alteration of the third phase indicating impaired excretion (Figure 9.2B, C). Eventually function reduces until uptake is little more than the background count and the appearances are those of a nonfunctioning kidney. At normal physiological urine flow, an obstructive curve may be obtained if there is inadequate hydration, a larger collecting system, poor function, or bladder interaction effects. Such false positives can be avoided if a maximal diuresis is achieved by performing renography in association with a diuretic.

Diuresis renography

The principles of diuresis renography were first proposed in the 1960s[2] and promoted by O'Reilly et al[3] as a simple method for differentiating patients with equivocal obstruction of the upper urinary tract. If a system is genuinely obstructed, flow is impaired at both high and low urinary flow rates (Figure 9.3A). In contrast, slow elimination due to urinary stasis alone will respond to an increase in the urinary flow rate with a rapid washout of tracer (Figure 9.3B). The increased flow is achieved with the sulfonamide 'loop' diuretic frusemide (furosemide). In a study of total urinary flow rates in 93 normal individuals, the resting flow, between 1 and

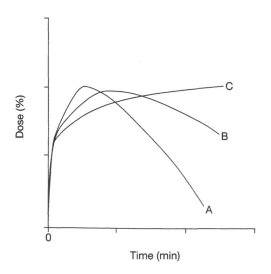

Figure 9.2   The renogram curve response to obstruction. A: Curve – demonstrating three phases of normal curve; B: effects of mild obstruction; C: effects of more severe obstruction.

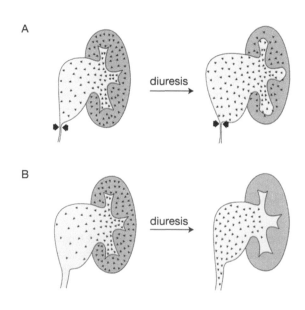

Figure 9.3   Principle of diuresis renography. (A) Obstructed: increased urine production leads to an accumulation of tracer. (B) Nonobstructed: increased urine production leads to a corresponding increased washout.

Figure 9.4 Mean urinary flow rate following frusemide injection.

3 ml/min, increased to an average of 24 ml/min following a 40 mg intravenous injection of frusemide, with some individuals attaining as much as 50 ml/min (Figure 9.4).[4] In the same study it was noted that the response to the diuretic became maximal 15 min after diuretic injection. It follows that, if maximum diuresis is required throughout a renogram, the diuretic should be injected 15 min before the radiopharmaceutical.[5,6]

Interpretation

A number of factors influence the effect of a diuresis on the renogram curve and must be considered when interpreting results (Figure 9.5).

Renal function

In adults, the level of renal function is a major determinant of the diuretic-induced flow rate. In a study to investigate the importance of renal function, linear relationships were observed between creatinine clearance,[7] glomerular filtration rate (GFR), effective renal plasma flow (ERPF)[4] and urinary flow rates following frusemide. These observations have immediate implications for the interpretation of the diuresis renogram. If single kidney GFR is < 15 ml/min, caution should be observed in interpretation of the diuresis renogram.

Hydration

Even in the presence of normal renal function, the response to diuretic may be suboptimal if the patient is not adequately

hydrated and flow is reduced (Figure 9.5B). Some authors have chosen not to rely on oral hydration alone and have suggested a forced diuresis with intravenous hypotonic saline prior to the study.[8]

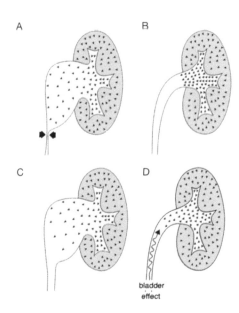

Figure 9.5 Causes of an 'obstructive' standard renogram curve. (A) True obstruction; (B) low flow; (C) large collecting system volume; (D) back pressure from bladder.

Collecting system volume

The primary application of diuresis renography is to determine whether a dilated upper urinary tract represents obstruction or merely stasis. Normally the increased flow following diuretic is sufficient to wash out the tracer accumulating in a dilated renal pelvis and confirm the absence of obstruction (Figure 9.5C). If, however, the collecting system is massively dilated, the increased flow may still be insufficient, despite a normal diuretic response and absence of obstruction.[9] Kletter and Nurnberger[10] observed when comparing diuresis renography with perfusion pressure–flow studies in 80 ureterorenal units that agreement between the two methods for diagnosing obstruction was 88% when collecting system volumes were <30 ml, but only 58% when the collecting system volumes exceeded 70 ml. Diuresis renography in the latter cases suggested obstruction not confirmed by perfusion pressure–flow studies.

Bladder effect

Interaction between the lower and upper urinary tract is commonly overlooked. Jones et al[11] demonstrated the influence of bladder filling on upper tract urodynamics by

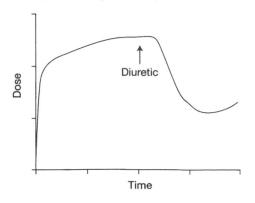

Figure 9.6 Classical responses of diuresis renography.

	Left	Right
Relative function	57%	43%
60 to 160 sec		
Uptake at 2 min:	11.5%	8.6% inj
Uptake at 3 min:	10.8%	8.5% inj
Time to peak	2.3%	2.3 min

Figure 9.7 Normal renogram curve.

repeating perfusion studies in 21 patients with the bladder empty and then full (Figure 9.5D). Interactive effects of a full or filling bladder on upper tract emptying can usually be abolished by asking the patient to void during the study, e.g. 10 min after the diuretic injection during F+20 renography. Continued data collection following voiding demonstrates changes in the upper tract urodynamics as a result of lower tract emptying. Certain groups of patients will require a renogram with an indwelling catheter if accurate reflection of upper/lower tract interaction is to be obtained.

Timing of the diuretic

The original description proposed injection of the diuretic 20 min after the radiopharmaceutical, referred to as F+20 diuresis renography. This enables the urodynamics through the upper tract to be studied without modification or manipulation. If rapid washout is observed, diuretic injection may be considered unnecessary, reducing the small but not insignificant inconvenience to the patient that results from diuretic injection. If the maximum possible diuresis is required from the outset, the diuretic should be injected 15 min before the radiopharmaceutical (F-15 diuresis renography) as previously discussed.[12] It reduces the 15–17% equivocal rate of F+20 diuresis renography to 3%.[5,13] Simultaneous injection of tracer and diuretic (F+0 renography) gives an alternative to the F-15 method which is more convenient and demonstrates results which are almost comparable in both children and adults.[14,15] When a variable injection time is adopted it is advisable for standardization purposes to label the renogram accordingly, e.g. F+15 or F-10.

Curve analysis

Three classic responses were described in the original account of F+20 diuresis renography (Figure 9.6: I–III).[3] An additional response has since been added (Figure 9.6: IV).[13]

I. Normal response before diuresis

A normal washout is obtained at resting flow rates before the diuretic is given (Figure 9.7). If the renogram is repeated after a diuretic injection it is possible that the system may decompensate and obstruct at diuretic flow rates. This is rare as it is unusual to have significant obstruction without dilatation and the latter should be detectable on the standard curve.

II. Obstructive response

The rising curve continues to rise despite injection of the diuretic, suggesting obstruction (Figure 9.8). Experimental evidence suggests that anything but an exponential clearance curve should be considered as evidence of obstruction.[9] Before accepting the conclusion of a definite obstructive response, the clinician must consider all possible reasons why it may be falsely positive as discussed previously: unrecognized dehydration, poor renal function, massive dilatation or a bladder effect. Hydration and bladder effects can be controlled. A volume effect can be predicted from imaging studies and the analogue images. From an estimate of the prevailing renal function, it is possible to guess at the likely urinary flow rate.[4] If single kidney glomerular filtration rate (SKGFR) is >16 ml/min, an obstructive response can be

	Left	Right
Relative function 60 to 160 sec	64%	36%
Uptake at 2 min:	12.9%	6.7% inj
Uptake at 3 min:	14.2%	9.2% inj
Time to peak	3.8 min	22 min

Composite

Figure 9.8 Example of type II diuresis renogram curve.

confidently assumed to be correct providing hydration, volume and bladder effects are excluded. If SKGFR is <16 ml/min, the result must be scrutinized. It may be obstructed, but there may have been insufficient increase in flow to wash out the tracer. Under these circumstances an F−15 study may be considered, but the increase in flow compared with the F+20 study is likely to be minimal when function is poor.

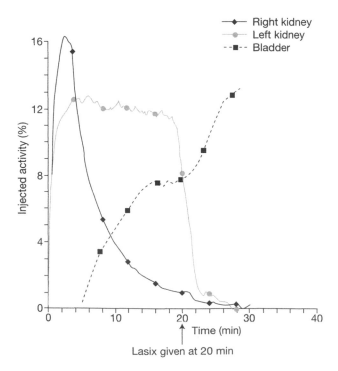

	Left	Right
Relative function 60 to 160 sec	42%	58%
Uptake at 2 min:	10.8%	15.1% inj
Uptake at 3 min:	13.2%	16.5% inj
Time to peak	5.0 min	3.4 min

Composite

Figure 9.9 Example of type IIIa nonobstructive diuresis renogram curve.

	Left	Right
Relative function	52%	48%
60 to 160 sec		
Uptake at 2 min:	8.3%	7.2% inj
Uptake at 3 min:	9.8%	9.7% inj
Time to peak	5.5 min	12 min

Composite

Figure 9.10 Example of type IIIb equivocal diuresis renogram curve.

IIIa. Nonobstructive response

An initially obstructive rising curve falls on injection of diuretic (Figure 9.9). It indicates that, at the diuretic flow rate achieved, the collecting system drains freely. Dilatation is the result of stasis rather than obstruction.

IIIb. Equivocal response

The initial obstructive rising curve on injection of diuretic neither washes out briskly nor continues to rise. The response is said to be equivocal (Figure 9.10). It must be established whether the result reflects a good diuretic response and a partially obstructed outlet or a suboptimal diuretic response and normal nonobstructed outlet. It may also represent a massively dilated system which an optimal diuretic response still cannot wash out.

This is the primary indication for an F–15 diuresis renogram. If there has been adequate hydration and the SKGFR is > 16 ml/min, then the equivocal response probably indicates subtotal obstruction. The increased flow rate of the F–15 renogram is sufficient to reduce the equivocal result to the 3% figure mentioned earlier.[5] The three responses of the F–15 renogram are shown in Figure 9.11. In the 3% who remain equivocal, it is policy to repeat the renogram in 3–6 months to establish if there has been deterioration in function. If function remains stable, there may be no need to intervene. If SKGFR is < 16 ml/min, then subtotal washout is an inconclusive result, probably due to subtotal diuretic response. An F–15 renogram may help but is unlikely to produce an enhanced diuresis when function is at this level or below. This equivocal result cannot be resolved further by

diuresis renography and the more invasive perfusion pressure–flow studies may be necessary to further clarify the situation.

IV. Delayed decompensation

The fourth response was first described by Homsy et al[16] as a 'delayed double peak pattern'. The initial washout in response to the diuretic is good, but then the curve flattens or even starts to rise (Figure 9.12). O'Reilly noted a further five cases on review.[13] The explanation rests with the steady increase in diuretic-induced urinary flow rate that does not peak until 15 min after injection. During the resting and early diuretic phases, the pertaining flow can be transported by the pelviureteric junction. Eventually, the flow rate reaches a level at which the system under stress can no longer transmit the urine load. It decompensates and further dilatation occurs. Outflow obstruction may even increase as a result. The balance is tipped and the amount of tracer entering the ROI drawn around the kidney exceeds elimination. The curve starts to rise once more. Other possible explanations must be considered before a firm diagnosis is made. A secondary infusion of radiopharmaceutical trapped in the forearm cannula might be persuaded into the circulation by arm movement: this should be avoided by adopting the technique of immediate flushing through the cannula with saline after the radiopharmaceutical injection. Vesicoureteric reflux could produce similar appearances but this and other interactive bladder effects can be excluded by asking the patient to void before completion of scanning or, better still, by placement of an indwelling catheter. If this fourth response is observed on

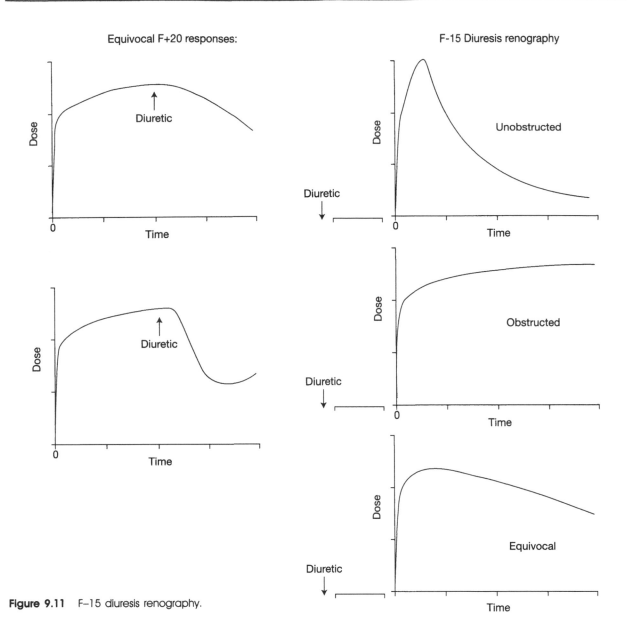

Figure 9.11 F–15 diuresis renography.

F+20 renography, it is the author's policy to proceed to an F–15 renogram as the increased diuretic flow rate should unmask obstruction if the explanation for this delayed response is correct. In the five cases recorded by O'Reilly,[13] performance of an F–15 diuresis renogram confirmed obstruction in three of the five cases. This response is indicative of true intermittent obstruction and should be treated appropriately.

Quantitative curve analysis

Some prefer a more quantitative assessment of the derived renogram curves than that based on curve pattern alone. Calculation of radionuclide clearance half-times is one option for which there are at least seven different methodologies.[17]

Output efficiency[18] and peak elimination rate[10] are alternatives. Unfortunately, these methods suffer from problems in defining the normal and obstructed ranges and such indices have a considerable range of equivocal results. The author's favoured approach is to study the curve pattern as a whole and therefore use all information available in reaching a diagnosis.

Perfusion pressure–flow studies

An alternative method for assessing obstruction, the perfusion pressure–flow study (PPFS), was proposed by Whitaker[6] in 1973 and gained popularity at about the same time as diuresis renography. Saline or contrast medium is perfused across the obstruction at a fixed flow rate, usually 10 ml/min.

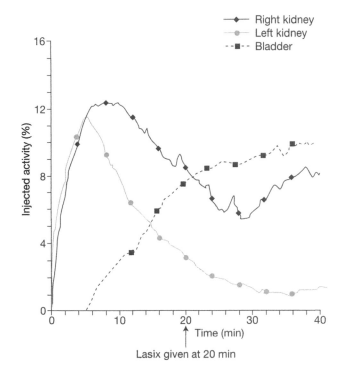

	Left	Right
Relative function 60 to 160 sec	53%	47%
Uptake at 2 min:	7.5%	6.5% inj
Uptake at 3 min:	9.6%	8.7% inj
Time to peak	5.4 min	8.5 min

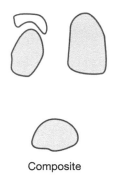

Composite

Figure 9.12 Example of type IV delayed decompensation diuresis renogram curve.

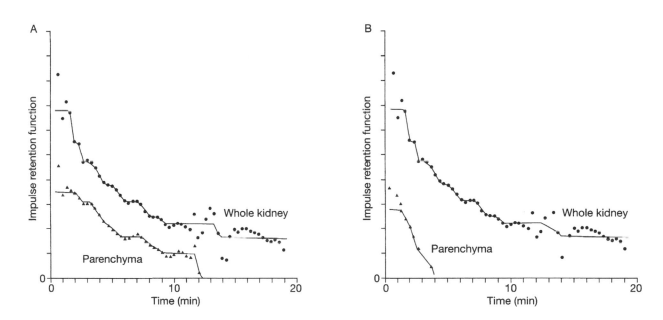

Figure 9.13 Parenchymal transit times. (A) Obstructed response. (B) Normal response.

Obstruction is assumed if the pressure in the infusate rises above 22 cmH$_2$O; a rise of less than 15 cmH$_2$O excludes obstruction.

The principle is entirely different from diuresis renography. The PPFS is a measure of outflow resistance to artificial perfusion of the renal pelvis and is unrepresentative of any other physiological parameters. Diuresis renography monitors increased but physiological urinary flow through the collecting system and is totally dependent on parameters such as the state of hydration and level of renal function.

It is therefore not surprising that agreement between the two methods is varied, ranging between 53% and 85% with both methods over- and underdiagnosing obstruction.[10,19–26] When assessing both methods, the important question is not whether the urinary tract can deal with a high urine flow rate, but whether the urinary tract can under normal physiological circumstances handle the volume presented to it without an adverse effect on renal function or producing symptoms. Every system has its maximal transmission rate above which it will decompensate. If physiological flow rates do not exceed this, it is of little significance.

Parenchymal transit time estimations

A modification of renography to further evaluate upper tract dilatation is the calculation of kidney transit times.[27,28] It is possible from stored renogram data to derive hypothetical curves which would result from a pulsed input of a unit quantity of tracer injected straight into the renal artery and subject to no recirculation. The process is termed 'deconvolution'. If significant obstruction is present, the transit times across both the whole kidney and parenchyma are prolonged (Figure 9.13). In good hands the technique is accurate and the complex processing involved simplified by modern computer availability. Unfortunately, the analysis remains involved and the availability of the simpler diuresis renogram has restricted the use of parenchymal transit time estimation.

Clinical application

The application of diuresis renography as described provides the clinician with a working diagnosis of obstruction. Its clinical significance (Figure 9.1) is determined retrospectively by the outcome of the clinical action taken as a result. The obstruction proves therefore to have been significant if 'relief' of the obstruction leads to resolution of symptoms, restoration or preservation of function, and resolution of secondary complications. A functionally 'proven' obstruction which over time remains asymptomatic and associated with no loss of function is almost certainly not significant. The clinical application is best illustrated by reference to the commonest cause of equivocal upper tract obstruction which occurs at the pelvi-ureteric junction.

Uretero-pelvic junction obstruction

Dilatation of the renal pelvis is usually discovered by intravenous urography or ultrasound in a patient being investigated for loin pain or haematuria (Figure 9.14) or may come to light as an incidental finding. The condition may be truly idiopathic, a neuromuscular defect at the pelvi-ureteric junction or associated with abnormalities such as aberrant

Figure 9.14 Left UPJ obstruction on intravenous urography.

lower pole vessels, kinks, adhesions or abnormal angulations. It may also be secondary to previous surgery, calculus disease or retroperitoneal scarring.

Diuresis renography is the first-line investigation and is central at each stage of the management process.

In a symptomatic patient with an obstructive renogram the treatment is surgical intervention. This is classically the dismembered Anderson–Hynes pyeloplasty. The obstructing segment of ureter is removed, dissected away from crossing lower-pole vessels if present and the dilated renal pelvis surgically reduced as necessary.

The relative function obtained by the study also helps determine the type of intervention. Because there are two kidneys and two upper tracts, reduction of function on one side may not be detected by the normal global parameters of renal function commonly employed. Without split function, the surgeon is unable to decide to what degree function must be preserved, e.g. whether a reconstructive pyeloplasty should be performed or whether a simple nephrectomy may be more appropriate. An important factor determining the type of intervention is often the amount of recoverable function of an obstructed kidney. DMSA scanning seems to be the most valuable noninvasive predictor of recoverable function.[29] An alternative method entails a 1–2-week decompression of the kidney by percutaneous nephrostomy or stenting. Repeat renography after this period provides a better estimate of recoverable function upon which management decisions can be based.

Outcome assessment

Following surgery, dilatation usually persists or may even progress as a result and therefore functional imaging is essential in follow-up. Renography combined with a measure of global function enables a comprehensive check on both urinary flow and individual kidney function.

Categorizing obstruction according to the F+20 and F-15 renographic responses described earlier, O'Reilly reported the outcome of 50 consecutive patients presenting with hydronephrosis. In those obstructed and undergoing surgery, a significant improvement in renal function was demonstrated in 96%.[30] Patients not obstructed on diuresis renography showed no deterioration in function over a 2-year follow-up period.[31] In a study of long-term follow-up of 50 patients evaluated by F-15 renography, similar results were obtained.[32] All patients with an obstructed F-15 renogram who underwent reconstructive surgery showed symptomatic and renographic improvement; 37 out of 39 unobstructed F-15 renogram patients remained unobstructed on a conservative follow-up policy. None of these experienced loss of split relative function in the kidney in question.

Obstructive diuresis renograms can be associated with preserved individual renal function on serial assessment, but expectant management may lead to a significant deterioration in ipsilateral function.[33] Lupton and Testa managed expectantly 23 patients with unilaterally obstructed diuresis renograms. All were managed conservatively for reasons of poor operative risk or well-preserved ipsilateral function and each had minimal or no symptoms. Either F+20 or F-15 renograms were performed and most had both at some time. The mean interval between serial scans was 10 months. There was deterioration in relative function > 10% in only four of the 23 patients. Of these, three subsequently underwent pyeloplasty. The preservation of function in the majority may reflect that, in this patient group, everyday flow rates do not reach diuretic-induced levels and obstruction only happens when the system is maximally stressed.

In a further study, 83 patients with hydronephrosis were investigated with pressure studies and renography and followed for a period of 17 years.[34] The decision to offer surgery was based primarily on symptom severity. Surgery was recommended in those patients under 50 years who were experiencing more than three episodes of pain per year. In this series 47 underwent pyeloplasty and 36 were treated conservatively. The investigation findings in this group are shown in Table 9.1.

Forty-nine percent of the conservatively treated patients had obstructed or equivocal diuresis renograms. The

Table 9.1 Distribution of pathological, equivocal and normal findings at manometry and isotope renography, and the peristaltic pattern in patients with and without subsequent pyeloplasty

	Pyeloplasty	No surgery
No. pts.	47	36
No. manometry pressure:	38	31
% High	59	16
% Equivocal	22	14
% Low	19	70
No. peristalsis	36	25
% Pathological	88	38
% Normal	12	62
No. renography findings	32	22
% Obstructed	69	27
% Equivocal	12	22
% Nonobstructed	19	50

outcome of follow-up is given in Table 9.2 which demonstrates fewer complications in the surgically treated group though still relatively few in the nonsurgical.

In addition, comparison of initial and late follow-up in the conservative group demonstrates no significant change in renographic assessment. This is not a randomized controlled study, but does raise the importance of considering all clinical and diagnostic information when deciding on patient management.

Every series is complicated by the inclusion of a small number of patients presenting with loin pain who demonstrate no obstruction as defined by either renographic or perfusion pressure flow studies (Figure 9.1 'Significant nonobstructed patients'). In such instances, it is the author's experience that pain may associate with distension of a particularly low compliant but unobstructed pelvis. If surgery is undertaken, results are often disappointing with continuation of presenting symptoms. Management becomes that of chronic visceral autonomic pain and identification of other possible causes.

Table 9.2 Complications during follow-up

	Pyeloplasty	No surgery
No. patients	41	28
Nephrectomy	5%	7%
Residual pain	7%	14%
Stone formation	5%	11%
Pyelonephritis	5%	7%
Hypertension	5%	7%

Table 9.3 Outcome of series of open dismembered pyeloplasty

Author	Year	Patients or kidneys	Success (%)
Poulsen et al[19]	1987	35	100
O'Reilly[31]	1989	30	83–93
MacNeily et al[35]	1993	75	85
McAleer and Kaplan[36]	1999	79	90
Austin et al[37]	2000	135/137	91
Houben et al[38]	2000	186/203	93
O'Reilly et al[30]	2001	24	96

Table 9.3 summarizes the results of additional series of patients undergoing the open dismembered Anderson–Hynes pyeloplasty.

In a recent poll of endourologists in the USA, it has become apparent that minimally invasive procedures have increased in popularity with 60% offering endopyelotomy and 25% laparoscopic pyeloplasty.[39] Endopyelotomy procedures performed either antegrade or retrograde have not matched the results of open pyeloplasty (Table 9.4).

Table 9.4 Series of endopyelotomy

Author	Year	Patients or kidneys	Success (%)
Schenkman and Tarry[40]	1998	8	88
Figenshau and Clayman[41]	1998	23	87
Faeber et al[42]	1995	32	81
Capolicchio et al[43]	1997	9	88
Motola et al[44]	1993	212	85
Giddens and Grasso[45]	2000	28	83

Even with endoluminal ultrasound to identify crossing vessels as the cause of the obstruction, endopyelotomy has started to give way to the dismembered pyeloplasty peformed laparoscopically. In a series of 41 patients success rates of 94% were obtained with laparoscopy compared

Table 9.5 Series of laparoscopic pyeloplasty

Authors	No.	Follow-up (months)	Success (%)
Bove et al[47]	11	21.3	91
Bentas et al (robotic)[48]	11	12	100
Klingler et al[49]	25	23.4	96
Sundaram et al (secondary ops)[50]	36	21.8	83
Parkin et al[46]	18	19	94
Siqueira et al[51]	19	14.4	94
Jarrett et al[52]	100	32.4	96

with 73% for ultrasound-assisted endopyelotomy.[46] This success rate for laparoscopic pyeloplasty mirrors other series and, though follow up is very short, is similar to results for the open operation (Table 9.5).

Urinary calculi

In adult urological practice urinary calculi are the most common cause of upper tract obstruction and therefore warrant consideration. The intravenous urogram or computerized tomography are usually involved in first-line diagnosis. The presence of obstruction is suggested from a dense nephrogram and delay in opacification of the collecting system. Ultrasound in conjunction with a plain abdominal film is advocated by some, but gives no information at all regarding function and does not exclude obstruction. A plain film with renogram for initial assessment has been advocated as an alternative to contrast studies.[53,54] In a series of 80 patients investigated with a MAG3 diuresis renogram and noncontrast helical CT within 12 hours of admission, patients were categorized according to renographic response: unobstructed, partially obstructed, totally obstructed or decompressed 'stunned' postobstruction.[55] The outcome of each of the groups is shown in Table 9.6.

Table 9.6 Functional categories in acute renal colic[55]

Category	% of patients	Outcome
Unobstructed	21	Discharged
Partially obstructed	32.5	Pain relief/decompression
Totally obstructed	24	Pain relief/decompression
Decompressed 'stunned' postobstruction	22.5	Discharged

This group demonstrated that KUB radiography, and even positive helical CT findings had a low positive predictive value for obstruction (in this study, 35%, 32% and 56%, respectively). Anatomic studies, including helical CT, should be followed by diuretic renography to diagnose and quantify obstruction and detect spontaneous decompression. Appropriate stratification of patients for emergency intervention, observation and medical therapy could greatly enhance medical management.

If a patient with a small or medium stone becomes symptom free, it is reasonable to allow the patient home in anticipation of the stone passing spontaneously. A normal diuresis renogram allows this decision to be made with confidence. There are a small group of patients who may be pain free yet have marked obstruction.[56] This may arise in cases where pain has persisted for more than 3–4 days but then ceased. Such cases were noted by Older et al[57] and Craven & Lecky,[58] who reported silent postobstructive renal atrophy on follow-up urography of patients with ureteric calculi. The patient should be reviewed regularly with a plain film and if the stone remains in place, a renogram requested. Increasing obstruction or a deterioration in split function on repeat scanning is an indication for intervention. In a study of 76 patients presenting with acute calculous obstruction, Kelleher et al[59] observed that, in all but two, ipsilateral split function returned to normal once the stone had passed or been removed.

Lower tract pathology and upper tract urodynamics

Lower tract dysfunction cannot be divorced from the upper tract. In patients with neuropathic bladders, reflux and chronic retention of urine, the effects on upper tract urodynamics may be profound. Mitchell[60] identified two types of chronic retention: those with low-pressure residuals and those with high-pressure residuals. It was noted that the latter group with 'high-pressure chronic retention' (HPCR) commonly developed associated upper tract abnormalities. If unheeded, severe hydronephrosis, uremia, hypertension and overflow incontinence would intervene. This group has been extensively studied. In the early stages of HPCR, upper tract function is normal. Ureteric peristalsis proceeds unhindered. As the hydrostatic pressure in the bladder rises, drainage of the upper tract is impaired and only proceeds in response to frusemide. Dilatation increases and is initially maximal in the supine position. When dilatation is sufficient to prevent the ureteric walls coapting between boluses, the disruption in flow becomes marked. This is reflected in obstructive renographic appearances, though simultaneous measurement of pressures in the bladder and upper tract in cases of HPCR demonstrate the pressure in the renal pelvis to be consistently lower.[61] Bladder drainage has a profound effect on the renogram, as demonstrated by George.[62] In management terms, renography at this late stage of HPCR is of academic interest only. More important is an isotopic GFR measurement to assess overall loss of function resulting from the chronic obstructive uropathy. It does serve, however, to stress the importance of considering the whole urinary tract when evaluating obstruction.

References

1. O'Reilly PH. Standardization of the renogram technique for investigating the dilated upper urinary tract and assessing the results of surgery. BJU Int 2003; 91: 239–43.

2. Rado JP, Bano C, Tako J. Radioisotope renography during furosemide (Lasix) diuresis. Nucl Med Commun 1968; 7: 212–21.

3. O'Reilly PH, Testa HJ, Lawson RS et al. Diuresis renography in equivocal urinary tract obstruction. Br J Urol 1978; 50: 76–80.

4. Brown SCW, Upsdell SM, O'Reilly PH. The importance of renal function in the interpretation of diuresis renography. Br J Urol 1992; 69: 121–5.

5. Upsdell SM, Testa HJ, Lawson RS et al. The uses and interpretation of modified diuresis renography. Contrib Nephrol 1990; 79: 103–7.

6. Whitaker RH. Methods of assessing obstruction in dilated ureters. Br J Urol 1973; 45: 15–22.

7. Upsdell SM, Leeson SM, Brooman PJ, O'Reilly PH. Diuretic-induced urinary flow rates at varying clearances and their relevance to the performance and interpretation of diuresis renography. Br J Urol 1988; 61: 14–8.

8. Sukhai RN, Kooy PP, Wolff ED et al. Predictive value of 99mTc-DTPA renography studies under conditions of maximal diuresis for the functional outcome of reconstructive surgery in children with obstructive uropathy. Br J Urol 1986; 58: 596–600.

9. Zechmann W. An experimental approach to explain some misinterpretations of diuresis renography. Nucl Med Commun 1988; 9: 283–94.

10. Kletter K, Nurnburger N. Diagnostic potential of diuresis renography: limitations by the severity of hydronephrosis and by impairment of renal function. Nucl Med Commun 1989; 10: 51–61.

11. Jones DA, Lupton EW, George NJ. Effect of bladder filling on upper tract urodynamics in man. Br J Urol 1990; 65: 492–6.

12. English PJ, Testa HJ, Lawson RS. Modified method of diuresis renography for the assessment of equivocal pelviureteric obstruction. Br J Urol 1987; 59: 10–4.

13. O'Reilly PH. Diuresis renography. Recent advances and recommended protocols. Br J Urol 1992; 69: 113–20.

14. Adeyoju AA, Burke D, Atkinson C et al. The choice of timing for diuresis renography: the F + 0 method. BJU International 2001; 88: 1–5.

15. Wong DC, Rossleigh MA, Farnsworth RH. F+0 diuresis renography in infants and children. J Nucl Med 1999; 40: 1805–11.

16. Homsy YL, Mehta PH, Huot D et al. Intermittent hydronephrosis: a diagnostic challenge. J Urol 1988; 140: 1222–6.

17. Conway JJ. 'Well-tempered' diuresis renography: its historical development, physiological and technical pitfalls, and standardized technique protocol. Semin Nucl Med 1992; 22: 74–84.

18. Chaiwatanarat T, Padhy AK, Bomanji JB et al. Validation of renal output efficiency as an objective quantitative parameter in the evaluation of upper urinary tract obstruction. J Nucl Med 1993; 34: 845–8.

19. Poulsen EU, Frokjaer J, Taagehoj-Jensen F et al. Diuresis renography and simultaneous renal pelvic pressure in hydronephrosis. J Urol 1987; 138: 272–5.

20. Hay AM, Norman WJ, Rice ML et al. A comparison between diuresis renography and the Whitaker test in 64 kidneys. Br J Urol 1984; 56: 561–4.

21. Whitaker RH, Buxton-Thomas MS. A comparison of pressure flow studies and renography in equivocal upper urinary tract obstruction. J Urol 1984; 131: 446–9.

22. Braren V, Bauriedel JK, Jones WB et al. Evaluation of normal and pathological ureteral dynamics: comparison of a radio-isotopic method with ureteral pressure/flow perfusion study. J Urol 1982; 127: 1014–6.

23. Senac MO Jr, Miller JH, Stonely P. Evaluation of obstructive uropathy in children: radionuclide renography vs. the Whitaker test. Am J Radiol 1985; 143: 11–5.

24. Gonzalez R, Chiou R. The diagnosis of upper urinary tract obstruction in children: comparison of diuresis renography and pressure flow studies. J Urol 1985; 133: 646–9.

25. Lupton EW, Richards D, Testa HJ et al. A comparison of diuresis renography, the Whitaker test and renal pelvic morphology in idiopathic hydronephrosis. Br J Urol 1985; 55: 119–23.

26. Kass EJ, Majd M et al. Comparison of the diuretic renogram and the pressure perfusion study in children. J Urol 1985; 134: 92–6.

27. Whitfield HN, Britton KE, Hendry WF et al. The distinction between obstructive uropathy and nephropathy by radioisotope transit times. Br J Urol 1978; 39: 433–6.

28. Britton KE, Nimmon CC, Whitfield HN et al. Obstructive nephropathy: successful evaluation with radionuclides. Lancet 1979; 1: 905–7.

29. Thompson A. The use of renal scintigraphy in assessing the potential for recovery in the obstructed renal tract in children. BJU International 2001; 87: 853–6.

30. O'Reilly PH, Brooman PJ, Mak S et al. The long-term results of Anderson-Hynes pyeloplasty. BJU International 2001; 87: 287–9.

31. O'Reilly PH. Functional outcome of pyeloplasty for ureteropelvic junction obstruction: prospective study in 50 consecutive cases. J Urol 1989; 142: 273–6.

32. Upsdell SM, Testa HJ, Lawson RS. The F–15 diuresis renogram in suspected obstruction of the upper urinary tract. Br J Urol 1992; 69: 126–31.

33. Lupton EW, Testa HJ. The obstructive diuresis renogram: an appraisal of the significance. J Urol 1992; 147: 981–3.

34. Kinn AC. Ureteropelvic junction obstruction: long-term followup of adults with and without surgical treatment. J Urol 2000; 164: 652–6.

35. MacNeily AE, Maizels M, Kaplan WE et al. Does early pyeloplasty really avert loss of renal function? A retrospective review. J Urol 1993; 150: 769–73.

36. McAleer IM, Kaplan GW. Renal function before and after pyeloplasty: does it improve? J Urol 1999; 162: 1041–4.

37. Austin PF, Cain MP, Rink RC. Nephrostomy tube drainage with pyeloplasty: is it necessarily a bad choice? J Urol 2000; 163: 1528–30.

38. Houben CH, Wischermann A, Borner G, Slany E. Outcome analysis of pyeloplasty in infants. Pediatr Surg Int 2000; 16: 189–93.

39. Marcovich R, Jacobson AI, Aldana JP et al. Practice trends in contemporary management of adult ureteropelvic junction obstruction. Urology 2003; 62: 22–5; discussion 5–6.

40. Schenkman EM, Tarry WF. Comparison of percutaneous endopyelotomy with open pyeloplasty for pediatric uretero-

pelvic junction obstruction. J Urol 1998; 159: 1013–5.

41. Figenshau RS, Clayman RV. Endourologic options for management of ureteropelvic junction obstruction in the pediatric patient. Urol Clin North Am 1998; 25: 199–209.

42. Faerber GJ, Ritchey ML, Bloom DA. Percutaneous endopyelotomy in infants and young children after failed open pyeloplasty. J Urol 1995; 154: 1495–7.

43. Capolicchio G, Homsy YL, Houle AM et al. Long-term results of percutaneous endopyelotomy in the treatment of children with failed open pyeloplasty. J Urol 1997; 158: 1534–7.

44. Motola JA, Badlani GH, Smith AD. Results of 212 consecutive endopyelotomies: an 8-year followup. J Urol 1993; 149: 453–6.

45. Giddens JL, Grasso M. Retrograde ureteroscopic endopyelotomy using the holmium:YAG laser. J Urol 2000; 164: 1509–12.

46. Parkin J, Evans S, Kumar PV et al. Endoluminal ultrasonography before retrograde endopyelotomy: can the results match laparoscopic pyeloplasty? BJU Int 2003; 91: 389–91.

47. Bove P, Ong AM, Rha KH, et al. Laparoscopic management of ureteropelvic junction obstruction in patients with upper urinary tract anomalies. J Urol 2004; 171: 77–9.

48. Bentas W, Wolfram M, Brautigam R et al. Da Vinci robot assisted Anderson-Hynes dismembered pyeloplasty: technique and 1 year follow-up. World J Urol 2003; 21: 133–8.

49. Klingler HC, Remzi M, Janetschek G et al. Comparison of open versus laparoscopic pyeloplasty techniques in treatment of uretero-pelvic junction obstruction. Eur Urol 2003; 44: 340–5.

50. Sundaram CP, Grubb RL 3rd, Rehman J et al. Laparoscopic pyeloplasty for secondary ureteropelvic junction obstruction. J Urol 2003; 169: 2037–40.

51. Siqueira TM Jr, Nadu A, Kuo RL et al. Laparoscopic treatment for ureteropelvic junction obstruction. Urology 2002; 60: 973–8.

52. Jarrett TW, Chan DY, Charambura TC et al. Laparoscopic pyeloplasty: the first 100 cases. J Urol 2002; 167: 1253–6.

53. Lundstam S, Wihed A, Suurkula M et al. Acute radiorenography during attacks of renal colic. J Urol 1983; 130: 855.

54. Embon OMGD, Shapira C, Koritny ES et al. Renal scintigraphy in initial evaluation of renal colic. Urology 1992; 39: 566–8.

55. Sfakianakis GN, Cohen DJ, Braunstein RH et al. MAG3–F0 scintigraphy in decision making for emergency intervention in renal colic after helical CT positive for a urolith. J Nucl Med 2000; 41: 1813–22.

56. Irving SO, Calleja R, Lee F et al. Is the conservative management of ureteric calculi of > 4 mm safe? BJU International 2000; 85: 637–40.

57. Older RA, Libshitz HI, Kelvin FM. Post-obstructive atrophy: often overlooked cause of unilateral small kidney. Urology 1976; 8: 517–9.

58. Craven D, Lecky JW. The natural history of post-obstructive renal atrophy shown by sequential urograms. Radiology 1971; 101: 555–60.

59. Kelleher JP, Plail RO, Dave SM et al. Sequential renography in acute urinary tract obstruction due to stone disease. Br J Urol 1991; 67: 125–8.

60. Mitchell. MSc Thesis: London; 1955.

61. Holden D, George NJR, Rickards D et al. Renal pelvic pressures in human chronic obstructive uropathy. Br J Urol 1984; 56: 565–70.

62. George NJR. High pressure chronic retention. In: O'Reilly PH, ed. Obstructive uropathy. Berlin: Springer; 1986: 247–61.

Antenatally detected hydronephrosis

10 Introduction

Amy Piepsz

Why separate obstruction in infants from obstruction in older children and adults?

Since the advent of fetal ultrasonography in the late 1970s, and the introduction of the systematic antenatal screening of hydronephrosis, the clinician is faced with an important population of infants with hydronephrosis. Dilatation of the fetal collecting system is observed in about 0.25% of pregnancies.[1] Beside entities such as urethral valves, vesico-ureteral reflux, hydro-ureteronephrosis or complicated duplex kidney, isolated pelvic dilatation will conceivably be the result of pelviureteric junction stenosis (PUJ). These neonates with PUJ are in good health and present no symptoms. The natural history of this condition, as well as its optimal management, are still a matter of debate. In contrast, obstruction in adults is often discovered on the basis of symptoms related to a heavy underlying pathology, and the controversy around the therapeutic attitude is less controversial.

A specific difficulty related to these young children is the initial immaturity of the renal morphology and function and the progressive changes that will occur during growth. Ignorance of these maturation patterns may result in serious errors of interpretation.

Moreover, several technical problems are related to this young age. Keeping the child quiet during any examination is a main concern, since movement may interfere with the quality of the test. A member of staff specifically trained in handling children is essential.

The small size of the kidneys, the thin cortical structure, the important overlap between collecting system and cortical area may all introduce difficulties in delineating the regions of interest, in correcting for non-renal tissue and in defining the cortical area. Similarly, the immature renal function is responsible for an unfavourable signal-to-noise ratio which may interfere with the precision of the measurements.

Finally, the responsibility of the clinician dealing with these young infants is great in this particular period of life, during which so many haemodynamic and urodynamic changes may interfere with the development of the kidney. Strategies of management are therefore aimed at preserving renal function and preventing the occurrence of severe infections.

Complete and partial obstruction

A traditional statement which is frequently used in the introduction of papers dealing with this clinical entity is that 'it is important to diagnose obstruction since obstruction left untreated will lead to loss of renal function'.

This is undoubtedly true in cases of total or subtotal obstruction. Urethral valves, for instance, constitute a neonatal emergency requiring a rapid surgical solution. Similarly, many situations observed in adults, such as stones or cancer with progressive invasion of the urinary tract, will lead to loss of renal function.

The antenatally detected PUJ is, in contrast, a partial obstruction and does not represent a surgical emergency. In most cases, this situation, even untreated, will not lead to loss of function.

Numerous experimental studies have been carried out in order to simulate the clinical model of antenatally detected PUJ. Chevalier et al[2,3] have demonstrated renal atrophy and apoptosis as a consequence of obstruction. It is clear, however, that the models created are subtotal or total obstruction. The consequences of these types of obstruction do not represent what is observed in children with PUJ. Josephson, a pioneer in the experimental approach of this pathology, has shown long-term preservation of renal function and anatomy despite the created obstruction.[4] The Ulm and Miller's model that he used creates a partial obstruction but again might not necessarily mimic the degree of narrowing seen in children.

Role of medical imaging

What is expected from medical imaging in PUJ is to allow the clinician to estimate the severity of the disease at diagnosis, to detect any degradation of renal morphology and function during follow-up, to decide on time about the management or the change in management of the patient and to estimate the results of the therapeutic approach.

A great number of parameters can be measured and the following chapters will try to clarify the respective importance of all these measurements. The size of pelvis and calyces in various physiological conditions will give timed information about the importance of hydronephrosis and the compliance of the system. Acceleration of kidney growth, on the contralateral side of the hydronephrotic kidney, may tell something about the functional behaviour of the dilated kidney. Invasive flow and pressure measurements have long been considered as the gold standard for obstruction. Level of function of the hydronephrotic kidney, as well as of the contralateral kidney, can presently best be measured by means of radionuclide methods. The quality of renal drainage is the other parameter provided by the renographic analysis, although the value of the information, in the case of poor drainage, is debatable. Histological studies are rare and concern exclusively operated patients. The biopsy findings speak for congenital creation and against progression of renal damage. In only a small number of kidneys did the renal microstructural changes contradict the successful expectancy course. The importance of some biological markers has still to be assessed. TGF-β1 in the urine might be a marker of fibrosis, and might therefore reflect the compliance of the pelvic wall.[5]

Radiological approach

The introduction of fetal ultrasonography has considerably modified the attitudes in PUJ, since it is now possible to develop strategies of management from the very first hours of life. As will be developed in Chapter 11, a considerable amount of information is currently available concerning the incidence of this entity or the acceptable cut-off values for a 'significant' increase in the anterior–posterior diameter. A related and essential topic is the adequate transmission of the information provided by fetal ultrasonography to the team who will take care of the child postnatally. Such a systematic approach is mandatory for any adequate prospective study.

Additional techniques for better definition of the morphology of the urinary tract are nevertheless useful in some situations and may help, for instance, in a better approach to infundibular stenosis or ureteral morphology, such as mid-ureteral stenosis. Intravenous urography, which has been the reference technique for many years, has now almost disappeared from the diagnostic strategy. This point, as well the recent introduction of magnetic resonance and CT scans, will be reviewed in Chapter 11.

Nuclear medicine

There has been significant progress in recent years in the information provided by the nuclear medicine renogram. The new tracers with high extraction rate, such as ^{99m}Tc

MAG3, I^{123} Hippuran or ^{99m}Tc EC have a better signal-to-noise ratio than with ^{99m}Tc DTPA, the latter tracer still being widely used. This is particularly important in young infants, in whom determination of parameters such as the differential renal function becomes significantly more accurate when using tracers with a high extraction rate. Details about techniques and pitfalls have been collected in recent consensus conferences and guidelines.[6,7]

Differential renal function is undoubtedly an important parameter, allowing estimation of the quality of renal parenchyma at diagnosis and during follow-up. By definition, however, this parameter has limitations and it would be significant progress to be able to define the single kidney function in absolute values and not simply by comparison with the contralateral kidney. The gamma camera parameters suffer, however, from a degree of inaccuracy, due to the numerous correction factors which have to be introduced, and no guidelines concerning this approach are presently available. Combining a blood sample method for overall GFR and a split function by means of renography may represent the best possible approach to single kidney function.

Estimation of renal transit will generally confirm a marked renal stasis, whatever the cause of hydronephrosis. Furosemide stimulation will try, in another step, to differentiate simple stasis from severe retention of tracer within the kidney. This is one of the main controversies that will be approached in Chapter 12. Similarly it is now considered that one should attempt to reach the best possible quality of drainage and therefore acquire late images performed after the effect of gravity and micturition. New parameters, such as output efficiency and NORA,[8,9] will allow us to quantify more objectively the performance of the furosemide stimulation. Cortical transit, which has been put forward because it may bypass the uncertainties related to the dilated cavities, has until now not proved to be efficient in the approach of antenatally detected hydronephrosis.

Finally, an alternative approach to the renogram might be the quantitation of renal function by means of ^{99m}Tc DMSA, even if no information on renal drainage is available using this technique. Because of the very high signal-to-noise ratio, it might be the most accurate way to estimate the differential renal function in infants. The constraint is, however, the need to acquire the data over a long period (24 h), in order to avoid any artificial accumulation of tracer within the collecting system.[10] As far as absolute DMSA uptake is concerned, the principle of this determination has been seriously questioned.[11] Moreover, no data are available concerning the day-to-day reproducibility of the method.

Pressure and flow measurements

Measuring pelvic outflow resistance during provocation has for a long time been a gold standard for obstruction.[12] The test has, however, not reached wide acceptance in young children, because of the invasiveness of the technique and the inaccuracy related to the administration of large, nonphysiological fluid volumes. Alternatively, the measurement of flow under a strictly constant pressure level might become a useful predictor in the future.[13]

Biological markers

The microstructure of the wall in and around the PUJ has been described and revealed as a consistent accumulation of collagen and elastin. The fibrosis of the pelvic wall may result in lower pelvic compliance and, as a consequence, in higher and more frequent pressure peaks. TGF-β1, a powerful promoter of collagen formation, is considerably raised in the tissue of PUJ walls that have this collagen deposition.[14] Urinary TGF-β1 could become a valuable marker of fibrosis combined with low pelvic compliance.

Can we define obstruction at initial diagnosis?

Stratifying the children with antenatally detected pelvic dilatation into two categories, those with and those without obstruction, is undoubtedly too simplistic a way to classify these patients. PUJ is in any case only a partially obstructed system and the degree of partial obstruction probably lies within a continuum, between slight and much more pronounced narrowing of the junction. Several factors, such as infection or position of the patient, can modify the degree of obstruction.

The size of cavities, as measured by means of radiological techniques, not only depends on the degree of narrowing, but also on factors such as compliance of the system, and therefore cannot serve as a marker of obstruction. Entities such as dilated vesico-renal reflux, obviously not related to obstruction, might reveal a similar degree of dilatation. The pitfalls related to pelvic pressure measurements have already been underlined. Differential function, as provided by the renogram, can be abnormally low as a consequence of obstruction, but additional factors such as associated renal dysplasia may explain an initial low function. Poor drainage under furosemide can be due simply to the reservoir effect of a dilated cavity. Finally, inspection of the pelviureteric junction during the pyeloplasty procedure will confirm, despite the narrowing of the junction, the still permeable lumen. The only definition of obstruction on which there is an agreement is 'the kidney which left untreated will show a deterioration of renal function'. This is unfortunately a retrospective diagnosis.

Can we predict deterioration of kidney function and anatomy?

More interesting is probably the question of whether or not we can predict deterioration of function and anatomy at initial evaluation. There are, however, no solid data demonstrating that the size of the renal cavity, the differential renal function, the level of pelvic pressure or the response to furosemide can pick up the patients at risk of deterioration. Lack of well-conducted prospective studies on nonoperated patients is probably responsible, at least partly, for the absence of clear replies to these questions. Other factors should also be prospectively evaluated. Noncompliant systems, as illustrated in Chapter 13, may represent a major risk factor and so it is worthwhile systematically evaluating the dosage of TGF-β1 as a marker of fibrosis and therefore of noncompliance.

What are the risks of a conservative nonsurgical attitude?

We have come far from the time when all children with PUJ were operated upon. Absence of symptoms, in those children antenatally detected, is certainly the main factor contributing to the choice of a nonsurgical attitude. The experimental and clinical work of some pioneers[4,15,16] has stimulated the clinicians to give the preference, in many circumstances, to a conservative attitude. Nevertheless, diverging opinions still exist and the controversy remains intense around the criteria for surgery and even the principle itself of no intervention in infants with PUJ.[17] Fear of loss of function, while the anomaly has been known since fetal life, is put forward.

A remarkably extensive compilation and critical review of the extremely heterogeneous literature has recently been published by Josephson.[18,19] Another huge compilation has also been published recently by Eskild Jensen et al.[20]

The most characteristic point coming out of these reviews is the lack of rigorous studies and the total absence of randomized studies on patients selected without initial prejudices. Series give contradictory results but are not comparable. One can only hope that well-designed studies, using techniques which are now well standardized, will be undertaken in the coming years, allowing the clarification of many unanswered questions.

In Chapter 12 Frøkiær will analyse the diverging results in the literature. In Chapter 13 Koff will present his own large experience over 10 years of a systematic conservative attitude.

In this introduction, I will simply put forward some of the main questions related to this controversy and some partial answers issued from the analysis made by Josephson in his recent compilation.

Is expectancy generally justifiable?

As a matter of fact, overall results are encouraging. According to Josephson's compilation,[18,19] 90% of 474 neonates allocated to watchful waiting were not operated on. Only 10% were subjected to delayed pyeloplasty, mostly because of an increase in pelvic size and/or decreasing differential renal function.

How often did symptoms occur in cases of expectancy?

Symptoms rarely occur. UTI is noted in about 5% of cases and is generally mild in nature. Renal colic seems to occur extremely rarely.

Does huge hydronephrosis foretell future function loss?

Josephson's survey[18] showed that half of the expectancies had an initial gross hydronephrosis. Nevertheless, in 88% of them, the nonoperative treatment could be carried through. On the whole, reports of increasing pelvic size were rare. Thus, so far, the presence of a gross hydronephrosis seems to have a limited prognostic value.

What is the risk of function loss during expectancy?

Again, according to Josephson's compilation,[18,19] expectancy was successful in 90% of the cases. Cross-over to delayed pyeloplasty was decided in about 10% of cases, the reason being either pelvic size increase or deterioration of differential function. These events mostly occurred during the first two years of life.

For those kidneys with an initial DRF less than 40%, expectancy led, according to Koff et al,[16] to improvement of

function in about 70% of cases. In those cases with deterioration of function, late pyeloplasty, performed without delay, generally restored the initial DRF values. Early pyeloplasty, in cases where DRF was less than 40%, probably did not result in a higher percentage of cases with restoration of function.

Does early surgery result in better preservation of split function than late surgery after deterioration of function?

The data available are essentially based on noncomparable series of patients. Patient series from the past are of no use for such an analysis, as they constitute a selected group of older and symptomatic cases. Clear answers can only come from well-designed prospective randomized studies.

What can be the long-term hazards of an expective attitude?

The experience on follow-up of conservatively treated patients is still limited in time and is not more than 10–15 years. In the past, however, when patients were addressed for PUJ discovered because of symptoms, DRF was often acceptable or almost normal, suggesting that the effect of symptoms on function was relatively modest.

Long-term follow-up on these patients is desperately needed, in order to evaluate more precisely the frequency and consequences of clinical symptoms, or the occurrence of complications such as severe tubular disease or stones.

Alternatively, is early surgery the solution to avoid any further complication?

Although not well documented, the occurrence of clinical complications is still possible in cases of pyeloplasty. Severe and recurrent infections due to multiresistant bacteria may follow the surgical procedure. Variable surgical complications, from minor events, such as leakage, to loss of renal function are possible in a minority of cases.

In cases of conservative treatment, how often should examinations be performed?

Those in favour of a conservative approach insist on the necessity of close follow-up, particularly during the first two years.[21] Ultrasound is certainly the instrument of choice to detect rapidly any significant alteration of pelvic size. The information about whether one can rely on repeated ultrasound to decide about performing a control of renogram is still required. In other words, can one assume an unchanged or improved function on the basis of a stable or improved hydronephrosis?

Conclusion

Antenatally discovered PUJ is still, after 20 years, a major field of controversy.

Expectancy and close follow-up have progressively gained wider acceptance, although the surgical approach, either systematic within the first months of life, or on the basis of variable morphological or functional parameters, is still the current preference for many clinicians. Progress in understanding the best approach to adopt can come only from well-designed prospective studies. Close follow-up of both groups of patients will be required anyway, since unexpected unfavourable developments are possible in both situations. Two extreme cases will illustrate this last statement.

Case 1

Antenatally detected right PUJ, closely followed by means of ultrasound and renography.

A renogram was performed at 10 months (Figure 10.1). Furosemide was injected together with the tracer (F0 test). The right kidney looks somewhat enlarged on the first 1–2 minutes. The split function is normal (left 49%, right 51%) despite a clear stasis in this right kidney, as seen at the end of the renogram ($NORA_{20}$ = 1.38). A late image was performed after the effects of gravity and micturition and showed a very satisfactory emptying of this right kidney ($NORA_{postmict}$ = 0.6). Overall glomerular filtration rate, measured by means of Cr-51 EDTA, was 95 ml/min/ 1.73 m^2. The conservative attitude was maintained.

The procedure was repeated 19 months later, at the age of 2.5 years. No particular clinical event was noted between the two renograms. The split function on the right side has now deteriorated considerably (left 84%, right 16%) while almost no emptying occurred on the late postmicturition image ($NORA_{postmict}$ = 3.08). Overall GFR was now 64 ml/min/ 1.73 m^2, despite the normal maturation which could be expected at that age.

Late pyeloplasty was performed 15 days later. One year later, only slight improvement of the right split function was observed (22%). There was no further improvement one year later.

Comment

Although it is well known that some deterioration may occur in cases where a conservative approach has been taken, it is rare to observe such an extreme loss of function.

Renogram performed at 10 months under furosemide stimulation (F0 test)

| 0–1 min | 1–2 min | 19–20 min | Postmicturition |

F0 test ...... 19 months later (2.5 years)

| 0–1 min | 1–2 min | 19–20 min | Postmicturition |

Figure 10.1 For legend, see text in Case 1, above.

Preoperative basic renogram

| 0–1 min | 1–2 min | 19–20 min | 19–20 min |

Preoperative frusemide test

| F + 0–1 min | F + 1–2 min | F + 19–20 min | Postmicturition |

Basic renogram, 6 months after pyeloplasty

| 0–1 min | 1–2 min | 19–20 min | 19–20 min |

Figure 10.2 For legend, see text in Case 2, below.

Case 2

Right PUJ detected by ultrasound performed at the age of 11 years, because of urinary tract infection. The renogram performed shortly after the diagnosis showed (Figure 10.2) an almost symmetrical split function (57% left, 43% right), as well as a renal stasis bilaterally, more pronounced on the right side. Furosemide was injected at the end of the renogram and the acquisition under furosemide showed a complete renal emptying on the left and a partial emptying on the side of the hydronephrosis. The postmicturition image revealed a good emptying of the right kidney: the residual activity in the right kidney was only 6% of the initial activity at the moment of injection of furosemide. Overall GFR (Cr-51 EDTA) was 108 ml/min/1.73 m^2.

Pyeloplasty was performed with the aim of preventing any possible renal damage. The operation was uneventful.

The renogram performed 6 months after surgery showed an almost complete disappearance of the right kidney on early parenchymal images (split function: 92% left, 8% right). There was no emptying of the right kidney after furosemide and micturition. Overall GFR was now 83 ml/min/1.73 m^2.

A new pyeloplasty was undertaken because of secondary PUJ stenosis. Control of the renogram 2 years later showed only partial improvement of the split function (76% left, 24% right). There was no further improvement of the split function.

Comment

Such an extreme loss of renal function related to pyeloplasty is rare, but can happen even in the hands of good paediatric surgeons.

References

1. Helin I, Persson PH. Prenatal diagnosis of urinary tract abnormalities by ultrasound. Pediatrics 1986; 78: 879–83.
2. Chevalier RL, Chung KH, Smith CD et al. Renal apoptosis and clustering following ureteral obstruction: the role of maturation. J Urol 1996; 156: 1474–9.
3. Chevalier RL, Gomez RA, Jones EE. Development determinants of recovery after relief of partial ureteral obstruction. Kidney Int 1988; 33: 775–9.

4. Josephson S. Experimental obstructive hydronephrosis in newborn rats. III. Long term effects on renal function. J Urol 1983; 129: 396–400.

5. Kim WJ, Yun SJ, Lee TS et al. Collagen-to-smooth muscle ratio helps prediction of prognosis after pyeloplasty. J Urol 2000; 163: 1271–5.

6. Prigent A, Cosgriff P, Gates GF et al. Consensus report on quality control of quantitative measurements of renal function obtained from renogram. International Consensus Committee from the Scientific Committee of Radionuclides In Nephrourology. Semin Nucl Med 1999; 29: 146–59.

7. Gordon I, Colarinha P, Fettich et al. Guidelines for standard and diuretic renography in children. Eur J Nucl Med 2001; 28: BP21–30

8. Chaiwatanarat T, Padhy AK, Bomanji JB et al. Validation of renal output efficiency as an objective quantitative parameter in the evaluation of upper urinary tract obstruction. J Nucl Med 1993; 34: 845–8.

9. Piepsz A, Tondeur M, Ham H. NORA: a simple and reliable parameter for estimating renal output with or without frusemide challenge. Nucl Med Commun 2000; 21: 317–23.

10. Piepsz A, Ham HR, Roland JH et al. Technetium-99m DMSA imaging and the obstructed kidney. Clin Nucl Med 1986; 11: 389–91.

11. Durand F, Prigent A. Can dimercaptosuccinic acid renal scintigraphy be used to assess global renal function? Eur J Nucl Med 2000; 27: 727–30.

12. Whitaker RH. Methods of assessing obstruction in dilated ureters. Br J Urol 1973; 45: 15–22.

13. Wahlin N, Magnusson A, Persson AEG. Pressure and flow measurements of hydronephrosis in children. A new approach to definition and quantification of obstruction. J Urol 2001; 166: 1842–7.

14. Seremitis GM, Maizels M. TGF-β1m RNA expression in the renal pelvis after experimental and clinical ureteropelvic junction obstruction. J Urol 1996; 156: 261–6

15. Ransley PG, Dhillon HK, Duffy PG et al. The postnatal management of hydronephrosis diagnosed by prenatal ultrasound. J Urol 1990; 144: 584–7.

16. Koff SA, Campbell KD. Nonoperative management of unilateral neonatal hydronephrosis. J Urol 1992; 148: 525–31.

17. Hanna MK. Antenatal hydronephrosis and ureteropelvic junction obstruction: the case for early intervention. Urology 2000; 55: 612–15.

18. Josephson S. Antenatally detected, unilateral dilatation of the renal pelvis: a critical review. 1. Postnatal non-operative treatment 20 years on – is it safe? Scand J Urol Nephrol 2002; 36: 243–50.

19. Josephson S. Antenatally detected, unilateral dilatation of the renal pelvis: a critical review. 2. Postnatal non-operative treatment – Long-term hazards, urgent research. Scand J Urol Nephrol 2002; 36: 251–9.

20. Eskild-Jensen A, Gordon I, Piepsz A, Frøkiær J. Congenital unilateral hydronephrosis. A review of the impact of diuretic renography on clinical treatment. J Urol 2005; 173: 1471–76.

21. Ulman I, Jayanthi VR, Koff SA. The long-term follow up of newborns with severe unilateral hydronephrosis initially managed nonoperatively. J Urol 2000; 164: 1101–5.

11 The radiological approach

Julie Ferzli, Jean-Nicolas Dacher

Introduction

Hydronephrosis is defined as a dilatation of the renal collecting system. Hydronephrosis should be differentiated from urinary tract obstruction as dilatation can be present without any obstruction. Congenital anomalies of the urinary tract represent 20% of all congenital malformations.[1] According to Peters,[2] obstruction is a condition of impaired urinary drainage which, if uncorrected, will limit the ultimate functional potential of the kidney.

The consequences of urinary tract obstruction vary in accordance with the age of the fetus (or child) at the onset of the disease, and with its natural history (transient vs permanent obstruction, occurrence of acute or chronic complications).

The renal parenchyma and the excretory system may be affected by obstruction. Thinning of the renal cortex, development of cysts, dilatation and histological changes of the pelvic and ureteric wall can be observed.

Detection of antenatal hydronephrosis on routine ultrasound examinations performed during the second and third trimesters of pregnancy has completely changed the postnatal management. Nevertheless, numerous cut-off values have been proposed for the antero-posterior diameter of the fetal renal pelvis as well as different classifications grading the fetal urinary tract dilatation in order to correlate prenatal findings with postnatal outcome.[3,4]

Optimal postnatal management begins with organized communication of the medical records of the fetus (images, reports, measurements) to the paediatric or surgical team who will take care of the newborn child. After birth, different imaging modalities are available including sonography, voiding cystourethrography, IV urography, pressure flow studies, diuresis renography and MRI. The main objectives of these various studies are to illustrate the anatomy of the urinary tract, to quantify the split renal function, and to assess the elimination curve of urine.

Some preliminary comments regarding the limitations of imaging should be made:

- Dilatation and excretion curves can fluctuate depending on hydration, bladder pressure and position of the child.
- Intermittent ureteropelvic junction (UPJ) obstruction can be missed by the usual tests and could remain a good indication for pressure–flow studies.

- In infants less than 6 weeks old, the renal immaturity alters the quality of contrast medium-based imaging studies.
- Information obtained from a single imaging study is limited. Follow-up examinations are of extreme importance in the context of obstruction.
- Follow-up examinations remain necessary after surgical relief of the obstruction.

Definition of fetal hydronephrosis

Measurement of the antero-posterior diameter of the renal pelvis on an axial scan of the fetal abdomen permits the detection of dilatation of the upper urinary tract (Figure 11.1).

A superior to 4 mm renal pelvis before 33 weeks gestational age (GA) or >7 mm after 33 weeks GA is a 100% sensitive criterion. However, the false-positive rate is very high in those conditions.[5]

Other values were proposed:[6]

- Prior to 24 weeks GA, the fetal urinary tract is normal if the renal pelvis AP diameter is 4 mm or less, calyces and ureters are nonvisible and the bladder is normal.
- After 24 weeks GA, the fetal urinary tract is abnormal if the renal pelvis AP diameter exceeds 10 mm, if the calyces are visible, if the ureter is dilated and if the bladder or the posterior urethra is enlarged and/or has a thickened wall.

Anderson et al[7] defined criteria for fetal hydronephrosis as follows: >4 mm before 24 weeks GA, >6 mm at 24–30 weeks GA, >8 mm after 31 weeks GA.

Fetal ultrasound can identify other predictors of outcome: involvement of one or both kidneys, evaluation of coexisting renal dysplasia (hyperechoic cortex, cysts), qualitative evaluation of the renal function from the assessment of lung development and the amount of amniotic fluid.

The abnormality should be characterized as much as possible by prenatal ultrasound, which in most cases cannot provide a complete urological diagnosis. This is the complementary role of postnatal evaluation, which is scheduled based on prenatal findings.

A

B

Figure 11.1 Third trimester ultrasound in a fetus with left hydronephrosis. A: Normal right kidney. Nondilated excretory system. Normally differentiated parenchyma. B: Axial scan of the left kidney showing a 22 mm AP diameter of the pelvis. UPJ obstruction was diagnosed postnatally.

Any fetus with hydronephrosis detected during the second trimester should be amenable to a follow-up study during the third trimester. The third trimester ultrasound seems to be the best predictor of postnatal uropathy. However, there is no direct correlation between the degree of dilatation and the renal function.[6,8]

Causes of fetal hydronephrosis

Various causes of fetal hydronephrosis have been described.[6,9–11] Transient and physiological hydronephrosis (extrarenal pelvis) represent respectively 48% and 15% of all cases. Recognition of these abnormalities is important to schedule appropriate postnatal follow-up.

When transient and physiological hydronephrosis have been eliminated, structural aetiologies are to be considered. The respective percentages of different uropathies vary in the literature according to the prenatal criteria of hydronephrosis, and the organization of postnatal follow-up. Thomas[11] showed that ureteropelvic junction (UPJ) obstruction and vesico-ureteral reflux (VUR) were the most frequent causes. Other causes are megaureter, duplicated ureters with or without ureterocele, posterior urethral valves and multicystic dysplastic kidney.

Ureteropelvic junction (UPJ) obstruction

UPJ obstruction is a quite complex and variable entity. This common obstruction of the urinary tract is thought to be due to an abnormal segment of the proximal ureter, a combination of muscular fibre disarray, excessive collagen deposition and abnormal intercellular conduction.

Kidney malrotation (e.g. horseshoe kidney) has been described as frequently associated with UPJ obstruction.[12] The natural history of UPJ obstruction is difficult to predict: pressure- or volume-dependent UPJ obstructions have been described.[13] Pressure-dependent obstructions roughly follow the hydrodynamics of a narrowed tube. Conversely, in volume-dependent obstruction, hydronephrosis aggravates abruptly when the renal pelvis reaches a given volume (Figure 11.2). The latter type can lead to intermittent obstruction, which is a challenging diagnosis. A crossing vessel (usually an artery) seems to be more frequently associated with intermittent UPJ obstruction.[14,15] Crossing vessels were described in 11–49% of kidneys with UPJ obstruction:[16] they are more commonly observed in adults and in older children than in infants or young children referred for prenatal diagnosis of hydronephrosis.

In cases of volume-dependent obstruction, when the critical volume of the pelvis has been reached, an obstructive kinking of the proximal ureter occurs which may be seen on

A

B

Figure 11.2 The unpredictible natural history of ureteropelvic junction obstruction. Prenatal diagnosis of moderately dilated excretory cavities had been made on the left side. A: First IVU performed at 1 year of age showed mild dilatation and no criteria of obstruction. B: Three years later the same child was referred for lumbar fossa pain. IVU (delayed film) showed severe UPJ obstruction.

imaging or at surgery. The multiform nature of UPJ obstruction explains why it is not possible to detect all cases prenatally: a fetus with a 'normal' pelvis can become a patient with an acute obstruction of the UPJ at any age of his/her life. In addition, diuresis renogram or functional MR cannot eliminate volume dependent UPJ obstruction if the critical volume of the pelvis has not been reached during the examination.

Vesico-ureteral reflux (VUR)

VUR is a common cause of fetal hydronephrosis (Figure 11.3). In addition, it is known to be associated in 20–50% of children presenting with an acute urinary tract infection even if they had no previous known renal disease.[17] VUR is known to be a significant risk factor for renal damage.

Whether primary or secondary to vesico-sphincteric disorders (voiding dysfunction, bladder outlet obstruction or neuro-genic bladder disorder), VUR usually results from an abnormal valve-like mechanism of the ureterovesical meatus.[18]

Prenatally detected VUR is more frequent in boys. This male predominance led to the theory of the transient fetal bladder outlet obstruction.[19,20] The spontaneous regression of prenatally detected VUR was widely described.

VUR is commonly associated with other urinary tract anomalies (UPJ obstruction, megaureter, kidney stone, duplicated ureter, ectopic ureter, bladder diverticulum).

Ureterovesical junction (UVJ) obstruction or megaureter

Obstructive (or primary) megaureter is the consequence of an abnormal peristalsis of the distal ureter leading to ureteral dilatation with or without pelvicalyceal dilatation (Figure 11.4).[21,22] The diagnosis may be suggested by prenatal

Figure 11.4 Single-shot fast spin echo T2-weighted image performed in a baby with left megaureter (prenatal diagnosis of ureterohydronephrosis). This picture was obtained after a less than 10 seconds sequence with no injection of contrast medium.

Figure 11.3 Postnatal examination in a baby boy who had had prenatal diagnosis of a moderate right hydronephrosis. Oblique film taken during a voiding cystourethrography showing right reflux into the lower pole of a duplicated kidney. Note the abnormal axis of the refluxing cavities.

ultrasound. A fibromuscular disorder with a relative increase in collagen fibres and reduction in muscular component is usually found on histopathological examination of the obstructive segment.[21] UVJ obstruction is sometimes associated with VUR. Secondary megaureter may be caused by VUR, ureteral valve, retrocaval ureter, ureteral stenosis, ureteral diverticulum, ureterocele or polyp.[23]

The natural history of UVJ obstruction is more conventional than that of UPJ obstruction: a progressive improvement occurs in the majority of cases and spontaneous healing is finally obtained. Surgery is considered in cases of severe obstruction, pain, or breakthrough infection. This natural history explains why primary megaureter is so rare in adults in contrast to UPJ obstruction, which remains quite common.

Duplicated ureter

The cause of hydronephrosis varies whether dilatation involves the upper or the lower pole ureter. Ectopic uretero-

cele is common in that context: it obstructs the lower extremity of the upper pole ureter. Prenatal diagnosis was shown to impact treatment since valuable function of the upper pole is frequently present at birth prior to any episode of infection.[24] Endoscopic incision found new supporters with the advent of prenatal diagnosis. This treatment is relevant when the upper pole presents significant residual function. A rare complication of ectopic ureterocele is urethral prolapse, which induces acute infravesical obstruction and requires urgent treatment. The main differential diagnosis of ectopic ureterocele is orthotopic ureterocele, which is frequently bilateral (Figure 11.5). Orthotopic ureterocele is not associated with a duplicated ureter and usually proves less obstructive than ectopic ureterocele. It is a relatively common cause of ureterohydronephrosis. US can easily demonstrate the thin-walled ureterocele within the bladder and make the differential diagnosis with megaureter.

Ectopic ureter is a variant of ectopic ureterocele. Obstruction and dilatation of the upper pole ureter are present. There is parallelism between the degree of ectopia and the severity of the upper pole dysplasia.

Vesico-ureteric reflux is frequently associated with lower moiety dilatation (Figure 11.3).

UPJ obstruction is a possible association that affects the lower pole more commonly than the upper pole.[25,26] The excellent results of prenatal diagnosis in the context of duplicated ureters have to be mentioned.[27]

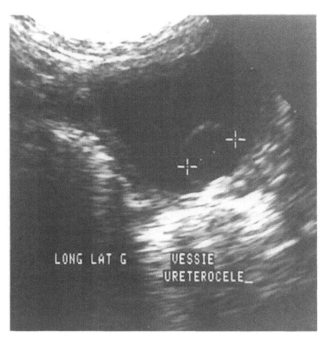

A

Figure 11.5 Prenatal diagnosis of bilateral uretero-hydronephrosis. Postnatally, ultrasound (A) showed a bilateral tiny ureterocele. No evidence of duplicated ureter. IVU (B) confirmed the diagnosis of bilateral orthotopic ureterocele, and showed functioning nonduplicated kidneys.

B

Posterior urethral valves (PUV)

Posterior urethral valves consist of abnormal mucosal folds between the urethral wall and the distal end of the veru montanum (Figure 11.6). Urethral obstruction is associated with bilateral ureterohydronephrosis and an enlarged thickened bladder in the most severe cases. There are various degrees of obstruction, hence various clinical presentations and renal or vesical consequences.[28,29] Antenatal ultrasound detection is the most common diagnostic modality. Radiographs aim to visualize urethral anatomy and to eliminate VUR.

Multicystic dysplastic kidney (MCDK)

Early obstruction of the embryonic urinary tract can lead to a multicystic dysplastic growth of the kidney, while later in pregnancy the same obstruction can induce hydronephrosis with corticomedullary dysplasia. Bilateral cases are fatal in utero, whereas unilateral cases present an excellent prognosis. This abnormality is not well known by physicians who treat adults as the multicystic kidney rapidly involutes and vanishes in most cases (Figure 11.7). In older children and adults, the lumbar fossa is found empty, and renal agenesis can be misdiagnosed.

Figure 11.6 VCUG in a baby boy with prenatal diagnosis of posterior urethral valves. Diagnosis has been confirmed by VCUG (suprapubic puncture). Note the patent urachus and vesicoureteric reflux.

Figure 11.7   Renal ultrasound in a baby with multicystic kidney. Involution has begun: the kidney is extremely thin and mainly constituted of noncommunicating cysts.

Antenatal ultrasound examination can make the diagnosis of MCDK, evaluate the contralateral kidney, and rule out most of the possibly associated anomalies.[30,31]

Postnatal investigations and management

Ultrasound

Ultrasound remains the cornerstone examination in the evaluation of infants and children with hydronephrosis. US has revolutionized diagnostic imaging of the urinary tract due to its constant developments, technical refinements and innovative applications.[32,33] Valuable information can be obtained in the absence of ionizing radiation, bladder catheter or intravenous injection of iodinated contrast medium. In the context of hydronephrosis, US examination should not be limited to an assessment of renal pelvis AP and ureteric diameters. A normal ultrasound examination includes the following elements: absence of thickened or fluctuating pelvis or ureter, nonvisible calyces, well-differentiated parenchyma, nonhyperechoic cortex, absence of cysts. Consecutive and comparative measurements of dilated segments, assessment of renal growth,[34] and assessment of the thickness and echogenicity of the renal parenchyma are all essential for management.

Grey-scale ultrasound cannot provide diagnostic criteria of obstruction.[35] However, two exceptions deserve to be mentioned: spontaneous perirenal urinoma was described pre- and postnatally as a mechanical consequence of increased intrarenal pressure, and calyceal dilatation was shown to be frequently associated with obstruction.

We would like to stress the importance of the postnatal ultrasound examination of newborns with prenatally detected hydronephrosis. High-quality management of children requires a high-quality US examination, which should preferably be performed by an experienced paediatric radiologist operating updated equipment with high frequency transducers. The timing of postnatal evaluation should be adapted to clinical status and prenatal findings. Postnatal US should be performed soon after birth in those rare infants with severe obstruction of the lower tract, which may be due to posterior urethral valves or ureterocele prolapse.[6] Day 4 of life is commonly chosen to perform the first postnatal US examination as the hydration status of the baby has normalized. Otherwise, it is convenient to examine the baby while still an inpatient with his/her mother at the maternity hospital. In patients with severe hydronephrosis, postnatal US can be coupled with voiding cystourethrography (VCUG). There is ongoing debate about the best strategy to apply in infants with antenatal mild to moderate pyelectasis. Ismaili et al.[36,37] demonstrated prospectively that US was an excellent screening tool (96% sensitivity and 97% negative predictive value) to predict significant nephrouropathies. These authors recommended performing two successive US scans (at day 4 and week 6 of life) and to stop investigations if both were normal. Longitudinal follow-up of children in the same institution with the same equipment by the same radiologist, guarantees optimal comparisons. Wide availability of prior examinations (showing measurements and scan planes in children as well as prenatal studies) is another factor for a high-quality follow-up; PACS (Picture Archiving Computerized System) proves useful in that domain.

Duplex Doppler was once thought to be an interesting diagnostic adjunct for obstruction. The hypothesis was that an increased resistive index (RI) in cortical and arcuate renal arteries would indicate obstruction.

Kesslet[38] and Lim[39] stated that resistive index could be a valid parameter for evaluation and follow-up of unilateral obstructive or nonobstructive hydronephrosis in children. Resistive indices were eventually used before and after administration of furosemide[40] as well as for renal functional evaluation.

In the context of congenital obstruction, those promising results were not confirmed, and Duplex Doppler only proved useful in school-age children with acute obstruction (e.g. with renal colic). Several reasons can explain the limited role of Duplex Doppler in obstruction: (1) the normal resistive index is physiologically higher in neonates than in older children; (2) co-operation (apnoea) of the patient is the key point of reliable measurement; (3) resistive index is unchanged in chronic obstruction.

Colour Doppler identification of a lower pole crossing vessel could be an interesting adjunct in children with UPJ obstruction,[16] and guide the treatment (open surgery vs retrograde interventional procedure). However, the technique should be applied with caution to avoid the risk of false-positive examinations.

A

Voiding cystourethrography (VCUG)

In a child with hydronephrosis, reflux should be eliminated prior to proceeding to any obstruction-focused examination. VCUG remains the gold standard imaging technique that permits the accurate diagnosis of VUR. The cyclic method should be employed to increase the sensitivity of the examination.[41,42] Sonocystography was recently described;[43] it does not deliver radiation, but it is a time-consuming and expensive technique that does not show the male urethra. It could be an elegant means to follow-up a child with a known reflux.[44,45] In this context, voiding urosonography could compete with radionuclide VCUG.[46]

Intravenous urography (IVU)

IVU is no longer justified in children with hydronephrosis and suspected obstruction. It delivers radiation, requires iodine contrast medium, and can be very time consuming. Moreover, it brings only a qualitative evaluation of renal function and obstruction.

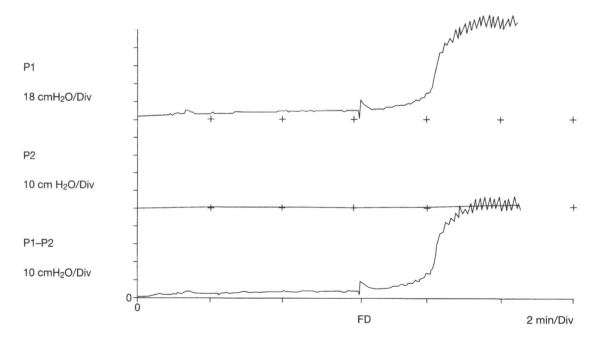

B

Figure 11.8   (A) Pressure–flow studies performed in a girl with left UPJ obstruction. Double puncture of the left renal pelvis had been performed under general anaesthesia. The excretory system was very dilated. (B) Constant flow perfusion of the upper urinary tract induced increase in renal (P1) and differential (P1–P2) pressures while bladder pressure did not change (P2). This test is no longer performed in our institution because it was deemed too invasive.

Pressure flow studies

These represent the genuine gold standard examination for obstruction. Since they were deemed invasive, these studies have progressively been abandoned by most groups. The principle was as follows: the child was placed in prone position under general anaesthesia in a radiology room, a catheter linked to a manometer was inserted into the bladder and two needles were guided percutaneously into the pelvic cavity (Figure 11.8A). One needle was used for constant flow infusion of contrast medium; the other one was used to record the pelvic pressure. A growing (supraphysiological, range 1–10 cc/s) flow was applied to the kidney and three pressure curves were simultaneously recorded: pelvis, bladder and differential (pelvic minus vesical) (Figure 11.8B). Obstruction was diagnosed when differential pressure rose above 15 cm of water. This test, first described by Whitaker,[47] remains interesting in identifying volume-dependent UPJ obstruction, vesical obstruction and obstruction in poorly functioning kidneys. Even though we had quite a good experience of these pressure–flow studies in our institution, we have progressively replaced them with the less-invasive dynamic studies (isotopes and MRI).

Figure 11.9 Right UPJ obstruction shown by MR (nonenhanced SSFSE sequence).

MR urography

Magnetic resonance is a newly described technique in the context of paediatric hydronephrosis.[48,49] The capabilities of MRI to illustrate the malformed urinary tract were extensively demonstrated (Figure 11.9). The anatomical study provided by MR is especially useful in neonates in whom intravenous urography is difficult due to the renal function immaturity. As compared with ultrasound, MR provides coronal images of the urinary tract (IVV-like view), which are usually very appreciated by surgeons. Single-shot fast spin echo (or turbo spin echo) sequences can show the dilated segments in multiple planes with no injection of contrast medium. MRI can also study the dilated excretory tract of a severely impaired kidney (or pole). Absence of any ionizing radiation is a significant advantage in this age range.

Moreover, the analysis of time–intensity curves generated from regions of interest drawn on sequential enhanced T1-weighted images was shown to approach the split renal function and excretory pattern.[48–52] Adequate sequences are fast field echo or fast spin echo ones with as short as possible TR and TE and a close to 90° flip angle. After administration of a low dose of gadolinium, the time–intensity curve comprises several successive segments (Figure 11.10). The first event is the vascular peak. Then, the curve reaches a baseline level, named 'p-level' (from peak trough). Thereafter, a gentle slope goes up to the glomerular peak (by 4 minutes after injection). Lastly, the curve goes down again as the contrast medium is excreted. A limitation of MR as compared with isotopic studies is the nonlinearity of the relation between the concentration of contrast medium and

the signal due to a possible T2 effect. This is the rationale for using a low dose of gadolinium chelate and as many T1-weighted sequences as possible.

Calculation of the differential renal function is based on the right-to-left ratio of two parameters drawn from the enhancing parenchyma.

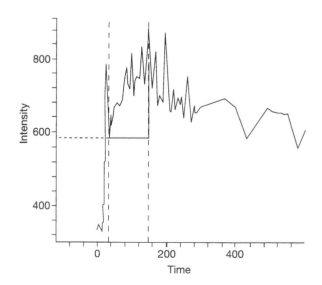

Figure 11.10 Typical time–intensity curve after injection of gadolinium. The region of interest was placed over the parenchyma.

Figure 11.11 Automatic segmentation of the renal volume on MR images (T1-weighted images with fat suppression after gadolinium enhancement).

- The area under the second segment of the slope, which represents the parenchymal transfer of contrast medium. This curve continues to ascend while more contrast material is extracted from the blood into the kidney than is excreted by the the kidney into the collecting system.
- The L/R ratio of functioning kidney volume (Figure 11.11).

Urinary excretion is assessed from the course of the excretory curve of the whole-kidney renogram as well as from the visually determined contrast material or tracer washout (Figure 11.12).

MRI is extremely promising in that field, but it still requires technical consensus and extensive evaluation prior to competing with the gold standard isotopic studies.

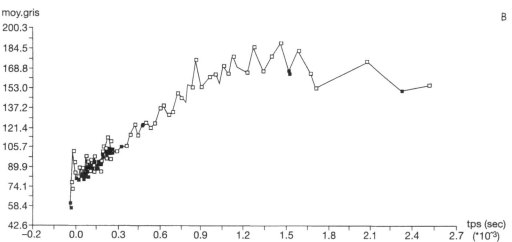

Figure 11.12 Normal excretory pattern on the right side (A). Obstructive pattern on the left side (B). Both curves were obtained in the same patient with unilateral left UPJ obstruction.

Conclusion

Pre- and postnatal ultrasound remains the cornerstone of the evaluation of fetuses and infants with hydronephrosis. The third trimester prenatal examination helps in selecting the newborns requiring postnatal studies with an optimal schedule. Postnatal ultrasound is usually performed by day 4, and should be repeated in many instances by 6 weeks of life. In children with prenatal diagnosis of hydronephrosis, two successive normal US examinations were shown to predict a low risk of significant nephrouropathy. VCUG should be performed to eliminate VUR in all infants with severe hydronephrosis as reflux may be associated with obstruction or cause the dilatation. Anatomical evaluation of obstructive uropathies should no longer be based on IVU. MR can provide the same information with no radiation and no contrast medium. In the near future, gadolinium-enhanced MRI could also compete with isotopic studies to evaluate the excretory pattern and the split renal function. An 'all in one' examination of children with hydronephrosis could hence be carried out.

References

1. Elder JS. Antenatal hydronephrosis. Fetal and neonatal management. Pediatr Clin North Am 1997; 44: 1299–321.
2. Peters CA. Urinary tract obstruction in children. J Urol 1995; 154: 1874–83.
3. Grignon A, Filion R, Filiatrault D et al. Urinary tract dilatation in utero. Classification and clinical applications. Radiology 1986; 160: 645–7.
4. Fernbach SK, Maizels M, Conway JJ. Ultrasound grading of hydronephrosis: Introduction to the system used by the Society for Fetal Urology. Pediatr Radiol 1993; 23: 478–80.
5. Corteville JE, Gray DL, Crane JP. Congenital hydronephrosis: Correlation of fetal ultrasonographic findings with infant outcome. Am J Obstet Gynecol 1991; 165: 384–8.
6. Toiviainen-Salo S, Garel L, Grignon A et al. Fetal hydronephrosis: is there hope for consensus? Pediatr Radiol 2004; 34: 519–29.
7. Anderson N, Clautice-Engel T, Allan R et al. Detection of obstructive uropathy in the fetus: Predictive value of sonographic measurements of renal pelvic diameter at various gestational ages. AJR 1995; 164: 719–23.
8. Avni FE, Hall M, Rypens F. The postnatal work-up of congenital uronephropathies. In Fotter R (ed) Pediatric Uroradiology. Springer: Berlin, Heidelberg, New York, 2001, pp 321–36.
9. Avni FE, Garel L, Hall M et al. Perinatal approach to anomalies of the urinary tract, adrenals, and genital system. In: Avni FE (ed) Perinatal Imaging from Ultrasound to MR Imaging. Springer: Berlin, Heidelberg, New York, 2002, pp 153–96.
10. Woodward M, Frank D. Postnatal management of antenatal hydronephrosis. BJU Int 2002; 89: 149–56.
11. Thomas DF. Prenatally detected uropathies: Epidemiological considerations. Br J Urol 1998; 81 (Suppl 2): 8–12.
12. Stephens FD. Ureterovascular hydronephrosis and the 'aberrant' renal vessels. J Urol 1982; 128: 984–7.
13. Koff SA, Hayden LJ, Cirulli C, Shore R. Pathophysiology of ureteropelvic junction obstruction: Experimental and clinical observations. J Urol 1986; 136: 336–8.
14. Dacher JN, Pfister C, Thoumas D et al. Shortcomings of diuresis scintigraphy in evaluating urinary obstruction: Comparison with pressure flow studies. Pediatr Radiol 1999; 29: 742–7.
15. Veyrac C, Baud C, Lopez C et al. The value of colour doppler ultrasonography for identification of crossing vessels in children with pelvi-ureteric junction obstruction. Pediatr Radiol 2003; 33: 745–51.
16. Rooks VJ, Lebowitz RL. Extrinsic ureteropelvic junction obstruction from a crossing renal vessel: demography and imaging. Pediatr Radiol 2001; 31: 120–4.
17. Galloy MA, Mandry D, Pecastaings M et al. Sonocystography: A new method for the diagnosis and follow-up of vesico-ureteric reflux in children. J Radiol 2003; 84: 2055–61.
18. Thomson AS, Dabhoiwala NF, Verbeek FJ et al. The functional anatomy of the ureterovesical junction. Br J Urol 1994; 73: 284–91.
19. Avni FE, Hall M, Damry N, Schurmans T. Vesicoureteric reflux. In Fotter R (ed). Pediatric Uroradiology. Springer: Berlin, Heidelberg, New York, 2001, pp 121–43.
20. Avni FE, Ayadi K, Rypens F et al. Can careful ultrasound examination of the urinary tract exclude VUR in the neonate? Br J Radiol 1997; 70: 977–82.
21. Sripathi V, King PA, Thomson MR, Bogle MS. Primary obstructive megaureter. J Pediatr Surg 1991; 26: 826–9.
22. Dixon JS, Canning DA, Gearhart JP et al. An immunohistochemical study of the innervation of the UVJ in infancy and childhood. Br J Urol 1994; 73: 292–7.
23. Avni FE, Hall M, Collier F, Schulman C. Anomalies of the renal pelvis and ureter. In Fotter R (ed) Pediatric Uroradiology. Springer: Berlin, Heidelberg, New York, 2001, pp 61–90.
24. Avni EF, Dacher JN, Stallenberg B et al. Renal duplications: the impact of perinatal ultrasound on diagnosis and management. Eur Urol 1991; 20: 43–8.
25. Wah TM, Weston MJ, Irving HC. Lower moiety pelvic-ureteric junction obstruction (PUJO) of the duplex kidney presenting with pyonephrosis in adults. Br J Radiol 2003; 76: 909–12.
26. Haliloglu M, Akpinar E, Akhan O. Lower-pole ureteropelvic junction obstruction with abnormal rotation in duplicated system. Eur J Radiol 2002; 41: 78–9.
27. Whitten SM, McHoney M, Wilcox DT et al. Accuracy of antenatal fetal ultrasound in the diagnosis of duplicated kidneys. Ultrasound Obstet Gynecol 2003; 21: 342–6.
28. Dacher JN. Abnormalities of the lower urinary tract and urachus. In Fotter R (ed) Pediatric Uroradiology. Springer: Berlin, Heidelberg, New York, 2001, pp 91–101.
29. Warren J, Pike JG, Leonard MP. Posterior urethral valves in

Eastern Ontario – a 30 year perspective. Can J Urol 2004; 11: 2210–5.

30. Mathiot A, Liard A, Eurin D, Dacher JN. Prenatally detected multicystic renal dysplasia and associated anomalies of the genito-urinary tract. J Radiol 2002; 83: 731–5.

31. Ranke A, Schmitt M, Didier F, Droulle P. Antenatal diagnosis of Multicystic Renal Dysplasia. Eur J Pediatr Surg 2001; 11: 246–54.

32. Riccabona M. Potential of modern sonographic techniques in paediatric uroradiology. Eur J Radiol 2002; 43: 110–21.

33. Riccabona M, Fritz G, Ring E. Potential applications of three dimensional ultrasound in the pediatric urinary tract: pictorial demonstration based on preliminary results. Eur Radiol 2003; 13: 2680–7.

34. Konus OL, Ozdemir A, Akkaya A et al. Normal liver, spleen, and kidney dimensions in neonates, infants, and children: evaluation with sonography. AJR 1998; 171: 1693–8.

35. Maizels M, Reisman ME, Flom LS et al. Grading nephro-ureteral dilatation detected in the first year of life: correlation with obstruction. J Urol 1992; 148: 609–14.

36. Ismaili K, Avni FE, Martin Wissing K, Hall M. Long-term clinical outcome of infants with mild to moderate fetal pyelectasis: validation of neonatal ultrasound as a screening tool to detect significant nephrouropathies. J Pediatr 2004; 144: 759–65.

37. Ismaili K, Avni FE, Hall M. Results of systematic voiding cystourethrography in infants with antenatally diagnosed renal pelvis dilatation. J Pediatr 2002; 141: 21–4.

38. Kessler RM, Quevedo H, Lankau CA et al. Obstructive vs nonobstructive dilatation of the renal collecting system in children: distinction with duplex sonography. AJR 1993; 160: 353–7.

39. Lim GY, Jang HS, Lee EJ et al. Utility of the resistance index ratio in differentiating obstructive from nonobstructive hydronephrosis in children. J Clin Ultrasound 1999; 27: 187–93.

40. Akata D, Haliloglu M, Caglar M et al. Renal diuretic duplex Doppler sonography in childhood hydronephrosis. Acta Radiol 1999; 40: 203–6.

41. Polito C, Moggio G, La Manna A et al. Cyclic voiding cystourethrography in the diagnosis of occult vesicoureteric reflux. Pediatr Nephrol 2000; 14: 39–41.

42. Papadopoulou F, Efremidis SC, Oiconomou A et al. Cyclic voiding cystourethrography: is vesicoureteral reflux missed with standard voiding cystourethrography? Eur Radiol 2002; 12: 666–70.

43. Darge K. Diagnosis of vesicoureteral reflux with ultrasonography. Pediatr Nephrol 2002; 17: 52–60.

44. Piaggio G, Degl'Innocenti ML, Toma P et al. Cystosonography and voiding cystourethrography in the diagnosis of vesicoureteral reflux. Pediatr Nephrol 2003; 18: 18–22.

45. Berrocal T, Gaya F, Arjonilla A, Lonergan GJ. Vesicoureteral reflux: diagnosis and grading with echo-enhanced cystosonography versus voiding cystourethrography. Radiology 2001; 221: 359–65.

46. Polito C, Rambaldi PF, La Manna A et al. Enhanced detection of vesicoureteric reflux with isotopic cystography. Pediatr Nephrol 2000; 14: 827–30.

47. Whitaker RH. Methods of assessing obstruction in dilated ureters. Br J Urol 1973; 45: 15–22.

48. Rohrschneider WK, Haufe S, Wiesel M et al. Functional and morphologic evaluation of congenital urinary tract dilatation by using combined static-dynamic MR urography: findings in kidneys with a single collecting system. Radiology 2002; 224: 683–94.

49. Rohrschneider WK, Haufe S, Clorius JH, Tröger J. MR to assess renal function in children. Eur Radiol 2003; 13: 1033–45.

50. Grattan Smith JD, Perez-Bayfield MR, Jones RA et al. MR imaging of kidneys: functional evaluation using F-15 perfusion imaging. Pediatr Radiol 2003; 33: 293–304.

51. Jones RA, Perez-Bayfield MR, Kirsch AJ, Grattan Smith JD. Renal transit time with MR urography in children. Radiology 2004; 233: 41–50.

52. Teh HS, Ang ES, Wong WC et al. MR renography using a dynamic gradient-echo sequence and low dose gadopentetate dimeglumine as an alternative to radionuclide renography. AJR 2003; 181: 441–50.

12 The nuclear medicine techniques

Jørgen Frøkiær, Anni Eskild-Jensen, Thomas Dissing

Introduction

Characteristically, urinary tract obstruction is associated with progressive hydronephrosis, parenchymal atrophy and impairment of renal functions. Hydronephrosis is common in paediatric urology, occurring in as many as 1.4% of fetuses and it may persist after birth.[1] However, hydronephrosis is not equivalent with obstruction and in the asymptomatic infant who has been diagnosed prenatally with hydronephrosis dilatation only persists in approximately 25% of the cases, consistent with a high degree of spontaneous resolution. This observation has therefore created a clinical enigma since a dilatation without progression and complications is clinically unimportant, whereas in an unpredictable minority of the dilatations it is important to detect obstruction to prevent renal function deterioration. At present there are no golden standard methods which in a satisfactory manner can establish or rule out whether a dilated kidney is obstructed. Moreover, there is no consensus on when a dilated kidney should be operated on and uniform criteria for when intervention is required are still lacking.

Postnatal management of children with unilateral hydronephrosis detected prenatally has remained a controversial topic for the past 10–15 years. During this period there has been a gradual paradigm shift away from early surgical intervention since preliminary reports indicated that hydronephrosis was not always associated with obstruction and could spontaneously improve or resolve with time. A major reason for this change in attitude is the result of an increasing academic interest in this condition where physicians have addressed a number of critical scientific questions based on clinical observations. An important contribution to this was based on studies observing that renal function did not deteriorate in infants and children with unilateral neonatal hydronephrosis suggesting that the urinary tract was not obstructed to a degree associated with progressive renal function impairment. It appeared that unilateral neonatal hydronephrosis could be a relatively benign condition and the risk of developing renal obstruction appeared relatively slight.[2] Because of diagnostic inaccuracy, the low risk of developing obstructive injury and the fact that many newborn kidneys with hydronephrosis rapidly improved function and dilation, it appeared safe to follow neonatal unilateral hydronephrosis closely and nonoperatively.

Consequently, identification of prenatal urinary tract dilatation by ultrasound (US) has challenged paediatric nephrologists, paediatric urologists, as well as radiologists and nuclear medicine physicians to find proper strategies to classify the infants who have a kidney that needs follow-up and/or surgery. The strategies for follow-up and treatment rely heavily on careful characterization of kidney function. The role of nuclear medicine and the techniques developed within this area during the past 15–20 years have provided key understanding of renal function development in infants with congenital unilateral hydronephrosis. Thus, one of the most important examinations to follow a hydronephrotic kidney is diuretic renography which is routinely performed to evaluate renal function and drainage of the kidney and ideally the purpose of diuresis renography is to establish or rule out whether a hydronephrotic kidney is obstructed or nonobstructed.

The purpose of this contribution is to present the value of state-of-the-art renography as an important tool for diagnosing renal function changes in cases with congenital unilateral dilatation of the renal pelvis. The decision-making process for those instances of urinary tract dilatation that require surgical correction and those that do not is based in part on the findings of diuresis renography. Thus, the development of renography during the past decade will be discussed and the role of renography in relation to short-term and long-term validation of renal function outcome after surgical and nonsurgical treatment of prenatally detected hydronephrosis will also be discussed.

Use of renography in infants and children with unilateral hydronephrosis

Gamma camera renography incorporates dynamic renoscintigraphy as a noninvasive method in both children and adults for evaluating hydronephrosis by the quantification of differential renal function (DRF) and drainage. However, children and infants are not small adults, and the recognition that specific precautions are required when examining renal function with the use of radionuclides in these individuals has generated several attempts to provide guidelines for renography with regard to both performance and interpretation. Diuretic renography was originally introduced based on the assumption that the radiopharmaceutical retained in a nonobstructed dilated system will be washed out when urine output is high, whereas the radiopharmaceutical will be retained in the renal pelvis if obstruction is present.[3] Despite the identification of an increasing number of perinatal cases with hydronephrosis recognized by the frequently routine use of prenatal ultrasonography the performance of renography differed among nuclear medicine practitioners and the surgical findings are occasionally discrepant from the diuretic renogram interpretation.[4] Thus, the need to develop by consensus a more uniform methodology was recognized for the first time in the early 1990s by the American Society of Fetal Urology and the Pediatric Nuclear Medicine Council of the Society of Nuclear Medicine, and a comprehensive standard method for diuretic renography entitled 'The well tempered diuretic renogram' was generated as guidelines for the following items: patient preparation (hydration and bladder catheterization), diuresis renography technique (radiopharmaceutical used, patient position during examination, data acquisition parameters, diuretic pharmaceutical and dosage, time of injection and regions of interest to monitor diuretic effect), and data analysis (percent differential renal function, curve pattern analysis and methods of measuring the diuretic response). Pooled diuresis renogram data were collected for analysis of the correlation with surgical results and clinical outcomes to determine the most appropriate information to be derived from the diuretic renogram in neonates with unilateral hydronephrosis.[5] Subsequently, another report was presented as a standardized approach to diuresis renography also for the paediatric population by the consensus committee of the Radionuclides in Nephrourology in order to improve reproducibility between centres, discourage unacceptable practice and stimulate further discussion between nuclear medicine and urology health care professionals who treat patients with dilated and obstructed upper urinary tracts.[6] The remaining great variation in techniques and interpretation of diuresis renography between different studies led to generation of another set of guidelines for standard and diuretic renography in children by The Pediatric Committee of the European Association of Nuclear Medicine with regard to: hydration, bladder status and effect of gravity, assessment of drainage, interpretation of drainage, selection of radiopharmaceutical, indications/contraindications and detailed recommendations regarding acquisition.[7] The overall aims with these guidelines have been to reduce variation and provide a common platform for the use of diuretic renography in infants and children with unilateral hydronephrosis. Moreover, the recognition that a child requires much longer examination time as an adult for the same examination dictates an appropriate appointment system to ensure that the staff has sufficient time to devote to the child and parent.[8]

The principle of renography is based on the intravenous injection of a radiopharmaceutical that is accumulated and

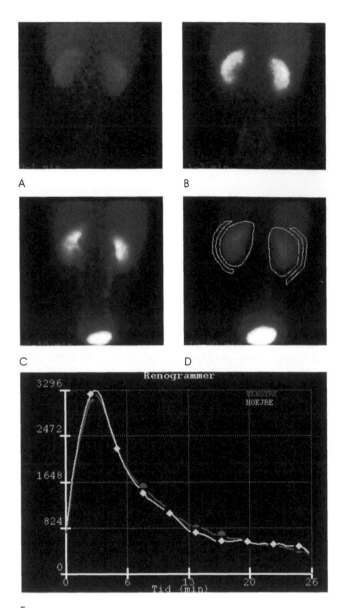

Figure 12.1 The principle of renography is based on the intravenous injection of a radiopharmaceutical that is accumulated and excreted by the kidneys, and which can be detected externally by a gamma camera providing a dynamic examination of the kidneys. A–D: Dynamic accumulation of MAG3 in the kidneys during different time frames of the study. A: Rapid accumulation in both kidneys is seen during the first minute. B: This is followed by a consolidated accumulation during the 1–3 min after injection. C: From 3–10 min there is visible drainage of urine (MAG3) passing via the ureters to the bladder. D: From 10–20 min accumulation of urine increases in the bladder in parallel with a reduction in renal activity. E: Dynamic curves of the change in activity within each kidney defined by the region of interest placed over each kidney.

excreted by the kidneys, and which can be detected externally by a gamma camera providing a dynamic examination of the kidneys. In practice two suitable radiopharmaceuticals are available for this purpose: ^{99m}Tc-diethylenetriaminepenta-acetic acid (^{99m}Tc-DTPA) which is handled by glomerular filtration and ^{99m}Tc-mercaptoacetyltriglycine (^{99m}Tc-MAG3) relying on tubular extraction.[9] ^{99m}Tc-MAG3 has the highest renal extraction fraction and target-to-background ratio and therefore provides the best image quality in children.[10,11] In addition, the usefulness of ^{99m}Tc-ethylenedicysteine (^{99m}Tc-EC) as a tubular agent with an even higher renal extraction has been documented.[12] The restricted commercial availability limits the use of this agent.

In infants and children renography is usually performed with the patient supine. After an intravenenous injection there is rapid renal accumulation of the radiopharmaceutical (Figure 12.1A). The renal handling of the radiopharmaceutical can be followed in a dynamic sequence and images can be constructed representing the renal activity at any given time. By defining regions of interest (ROI) around the kidneys (Figure 12.1D) a renogram can be constructed based on the time–activity curves of radioactive decay within the defined areas (Figure 12.1E). Thereby the arrival, transit and excretion of radioactive tracer from the kidneys can be monitored in a dynamic sequence allowing estimation of relative uptake as differential renal function (DRF) and excretion (drainage). DRF expressing the percentage of the sum of left and right kidney function can be calculated using two well-accepted algorithms, i.e. the integral method and the Patlak–Rutland method, the latter adjusting for intravascular background activity as well.[7,13]

The renogram curve can be divided into three phases (Figure 12.2).[14] During the first few seconds after injection, the curve rises rapidly reflecting the speed of injection and the vascular supply to the kidney (vascular phase). The second phase lasting 2–3 minutes after injection represents tracer accumulation within a kidney but no excretion is initiated (parenchymal phase). The increase in renal activity during this period represents the DRF. The third phase is initiated when the tracer starts to leave the kidney, which is after 2–5 minutes in the normal kidney (drainage phase). Importantly, the peak of the renogram curve (T_{max}) does not represent the moment when the tracer starts to leave the kidney, but merely the equilibrium between uptake and excretion.

Drainage reflects excretion, or disappearance, of the radiopharmaceutical from the kidney. Assessment of drainage can be done qualitatively and quantitatively. By simply inspecting the renogram curve a qualitative evaluation is done regarding the following characteristics: an early peak followed by a rapidly descending phase is typical for normal excretion. An important delay in excretion is characterized by a continuously ascending curve. Several techniques have been proposed for quantitating the transit of tracer through the kidney. These range from simple descriptive parameters, such as the time to reach the maximum of the renogram curve or mathematical quantification by some recently developed methods (pelvic excretion efficiency (PEE), output efficiency (OE) and normalized residual activity (NORA)).[15–18] When dilatation of the collecting system exists, the standard renogram is generally characterized by a continuously rising curve, reflecting poor drainage of the kidney. In this condition, furosemide should be administered which increases urinary flow and may distinguish between good, intermediate and poor drainage. Assuming that the tracer retained in the dilated nonobstructed system will be washed out when urine production is high, whereas it will be retained despite increasing diuresis in cases of obstruction. Several protocols exist giving the diuretic before (F–15), simultaneous with (F0) or after the radiotracer (F+20) and there is no current evidence that one method is superior to the others.[7] Importantly, it has recently been demonstrated that the quality of drainage obtained during the F+20 and F0 procedures can easily be compared using both OE and NORA.[19] A very similar quality of drainage was reached for both procedures when considering only the postmicturition image (PMI) (for detailed description of the PMI see below). Thus, it remains mandatory to obtain a PMI irrespective of the timing of the furosemide injection and despite the use of tracers with a high extraction rate

Pitfalls in the interpretation of renography

Since diuretic renography is an important and frequently used investigation in guiding the treatment and follow-up of children with congenital hydronephrosis it is also important to know the pitfalls.[20] Valuable and reproducible information on DRF and drainage can be obtained provided the investigation is performed in a standardized manner. It is mandatory that DRF is calculated before the tracer excretion is initiated, i.e. within the first 2 minutes of the renogram. Choosing any other timeframe will underestimate the DRF of the non-

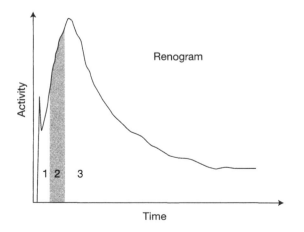

Figure 12.2 Theoretical renogram consisting of three different phases. Phase 1 (vascular phase); phase 2 (parenchymal phase) and phase 3 (drainage phase).

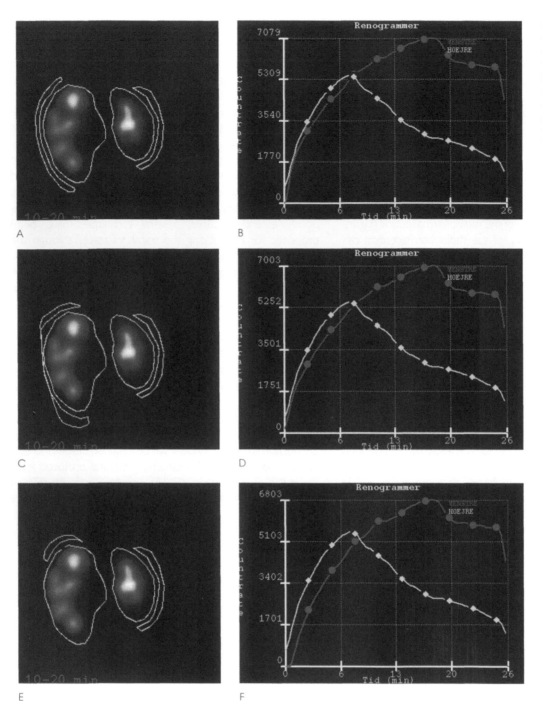

Figure 12.3 The accuracy of the DRF estimate depends on the method of background subtraction. As can be seen from this figure placement and size of the background area has a significant impact on DRF.

dilated contralateral kidney and thereby overestimate DRF of a hydronephrotic kidney. If furosemide is given early (F-15 or F0) the intrarenal transit of the tracer may be accelerated and thereby excretion to the pelvis in which case the timeframe for DRF calculation should be adjusted.[21]

When calculating DRF, activity in the extrarenal tissue (background activity) included in the renal ROI must be subtracted, and the accuracy of the DRF estimate depends on the method of background subtraction (Figure 12.3). Subtracting activity in an area surrounding the kidney outline

size normalized to the renal ROI is probably the most adequate method (Figure 12.3A, B).[13] Large hydronephrotic kidneys may not allow space for this approach in which case a background area above and below the kidney is recommended[7] and as demonstrated in Figure 12.3, location and size of the background area has significant impact on the DRF (Figure 12.3A–F).

A DRF between 45–55% is considered to be within the normal range.[7,13] There is no definition of a 'significant' reduction or increase in DRF. Although the methodological variation is likely less than 3% provided good signal-to-noise ratio[22] the physiological variation may be higher, especially in the infant. Thus, the estimation of DRF will depend on good tracer extraction which improves with succeeding renal maturation.[23] As DRF measures relative function hydronephrotic kidney changes may reflect changes in function of the opposite kidney, either due to contralateral compensatory functional increase or bilateral renal disease.

There are also a number of potential pitfalls with regard to interpretation of the renogram. Classically, drainage is described using the $T^1/_2$ time defined as the time for half of the accumulated tracer to leave the pelvis, reflecting only the rate of change of activity in the dilated pelvis.[24] When the $T^1/_2$ time is short, impaired drainage is excluded. Prolonged $T^1/_2$

Figure 12.4 A: Control ultrasonography of a left kidney in a 17-month-old child with left prenatally diagnosed hydronephrosis demonstrating persistent severe dilatation of the left renal pelvis. B: Images, and C: diuretic renography curves (including a PMI) of an F0 MAG3 study at 18 months of age. The left kidney DRF is 56%. The images show micturition during the 0–20-min study and between the 20-min image and the postmicturition and posterect image (PMI) which was obtained 45 min after MAG3 administration.

time, however, is not synonymous with obstruction to urine outflow and several variables will influence the shape of the renogram curve, including the timing of diuretic administration.[25,26] A diagnosis of obstruction should therefore not be made simply on the basis of compromised drainage on the renogram curve.

Poor hydration will lead to tracer stasis in the pelvis because of inadequate urine production and decreased furosemide response.[5] Consequently, it is crucial that the child is well-hydrated and fluid intake prior to the investigation is therefore recommended.[7,20] Poor pelvic emptying may be apparent because of a full bladder and because gravity is having no effect in the supine position.[15,27,28] By evaluating pelvic activity after bladder emptying and maintaining the patient temporarily erect before terminating the investigation to allow a normal gravitational effect, i.e. obtaining a so-called PMI (Figure 12.4), drainage from a nonobstructed dilated pelvis may be evaluated and improved compared to the interpretation based on the investigation without including the PMI in the evaluation.[17]

Poor renal function may affect the descending part of the renogram and cause insufficient or slow pelvic filling. Therefore renal function should be integrated in the interpretation of drainage and simple methods which are less influenced by renal function, such as PEE, OE and NORA have recently been developed.[15–18] The size of the pelvis may also influence the shape of the renogram curve (Figure 12.5).[29] Accumulation of tracer is likely in the more severely dilated pelvis due to 'reservoir effect'. In general, the larger the pelvis the more dilution of tracer is expected and the more cautious the interpretation of prolonged drainage should be. Therefore it is important to take into consideration that drainage is dependent on both flow rate (urine production) and volume of the renal pelvis as indicated (Figure 12.5C).

Overall it is recommended that in asymptomatic children with unilateral ureteropelvic junction dilatation drainage should not be assessed using half-time. Instead, techniques considering renal function, gravity and an empty bladder are recommended, such as renal OE, PEE or NORA.

Defining obstruction

Obstruction and hydronephrosis are closely associated, although obstruction is not easily defined physiologically. It is obvious that hydronephrosis is a descriptive clinical term defined as distension of the pelvis and calices of the kidney with accompanying atrophy of the renal parenchyma (Figure 12.6). Consequently, diagnosing hydronephrosis is not difficult. In contrast, obstruction is poorly defined and difficult to diagnose. Recognizing that obstruction inevitably will impair renal function, the best considered is the retrospective unequivocal definition proposed by Koff as any restriction to urine flow, that left untreated, will cause progressive renal

Figure 12.5   The size of the pelvis may influence the shape of the renogram curve. Accumulation of tracer is likely in the more severely dilated pelvis due to 'reservoir effect'. In general the larger the pelvis the more dilution of tracer is expected and the more cautious the interpretation of prolonged drainage should be. The plateau curve in C does not represent 'a true' obstruction, but an equilibrium. It is important to take into consideration that drainage is dependent on both urinary flow rate and pelvis volume.

deterioration.[30] Indeed, this definition unmasks the insufficient knowledge of the natural history of an obstruction in terms of kidney function. Understanding the natural history requires a conservative attitude towards these patients. The need for this was recognized more than 20 years ago, when Samuelson and colleagues in an elegant study, examined renal function in children with unilateral hydronephrosis in response to surgical or nonsurgical treatment and found that GFR remained normal at follow-up despite treatment regimen.[31] The study indicated that the parenchymal function in unilateral idiopathic hydronephrosis in children more than 1 year old usually is normal, but may deteriorate due to urinary tract infection. Consistent with this, additional studies consisting of more patients were performed supporting the observation that renal function does not deteriorate in the majority of cases with unilateral congenital hydronephrosis.[32,33] Thus many cases with dilatation may be due to a so-called balanced obstruction/hydronephrosis where renal function does not deteriorate. However, it is yet unclear, to what extent obstruction depletes the renal functional potential of a hydronephrotic kidney, which is especially relevant for the neonatal hydronephrotic kidney (Figure 12.6). Therefore, an extended version of the definition of obstruction proposed by Koff has been forwarded as 'A condition of

Figure 12.6   The relative time course for renal function during obstruction. Obstruction will be followed by a reversible phase referred to as 'obstructive uropathy'. If correction is performed at this stage of obstruction impairment of kidney function may be minimal or prevented. However, if obstruction persists, impairment of renal function is irreversible with the onset of obstructive nephropathy and correction will not restore renal function, with the potential risk of further deterioration.

Figure 12.7   Unilateral dilation of the renal pelvis in the neonate may be caused by prenatal obstruction of different severities. Consequently, this may impair nephrogenesis with the development of different degrees of hydronephrosis or in the most severe cases in dysplastic kidneys.

Table 12.1 Summary of the results of key publications based on patients with unilateral dilatation of the urinary tract from the past 10 years with regard to the number of operated patients and criteria for surgical intervention

	Study population (no. cases)	% operated at study entry	% operated after observation	Criteria for surgical intervention
Cartwright et al	72 (90% prenatal)	43	15	DRF <35% or decreasing, symptoms, not specified
Freedman et al	160 with delayed drainage curve	12.5	3.5	DRF <40%
Cornford et al	316 with delayed drainage curve	8	7	DRF <40% or decreasing, increasing HN, symptoms
Dhillon et al	148*	26	22	DRF <40%, symptoms, social reasons
Takla et al	51 prenatal	12	37	DRF <35% or decreasing, delayed drainage
Subramaniam et al	100 prenatal	51	26	DRF <40% or decreasing, symptoms
Ulman et al	104 prenatal SFU[38] grade 3–4 HN	none	22	decreasing DRF, increasing HN
Thorup et al	100 prenatal	34	23	DRF <40% or decreasing, symptoms

*Including unilateral (77), bilateral (66 kidneys) or solitary hydronephrotic kidneys.
HN: hydronephrosis.

impaired urinary drainage that if uncorrected will limit the ultimate functional potential of a developing kidney'.[34] This may particularly be true in cases with neonatal obstruction of the kidney where a prenatal obstruction may have impaired nephrogenesis resulting in varying degrees of hydronephrosis and in the most severe cases in renal dysplasia (Figure 12.7).

The impact of renography in clinical decision making

Prenatal hydronephrosis is found in approximately 0.25% of pregnancies.[35] At present the natural history of congenital hydronephrosis is still incompletely understood. It may therefore be important to distinguish the degree of hydronephrosis when evaluated since spontaneous resolution takes place in approximately 50% of the cases with mild hydronephrosis whereas spontaneous resolution is seen only in 15% of patients with moderate hydronephrosis and in none with severe hydronephrosis.[36] Consequently, no intervention is required in the majority of cases, but functional evaluation is necessary in a relatively large number of children depending on the study population, criteria for intervention, follow-up regimen, selection bias and differences in referred cases to the respective departments. In a recent review of the literature[37] it was established that 0–51% of the cases were operated at study entry or after the first evaluation, consistent with an enormous variation of selection criteria (Table 12.1). Approximately 25% were operated after a period of observation using symptoms, decreasing or persistence of low DRF, deteriorating drainage pattern or increasing dilatation as indications for surgery, supporting the view that there is no

consistency in the criteria for treatment. Commonly, a decreased DRF at initial assessment is often used as a sign of obstruction and thereby an indication for surgery. This indication has been questioned in a study where all hydronephrotic kidneys were subjected to nonoperative follow-up despite the initial level of DRF.[38] This study demonstrated that 27 neonates (38%) of the 71 with long-term follow-up had an initial DRF <40% and 15 of these required surgery due to decreasing DRF and/or increasing hydronephrosis. Thus, only a little more than half of the cases with initial DRF <40% were 'truly' obstructed in this study. Overall 22% of 104 children underwent surgery because of decreasing DRF and/or increasing hydronephrosis. An important finding was that the number of infants requiring surgery was higher in the group with initial reduced function suggesting a susceptible group who require closer follow-up.

The primary goal of surgical intervention is to maintain or improve renal function, but this is not always achieved. As demonstrated in Table 12.1 where renal function is related to indications for surgery it is evident that it is difficult to compare the individual studies. The overall impression is that improvement does not occur when surgery is done because of initial decreased DRF. The retrospective study by Calisti et al[39] is the only exception. The findings of this particular study were that reversible renal damage seems to be associated with extrinsic obstructions from polar vessels, which are predominant among symptomatic, later detected cases, whereas a congenital, irreversible loss of function accompanies intrinsic obstructions, typical of prenatally diagnosed cases. Kidneys with very low DRF may maintain or improve function on conservative observation indicating that surgery may be unnecessary in some kidneys with initial decreased function and that the first MAG3 diuretic renogram cannot predict renal function.[38] A hydronephrotic kidney with a DRF below

40% may have developed like this in utero and no surgical intervention can be expected to produce a 'normal' kidney. With regard to whether improvement of renal function is related to age at surgery, it remains unclear if the chance of postoperative functional restitution is greater in the younger age compared to later intervention. Important information about the time interval between functional deterioration and surgical intervention is missing in these studies which may be more important than age at surgery for the functional outcome.[7,15,17,27,28,37]

It has been hypothesized that kidneys with an initial low function have a higher risk of deteriorating than those with normal function. And in a recent study a higher fraction of kidneys with initial DRF below 40% required surgical intervention (35%) than kidneys with initial DRF >40% (14%) suggesting a closer follow-up in these cases.[38]

Diuretic renography plays an important role in the clinical decision making. Clinically, it is important to subject neonates with unilateral dilation of the renal pelvis to a consistent regimen taking advantage of as much information as possible. The Danish Societies of Nuclear Medicine, Radiology, Pediatric Urology and Pediatrics have reached consensus regarding this, which may work as a useful guide to decision making in neonatal cases with unilateral dilatation of the renal pelvis (Figures 12.8 and 12.9).

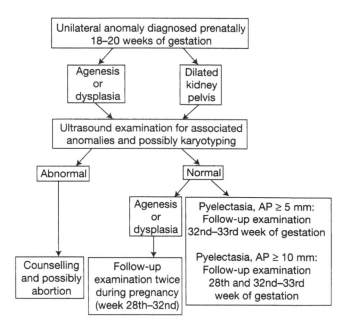

Figure 12.8 Flow chart representing the diagnostic strategy for a fetus diagnosed with a unilateral anomaly in week 18 during pregnancy representing a summary of the overall consensus strategy provided by The Danish Societies of Nuclear Medicine, Radiology, Pediatric Urology and Pediatrics.

Figure 12.9 Flow chart representing the diagnostic and treatment strategy for neonates with prenatally diagnosed unilateral dilatation of the urinary tract representing a summary of the overall consensus strategy provided by The Danish Societies of Nuclear Medicine, Radiology, Pediatric Urology and Pediatrics.

Interpretation of renal drainage

Diuretic renography may be undertaken in many different ways according to existing guidelines[7] and the hydronephrotic kidney drainage curve is often used when deciding whether to operate or not. Useful information may be obtained in the immature hydronephrotic kidney where agreement exists about the definition of good drainage.[18,40] However, as opposed to the older symptomatic child the definition of obstruction based on an impaired drainage curve cannot be transferred to the asymptomatic infant kidney with an enlarged collecting system and/or renal immaturity.[20] Further, the risk of inappropriate data acquisition, processing and interpretation may lead to erroneous conclusions in this population. Therefore the use of diuretic curve interpretation alone has become less popular and some institutions no longer consider the drainage pattern in decision making.[38,41,42]

When interpreting and comparing diuretic drainage curves standardization of investigational procedures, as well as the use of drainage facilitating techniques, are important. Unfortunately few studies provide information on these matters.[7] Often the diuretic renogram is performed without considering bias induced by differences in hydration, kidney function, pelvic size, gravity and bladder filling. It is therefore difficult, and at times impossible to compare findings between studies. Nevertheless, a number of studies indicate that $T^1/_2$ time is not useful as an absolute parameter for predicting the functional course.[17,38,40,43] A significant fraction of kidneys followed nonoperatively which maintain or improve renal function have prolonged $T^1/_2$ time and compromised drainage[38,40,44,45] regardless of the use of drainage-facilitating techniques as recommended by the EAMN guidelines.[17] Drainage patterns are not stable and variability on sequential diuretic renography without surgical intervention is documented in a large fraction of hydronephrotic kidneys.[17,40] Therefore impaired drainage may not be a persistent finding when the diuretic renography is repeated[17] and may improve spontaneously on follow-up along with resolution or improvement of hydronephrosis and renal maturation.[38,44,46]

The percentage of cases with compromised drainage depends on the selection of the study population. Kuyvenhoven et al[47] found poor drainage in 16% of hydronephrotic children younger than 3 months measuring output efficiency on a postvoid and gravity-assisted view whereas Amarante et al[17] found 44% with poor drainage using similar methods. The number of cases with compromised drainage also depends on pelvic size and a mathematical model shows that drainage can be significantly influenced simply by changing the pelvic volume.[29] A poor drainage response is not synonymous with ongoing obstruction but may be associated with severe hydronephrosis, which according to the results by Dhillon et al. may signify an increased risk[42] and therefore should be followed more carefully.

Although surgery may not improve renal function, drainage is usually improved. In the study by Gordon et al. the percentage of obstructed drainage curves in children operated because of decreased or decreasing function was reduced from 72% to 33%.[40] In the studies by Ransley and colleagues and by Ulman and Koff, improved drainage and decreased hydronephrosis were found in all postoperative cases.[38,48] Salem et al. also observed improved drainage postoperatively in kidneys which preoperatively had prolonged $T^1/_2$ time,[49,50] whereas Piepsz and colleagues demonstrated that most kidneys remained dilated postoperatively and that prolonged drainage reflected stasis in the dilated cavities.[51] Although improvement or normalization in drainage and $T^1/_2$ time has been used as an indicator of surgical success[52] this is highly questionable as the postoperative drainage curves depend on the postoperative pelvic size (Figure 12.5A–C).

How often should renography be performed and for how long should assessment be continued?

The optimal schedule for serial investigations remains controversial and unknown. The study by Ulman et al indicated that close follow-up during the first 2 years (especially early in life) with diuretic renography and ultrasound may improve functional outcome.[38] At the other extreme, kidneys with prenatal diagnosis that are lost to follow-up are not likely to recover function after delayed surgery.[53,54] When evaluating and comparing existing studies maturational improvement in renal function is not accounted for. This would only be enlightened in a randomized prospective study. An important message to take home from the numerous studies is that there is a time frame for reversal, but this may be individual and remains unknown as reversal of function is only obtained in a fraction of kidneys. Therefore, it may be speculated that the population of prenatal diagnosed unilateral hydronephrosis consists of kidneys with prenatal damage and no potential for recovery despite operation, kidneys that will improve their function spontaneously during growth and maturation, and kidneys with ongoing obstruction that may regain function by timely surgical relief. Unfortunately no studies so far have managed to provide methods that can identify these potential subgroups and thereby guide the follow-up regimen. Interestingly, a recent study comprising data from the US-based so-called Nationwide Inpatient Sample analysed the trends in surgical correction of paediatric ureteropelvic junction obstruction.[54] The conclusion of this study was that practice patterns in paediatric pyeloplasty evolved between 1988 and 2000. Although mean age at surgery decreased in the population during the study period, a significantly smaller proportion of procedures are being performed during the first 6 months of life. This finding suggests that patients with a diagnosis of prenatal hydronephrosis are increasingly being observed instead of undergoing surgery in the newborn period and infancy.[54] One important reason for this may be related to the use of renography as a routine method for monitoring renal function combined with proper diagnostic strategies as outlined previously in this chapter (Figures 12.8 and 12.9).

The results and prevailing procedures underscore that randomized standardized clinical trials are still missing despite 20 years of publishing mostly retrospective investigations into congenital hydronephrosis. The frequency of sequential diuretic renography is controversial and based on empirical and individual practice. In most studies the schedules for initial and repeated investigations are not described in detail. Some centres use fixed intervals between investigations,[48,55] others a more individual schedule based on the value of DRF.[38]

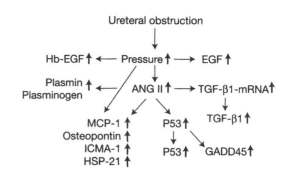

Figure 12.10 Major steps in the ANG II regulating pathways in the kidney in response to unilateral obstruction of the ureter. Obstruction results in a pressure increase which in turn will increase the expression of the intrarenal renin-angiotensin system, including an enhanced production of ANG II. This leads to activation of a series of molecular changes which are proinflammatory, pro-apoptotic and plays a pivotal role for the development of fibrosis and progressive obstructive nephropathy. ANG II, angiotensin II; EGF, epidermal growth factor, Hb-EGF, heparin-binding epidermal growth factor, TGF-β-1, transforming growth factor β-1; MCP-1, monocyte chemoattractant protein-1; ICMA-1, intercellular adhesion molecule-1; HSP-21, heat shock protein-21; P53, tumour suppressor protein P53; GADD45, growth-arrest and DNA damage-inducible gene 45; ↑, increase; ↓, decrease.

Can the number of renographic investigations be reduced based on sequential and stationary ultrasound findings?

It has been suggested that the size of the dilated pelvis may correlate to the risk of functional deterioration.[56] If so, the number and frequency of renographic assessments may be guided by the size of the pelvis. The risk of functional deterioration appears to be low in the case of SFU grade 1–2[57] or an anterior-posterior pelvic diameter <12–15 mm[41,48,57] unless severe prenatal hydronephrosis or severely dilated calices.[42] In the case of more severe dilatation controversy exists as Dhillon et al. recommended immediate surgery if the anterior-posterior pelvic diameter exceeds 50 mm whereas others found no association between severe hydronephrosis and functional deterioration.[38,43]

Although a few studies have suggested a correlation between functional deterioration and the degree of prenatal dilatation or increasing postnatal dilatation the predictive potential of these parameters remains unknown[59,60] and further studies are needed to clarify the potential of guiding postnatal treatment and follow-up based on pre- and postnatal dilatation.

Evidence-based development of new diagnostic strategies

Thorough evaluation of hydronephrosis in the fetus or neonate requires an understanding of fetal and neonatal renal physiology, the transition from an intrauterine to extrauterine environment, and renal structural and functional maturation. In a recent National Institutes of Health sponsored workshop on congenital urinary tract obstruction it was concluded that the natural history of obstructive nephropathy should be defined by developing biomarkers in humans and animal models to generate measures of injury and functional impairment, including imaging techniques such as renography.[61] Thus, to clarify the natural history of congenital hydronephrosis animal models have contributed immensely to improve the knowledge and understanding on renal function development in response to congenital obstruction. It has been established that the resulting kidney damage is not a simple result of mechanical urine flow impairment but rather a complex syndrome involving alterations in glomerular haemodynamics and tubular function caused by the interaction of a variety of cytokines and vasoactive factors (for review see references 61 and 62). From numerous studies it is evident that the renin-angiotensin system (RAS) plays a pivotal role for the pathophysiological changes observed in response to an obstruction (Figure 12.10). Provided that a persisting unilateral ureter obstruction in a child will be associated with an enhanced expression of the RAS and an unobstructed hydronephrosis will not be associated with an increased expression of the RAS, several attempts have been done to use blockade of the RAS system in combination with renography in a predictive manner with the aim to confirm or rule out the presence of urinary tract obstruction in cases with unilateral hydronephrosis.[61] So far, these investigations have failed to convincingly demonstrate that blockade of the RAS in combination with renography provides results to discriminate whether a dilated system is obstructed. This may reflect the complex nature of urinary tract obstruction. In addition to the RAS, numerous other pathways important for renal functions are turned on in the obstructed kidney, including growth factors such as TGF-β and epidermal growth factor, endothelin and several cytokines.[63]

Moreover, animal studies have provided evidence that severe hydronephrosis does not always cause renal function loss or progressive dilatation during long-term follow-up.[64,65] In a neonatal pig model with unilateral partial obstruction and grade 3–4 hydronephrosis early renographic evaluation including DRF and pelvic size did not predict the functional outcome.[65,66] These results support the view of the clinical studies demonstrating that renal function deterioration is not impaired even at severe dilatations.[67] It has been hypothesized that the extrarenal pelvic dilatation may serve to protect the renal parenchyma from functional deterioration caused by overdistension and a rise in pressure. This so-called 'equilibrium theory' refers to an equilibrium between outflow restriction, urine production and pelvic reservoir capacity, as discussed in Chapter 13. The compliance, contractility and capacity of the renal pelvis may therefore play an important role in determining the prognosis of kidney function and due to mechanical properties allow increasing urine volumes to be contained without a concomitant increase in pelvic pressure.[64]

References

1. Grignon A, Filion R, Filiatrault D et al. Urinary tract dilatation in utero: classification and clinical applications. Radiology 1986; 160: 645–7.

2. Koff SA, Peller PA, Young DC, Pollifrone DL. The assessment of obstruction in the newborn with unilateral hydronephrosis by measuring the size of the opposite kidney. J Urol 1994; 152: 596–9.

3. O'Reilly PH, Lawson RS, Shields RA, Testa HJ. Idiopathic hydronephrosis – the diuresis renogram: a new non-invasive method of assessing equivocal pelvioureteral junction obstruction. J Urol 1979; 121: 153–5.

4. Conway JJ, Maizels M. The 'well tempered' diuretic renogram: a standard method to examine the asymptomatic neonate with hydronephrosis or hydroureteronephrosis. A report from combined meetings of The Society for Fetal Urology and members of The Pediatric Nuclear Medicine Council – The Society of Nuclear Medicine [see comments]. J Nucl Med 1992; 33: 2047–51.

5. Conway JJ. 'Well-tempered' diuresis renography: its historical development, physiological and technical pitfalls, and standardized technique protocol. Semin Nucl Med 1992; 22: 74–84.

6. O'Reilly P, Aurell M, Britton K et al. Consensus on diuresis renography for investigating the dilated upper urinary tract. Radionuclides in Nephrourology Group. Consensus Committee on Diuresis Renography. J Nucl Med 1996; 37: 1872–6.

7. Gordon I, Colarinha P, Fettich J et al. Guidelines for standard and diuretic renography in children. Eur J Nucl Med 2001; 28: BP21–BP30.

8. Gordon I. Issues surrounding preparation, information and handling the child and parent in nuclear medicine. J Nucl Med 1998; 39: 490–4.

9. Rehling M. Measuring renal function. In: Peters M (ed). Nuclear Medicine in Radiological Diagnosis. London: Martin Dunitz, 2003: 163–179.

10. Eshima D, Taylor A Jr. Technetium-99m (99mTc) mercapto-acetyltriglycine: update on the new 99mTc renal tubular function agent. Semin Nucl Med 1992; 22: 61–73.

11. Gordon I, Colarinha P, Fettich J et al. Guidelines for standard and diuretic renography in children. Eur J Nucl Med 2001; 28: BP21–BP30.

12. Kabasakal L, Atay S, Vural VA et al. Evaluation of technetium-99m-ethylenedicysteine in renal disorders and determination of extraction ratio. J Nucl Med 1995; 36: 1398–403.

13. Prigent A, Cosgriff P, Gates GF et al. Consensus report on quality control of quantitative measurements of renal function obtained from the renogram: International Consensus Committee from the Scientific Committee of Radionuclides in Nephrourology. Semin Nucl Med 1999; 29: 146–59.

14. O'Reilly PH, Shields RA, Testa HJ. Renography. In: O'Reilly PH, Shields RA, Testa HJ (eds). Nuclear Medicine in Urology and Nephrology. London: Butterworths, 1986: 9–25.

15. Anderson PJ, Rangarajan V, Gordon I. Assessment of drainage in PUJ dilatation: pelvic excretion efficiency as an index of renal function. Nucl Med Commun 1997; 18: 823–6.

16. Piepsz A, Tondeur M, Ham H. NORA: a simple and reliable parameter for estimating renal output with or without frusemide challenge. Nucl Med Commun 2000; 21: 317–23.

17. Amarante J, Anderson PJ, Gordon I. Impaired drainage on diuretic renography using half-time or pelvic excretion efficiency is not a sign of obstruction in children with a prenatal diagnosis of unilateral renal pelvic dilatation. J Urol 2003; 169: 1828–31.

18. Kuyvenhoven JD, Ham HR, Piepsz A. Influence of renal function on renal output efficiency. J Nucl Med 2002; 43: 851–5.

19. Donoso G, Kuyvenhoven JD, Ham H, Piepsz A. 99mTc-MAG3 diuretic renography in children: a comparison between F0 and F+20. Nucl Med Commun 2003; 24: 1189–93.

20. Eskild-Jensen A, Gordon I, Piepsz A, Frokiaer J. Interpretation of the renogram: problems and pitfalls in hydronephrosis in children. BJU Int 2004; 94: 887–92.

21. Donoso G, Ham H, Tondeur M, Piepsz A. Influence of early furosemide injection on the split renal function. Nucl Med Commun 2003; 24: 791–5.

22. Piepsz A, Tondeur M, Ham H. Relative 99mTc-MAG3 renal uptake: reproducibility and accuracy. J Nucl Med 1999; 40: 972–6.

23. Lythgoe MF, Gordon I, Anderson PJ. Effect of renal maturation on the clearance of technetium-99m mercaptoacetyltriglycine. Eur J Nucl Med 1994; 21: 1333–7.

24. Kass EJ, Fink-Bennett D. Contemporary techniques for the radioisotopic evaluation of the dilated urinary tract. Urol Clin North Am 1990; 17: 273–89.

25. Gordon I. Diuretic renography in infants with prenatal unilateral hydronephrosis: an explanation for the controversy about poor drainage. BJU Int 2001; 87: 551–5.

26. Amarante J, Anderson PJ, Gordon I. Impaired drainage on diuretic renography using half-time or pelvic excretion efficiency is not a sign of obstruction in children with a prenatal diagnosis of unilateral renal pelvic dilatation. J Urol 2003; 169: 1828–31.

27. Jones DA, Lupton EW, George NJ. Effect of bladder filling on upper tract urodynamics in man. Br J Urol 1990; 65: 492–6.

28. Gordon I, Mialdea-Fernandez RM, Peters AM. Pelviureteric junction obstruction. The value of a post-micturition view in 99mTc DTPA diuretic renography. Br J Urol 1988; 61: 409–12.

29. Gordon I. Diuretic renography in infants with prenatal unilateral hydronephrosis: an explanation for the controversy about poor drainage. BJU Int 2001; 87: 551–5.

30. Koff SA. Problematic ureteropelvic junction obstruction. J Urol 1987; 138: 390.

31. Samuelson U, Granerus G, Bjures J et al. Renal function in idiopathic hydronephrosis in children. Follow-up after conservative and surgical treatment. Scand J Urol Nephrol 1984; 18: 135–41.

32. Koff SA, Campbell K. Nonoperative management of unilateral neonatal hydronephrosis. J Urol 1992; 148: 525–31.

33. Koff SA, Campbell KD. The nonoperative management of unilateral neonatal hydronephrosis: natural history of poorly functioning kidneys. J Urol 1994; 152: 593–5.

34. Peters CA. Urinary tract obstruction in children. J Urol 1995; 154: 1874–83.

35. Helin I, Persson PH. Prenatal diagnosis of urinary tract abnormalities by ultrasound. Pediatrics 1986; 78: 879–83.

36. Feldman DM, DeCambre M, Kong E et al. Evaluation and follow-up of fetal hydronephrosis. J Ultrasound Med 2001; 20: 1065–9.

37. Eskild-Jensen A, Gordon I, Piepsz A, Frokiaer J. Congenital unilateral hydronephonephrosis: A review of the impact of diuretic renography on clinical treatment. J Urol 2005; 173: 147–6.

38. Ulman I, Jayanthi VR, Koff SA. The long-term followup of newborns with severe unilateral hydronephrosis initially treated nonoperatively. J Urol 2000; 164: 1101–5.

39. Calisti A, Perrotta ML, Oriolo L et al. Functional outcome after pyeloplasty in children: impact of the cause of obstruction and of the mode of presentation. Eur Urol 2003; 43: 706–10.

40. Gordon I, Dhillon HK, Gatanash H, Peters AM. Antenatal diagnosis of pelvic hydronephrosis: assessment of renal function and drainage as a guide to management. J Nucl Med 1991; 32: 1649–54.

41. Subramaniam R, Kouriefs C, Dickson AP. Antenatally detected pelvi-ureteric junction obstruction: concerns about conservative management. BJU Int 1999; 84: 335–8.

42. Dhillon HK. Prenatally diagnosed hydronephrosis: the Great Ormond Street experience. Br J Urol 1998; 81: 39–44.

43. Zaccara A, Marchetti P, la SE et al. Are preoperative parameters of unilateral pyelo-ureteric junction obstruction in children predictive of postoperative function improvement? Scand J Urol Nephrol 2000; 34: 165–8.

44. Freedman ER, Rickwood AM. Prenatally diagnosed pelvi-ureteric junction obstruction: a benign condition? J Pediatr Surg 1994; 29: 769–72.

45. Palmer LS, Maizels M, Cartwright PC et al. Surgery versus observation for managing obstructive grade 3 to 4 unilateral hydronephrosis: a report from the Society for Fetal Urology. J Urol 1998; 159: 222–8.

46. Takla NV, Hamilton BD, Cartwright PC, Snow BW. Apparent unilateral ureteropelvic junction obstruction in the newborn: expectations for resolution. J Urol 1998; 160: 2175–8.

47. Kuyvenhoven JD, Ham HR, Piepsz A. Re: Impaired drainage on diuretic renography using half-time or pelvic excretion efficiency is not a sign of obstruction in children with a prenatal diagnosis of unilateral renal pelvic dilatation. J Urol 2004; 171: 806.

48. Ransley PG, Dhillon HK, Gordon I et al. The postnatal management of hydronephrosis diagnosed by prenatal ultrasound. J Urol 1990; 144: 584–7.

49. Salem YH, Majd M, Rushton HG, Belman AB. Outcome analysis of pediatric pyeloplasty as a function of patient age, presentation and differential renal function. J Urol 1995; 154: 1889–93.

50. Chung S, Majd M, Rushton HG, Belman AB. Diuretic renography in the evaluation of neonatal hydronephrosis: is it reliable? J Urol 1993; 150: 765–8.

51. Piepsz A, Kuyvenhoven JD, Tondeur M, Ham H. Normalized residual activity: usual values and robustness of the method. J Nucl Med 2002; 43: 33–8.

52. Pohl HG, Rushton HG, Park JS et al. Early diuresis renogram findings predict success following pyeloplasty. J Urol 2001; 165: 2311–15.

53. Chertin B, Fridmans A, Knizhnik M et al. Does early detection of ureteropelvic junction obstruction improve surgical outcome in terms of renal function? J Urol 1999; 162: 1037–40.

54. Nelson CP, Park JM, Dunn RL, Wei JT. Contemporary trends in surgical correction of pediatric ureteropelvic junction obstruction: Data from the Nationwide Inpatient Sample. J Urol 2005; 173: 232–6.

55. Eskild-Jensen A, Munch JT, Olsen LH et al. Renal function may not be restored when using decreasing differential function as the criterion for surgery in unilateral hydronephrosis. BJU Int 2003; 92: 779–82.

56. Dhillon HK. Imaging and follow up of neonatal hydronephrosis. Curr Op Urol 1995; 5: 75–8.

57. Fernbach SK, Maizels M, Conway JJ. Ultrasound grading of hydronephrosis: introduction to the system used by the Society for Fetal Urology. Pediatr Radiol 1993; 23: 478–80.

58. Thorup J, Jokela R, Cortes D, Nielsen OH. The results of 15 years of consistent strategy in treating antenatally suspected pelvi-ureteric junction obstruction. BJU Int 2003; 91: 850–2.

59. Hafez AT, McLorie G, Bagli D, Khoury A. Analysis of trends on serial ultrasound for high grade neonatal hydronephrosis. J Urol 2002; 168: 1518–21.

60. Barker AP, Cave MM, Thomas DF et al. Fetal pelvi-ureteric

junction obstruction: predictors of outcome. Br J Urol 1995; 76: 649–52.

61. Chevalier RL, Peters CA. Congenital urinary tract obstruction: Proceedings of the State-Of-The-Art Strategic Planning Workshop – National Institutes of Health, Bethesda, Maryland, USA, 11–12 March 2002. Pediatr Nephrol 2003; 18: 576–606.

62. Wen JG, Frokiaer J, Jorgensen TM, Djurhuus JC. Obstructive nephropathy: an update of the experimental research. Urol Res 1999; 27: 29–39.

63. Chevalier RL. Biomarkers of congenital obstructive nephropathy: past, present and future. J Urol 2004; 172: 852–7.

64. Koff SA. The beneficial and protective effects of hydronephrosis. APMIS Suppl 2003; 109: 7–12.

65. Eskild-Jensen A, Christensen H, Lindvig M et al. Renal functional outcome in unilateral hydronephrosis in newborn pigs. J Urol 2000; 163: 1896–900.

66. Eskild-Jensen A, Jacobsen L, Christensen H et al. Renal function outcome in unilateral hydronephrosis in newborn pigs. II. Function and volume of contralateral kidneys. J Urol 2001; 165: 205–9.

67. Homsy YL, Tripp BM, Lambert R et al. The captopril renogram: a new tool for diagnosing and predicting obstruction in childhood hydronephrosis. J Urol 1998; 160: 1446–9.

13 The point of view of the urologist

Stephen A Koff

Introduction

With refinement in ultrasound technology over the past 15 years, a near epidemic of hydronephrosis identified antenatally has created an unparalleled management dilemma for paediatric urologists. At issue is the concept, still extant despite natural history studies to the contrary,[1-3] that hydronephrosis is a pathological process, caused by a partial obstruction that was present in utero and is possibly still present after birth, that damages the kidney or reduces its functional potential. Although not well appreciated among paediatric urologists, a direct challenge to this concept was clearly posed by studies[4-12] on the physiology of partial obstruction-induced hydronephrosis and on the physical attributes and behaviour of the partially obstructed renal pelvis. When these are reviewed with a contemporary eye towards hydronephrosis in the newborn, they point to exactly the opposite conclusion: hydronephrosis is not a pathological process but actually a compensating physiologic mechanism by which the renal pelvis protects the kidney from high pressures and renal damage. In fact, hydronephrosis, especially when it involves the already stretchy and distensible pelvis of the infant appears to not only be uniquely beneficial but to paradoxically mislead the unwary in to misdiagnosing obstruction. Herein we present a counterargument which by describing the physiological bases of these beneficial and protective effects of hydronephrosis has important implications for a more contemporary clinical management of this challenging group of patients.

Chronic partial upper urinary tract obstruction (CPUUTO)

CPUUTO is a common form of problematic renal obstruction in young children and is of great clinical concern because it is often difficult to diagnose, especially in infancy, and untreated may progressively damage the kidney. It must be distinguished from total obstruction which causes little diagnostic confusion because it is rapidly injurious and often destroys the kidney prior to birth. Although hydronephrosis is an easy to recognize consequence of partial obstruction, its diagnostic specificity is limited because it may be the consequence of many nonobstructive conditions, such as reflux. Uniquely, CPUUTO is an extremely difficult form of obstruction to characterize physiologically, because the parameters which usually define obstruction in other organ systems are not valid in its diagnosis.[12]

Renal pelvic pressure is usually normal. If it were not normal then the diagnosis of chronic partial obstruction would be very easy. One would simply place a needle in the renal pelvis and note the elevated pressure. Whitaker's test would never have needed to be invented or performed.

Renal pelvic volume increases in CPUUTO but seemingly puzzling often stabilizes and does not enlarge further.

The outflow rate across the UPJ is normal in chronic partial obstruction and is almost always the same as the inflow rate. Were it less, even if it was reduced by only a small amount, the renal pelvis would expand rapidly by this differential rate, and would overdistend rapidly.

In the face of all these normal measurements, the mechanism for hydronephrosis appears to be genuinely puzzling and one must ponder the seemingly simplistic question. If pelvic pressure is normal in CPUUTO, why doesn't the renal pelvis just shrink to a smaller volume?

The pathophysiology of chronic partial upper urinary tract obstruction

The answer to this query requires an understanding of the physiology of CPUUTO and the nature of equilibrium in hydronephrosis which is best accomplished by observing the behaviour of a partially obstructed kidney in an animal model. When an incompletely occluding ligature was placed just below the UPJ in dogs,[7,8] pelvic volume was observed to increase initially in all (Figure 13.1) but thereafter some pelves reached an equilibrium and enlarged no further while others decreased in volume (Figure 13.2). The elevated pressures in the renal pelvis seen immediately after creation of obstruction decreased progressively over time to normalize after several

Figure 13.1 Pelvic volume changes occurring *early* after partial upper ureteral ligation (after Koff[7]).

Figure 13.3 Normalization of pelvic pressures in chronic partial upper ureteral obstruction.

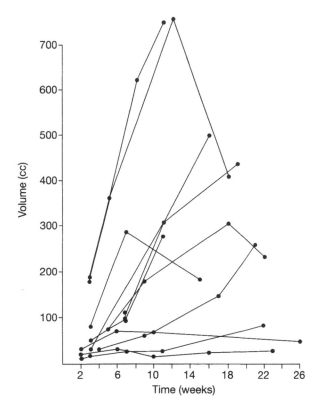

Figure 13.2 Pelvic volume changes occurring *late* after partial upper ureteral ligation.

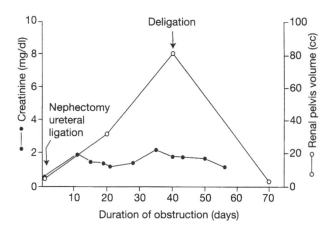

Figure 13.4 Changes in renal function and renal pelvis volume after partial upper ureteral ligation and contralateral nephrectomy.

weeks (Figure 13.3). The protective effect of hydronephrosis can begin to be seen in a one-kidney canine model in which nephrectomy and creation of contralateral partial obstruction occurred simultaneously, when changes in renal function, measured by serum creatinine (a reasonably accurate reflec-

tion of solitary kidney function in a one-kidney model) and pelvic volume were observed over time (Figure 13.4). Creatinine remained fairly stable despite a partial UPJ obstruction which is significant enough to cause progressive hydronephrosis exceeding 80 ml (normal = <3 cc). After release of obstruction although pelvic volume returns towards normal, renal function remains unaffected. It appears as if the hydronephrosis has in some way protected the renal parenchyma from functional deterioration even in the presence of a significant partial UPJ obstruction. However, not all kidneys subjected to the same degree of partial UPJ obstruction will be so lucky. In some cases even a large hydronephrosis will be unable to protect some kidneys from progressive renal functional deterioration (Figure 13.5).

Figure 13.6 Pressure–volume relationships obtained by pelvimetric study of a kidney at two stages of hydronephrotic dilation (after Koff[7]).

Figure 13.5 Variable effect of hydronephrosis on renal function in six dogs undergoing partial upper ureteral obstruction and contralateral heminephrectomy.

These observations suggest that hydronephrosis induced by partial UPJ obstruction permits the same degree of obstruction to cause progressive dilation of the pelvis and renal impairment of renal function at low pelvic volumes but not at high pelvic volumes. How the partially obstructed hydronephrotic kidney exerts these beneficial and protective effects requires further analysis.

Determinants of progression and equilibrium in hydronephrosis

Once a partial obstruction is created the factors which determine whether the dilation will progress or equilibrate are multiple and interrelated. They include the mass and health of the renal parenchyma, volume of urine produced, physical properties of the renal pelvis and, of course, the actual tightness of obstruction which influences urinary outflow. Of these, the behaviour and physical properties of the renal pelvis, its compliance, contractility and capacity have received scant attention, perhaps because their significance is not intuitively obvious, yet they may well be the most important factors in determining the fate of the partially obstructed kidney.

The physical properties of the renal pelvis have been assessed experimentally by pelvimetric examination which defines pelvic pressure–volume relationships during filling.[9,10,12] This test is similar to a cystometric examination and involves filling the renal pelvis with fluid at a constant rate

while monitoring changes in pelvic pressure during temporary occlusion of the UPJ. Typical pelvimetric curves have characteristic shape and are similar to cystometric curves (Figure 13.6). They are comprised of a slowly rising low-pressure filling or accommodation phase during which the pelvic smooth muscle relaxes and accommodates to increasing volume. This is followed by a more rapidly rising overdistension phase during which the smooth muscle exceeds its relaxation potential, is overstretched and reflects elastic and connective (viscoelastic) tissue stretching within the pelvis wall. The transition point between these two phases defines the physiological capacity volume (VC) of the renal pelvis and this inflection point is usually easily identified. Below this capacity volume (VC), pressures are generally within the normal range and do not exceed 20 cm water. Above VC, pressures rise rapidly to exceed normal and quickly reach levels that are potentially damaging to the kidney. The slope of the overdistension phase may be measured as dP/dV (Figure 13.6).

The pressure–volume relationships of progressive hydronephrosis in the partially obstructed kidney have been studied and characterized experimentally and clinically[9,10,12] by initially creating a partially obstructing ligature around the upper ureter, and then performing serially pelvimetric studies during progression and resolution of hydronephrosis. Study of many normal, obstructed hydronephrotic kidneys as well as hydronephrotic kidneys after release of obstruction revealed a very similar shaped pelvimetric curve with the inflection point defining capacity volume, VC, easily recognizable (Figure 13.6).

As hydronephrosis progresses and the renal pelvis enlarges the serial curves evolve and reflect two distinct events that are simultaneously occurring. As the pelvis enlarges, the slope of the overdistension curve decreases, and the capacity volume, VC, increases. Together, these two factors determine to a great extent the behaviour and prognosis of the partially obstructed hydronephrotic kidney. As hydronephrosis progresses, the larger pelvis will have a greater capacity reservoir volume, VC , which functions increasingly as a volume

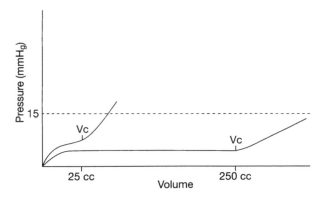

Figure 13.7 Pelvimetric changes during progressive hydronephrosis demonstrate an increase in pelvis capacity, VC, and a decrease in the slope of the overdistension portion of the curve.

buffer to protect the pelvis from overdistension. Likewise, a lower slope to the overdistension curve, implies that pressure in the pelvis will rise more slowly once volume expands, overstretches, as the capacity of the pelvis (VC) is exceeded. Depending on the rate and extent of volume expansion, these factors may delay, mitigate or even prevent altogether the development of pressure-induced renal parenchyma damage (Figure 13.7).

The clinical implications of these physiological phenomena are significant. They explain how pressures rise faster and reach higher levels in kidneys with small renal pelves than large pelves. This is the reason that kidneys with small or confined intrarenal pelves are more vulnerable to obstruction than kidneys with large pelves. Also explained is why the presence of infection in the obstructed hydronephrotic kidney magnifies renal injury by causing the pelvis to thicken, lose its compliance and elasticity and develop higher pressures more rapidly. They also provide insights into the mechanisms which allow the renal pelvis to maintain a state of hydronephrotic dilation despite normal pressures and allow it to reach a state of equilibration despite persisting partial obstruction.

Why doesn't the partially obstructed hydronephrotic kidney shrink to a more normal pelvic size when pelvic pressure is normal?

The answer to this seemingly simple question provides a key to understanding the pathophysiology of progressive hydronephrosis in partial UPJ obstruction. Intermittent diure-

sis is a driving force for progression of hydronephrosis and two physical properties of the renal pelvis determine its fate. These are: (1) hysteresis, a mechanical property by which the force needed to create a deformation is always greater than the force needed to maintain that deformation, and (2) stress relaxation, an attribute of the pelvic wall which enables it to slowly enlarge or creep under stress, rather than to tear or disrupt.

It is important to recognize in chronic partial obstruction that the hydronephrotic renal pelvis is rarely overdistended. Pelvic volumes vary and depend on the state of hydration and urine production. The instigating event in progressive hydronephrosis appears to be an imbalance between urine production into the pelvis and urine outflow from the pelvis. With extrinsic obstructions, the imbalance is caused by an aberrant vessel or band or kinking which reduces the lumen of the UPJ and causes fluid accumulation. In contrast, for intrinsic UPJ obstructions which fix the luminal calibre of the UPJ and do not allow it to dilate, imbalance occurs during diuresis. In either case, the consequence of urine imbalance is pelvic volume expansion. As the pelvis enlarges, its pressure is determined by the particular pelvimetric relationship that exists at that point in time. During volume expansion, pathological pressures generally do not develop and are not sustained as long as the pelvic smooth muscle relaxes sufficiently to accommodate to the increased volume. However, beyond a point, continued pelvic volume expansion will overstretch the pelvis and lead to progression of hydronephrosis.[4-6]

Physiologically, the overstretched pelvis will develop pathologically high pressures which will negatively affect renal function. The most obvious functional change will be a decrease in urine production which may cease if pressures get too high. Once urine production decreases or stops, the pelvis will stop enlarging and will eventually begin to decrease in size as urine flows out across the UPJ and through alternative lymphatic and tubular backflow channels. However, if the overdistension has altered the integrity of the pelvic wall, then progression of hydronephrosis will result, because once the pelvis enlarges beyond its accommodative limits the viscoelastic tissues stretch under stress and are deformed to a new maximum volume. This will reset the pressure–volume relationships within the pelvis and will shift the pelvimetric curve to the right (Figure 13.8). The consequence of this will be that at any pelvic volume the pressure within the pelvis will be slightly less than before. In addition, the pelvis will now also have a slightly larger maximum capacity volume, VC. This reflects hysteresis because while it took excessive pressure (force) to overstretch and enlarge the pelvis, it now takes less pressure (force) to maintain the enlarged pelvis in its new slightly overstretched state. The new pelvimetric curve relationships become operative immediately and they determine the pressure that exists at each and every increment of smaller pelvic volume (Figure 13.8). The answer to the above query becomes apparent: the pelvis does not shrink to a normal size when pressures are normal because *pressure*

Figure 13.8 Mechanism for progressive hydronephrosis in partial obstruction. Pelvic overdistension shifts pressure–volume relationships to a new pelvimetric curve which remain fixed until a new episode of overdistension occurs (after Koff).

does not determine volume within the renal pelvis. Rather, *pressure is determined by volume* in the pelvis according to the pressure volume pelvimetric relationship in the pelvis; pressure at each increment of volume reflects the smooth muscle and viscoelastic properties of the pelvis wall.

Figure 13.8 reveals the pressure–volume relationships in an expanding partially obstructed hydronephrotic kidney and it displays a series of pelvimetric curves. Each curve reflects a pressure–volume relationship that remains constant until the next episode of pelvic overdistension. In essence, the process of hydronephrotic expansion in partial obstruction involves a series of small episodes of renal pelvic overdistension. Not all diuretic or obstructive episodes will be of sufficient duration or degree to produce overdistension, but when overstretching does occur it will shift the pelvimetric curve to the right and cause progression of hydronephrosis.

Despite the pathophysiology required to create progressive hydronephrosis, hydronephrosis per se should not be viewed as pathological or harmful. It is actually protective, and its salutary effects are seen when the pelvimetric curve is examined more carefully. Figure 13.3 illustrates that partial obstruction initially causes high and potentially damaging pelvic pressures. But, with increasing hydronephrosis, the maximum pressures within the partially obstructed (canine) kidney decrease toward normal and after about 6–10 weeks remain within the normal range. This is because the enlarged renal pelvis now has a larger maximum capacity and can take in significantly more urine volume before pelvic overdistension occurs. In addition, the rate at which pressures rise within the pelvis is less than before because the slope of the overdistension curve has decreased. This implies that a longer period of imbalance between inflow and outflow will be tolerated before the pelvis exceeds its accommodative limit and before pressures reach pathological levels; theoretically, if the pelvis enlarges sufficiently, pressures may never become pathologically high.

Taken together, the biological changes occurring in the hydronephrotic renal pelvis enable it to become large enough to reduce the likelihood for pelvic overdistension but should overdistension occur they blunt the pelvic pressure rise to keep it from reaching damaging levels. As a result when the pelvis is extremely compliant and stretchy as exists in the newborn, hydronephrosis actually may prevent a partial urinary obstruction from causing progressive hydronephrosis and renal damage by inducing a state of equilibrium between outflow restriction, urine production and pelvic reservoir capacity. This truly is a beneficial and protective effect, an effect that paediatric urologists who almost daily face the clinical management dilemma of hydronephrosis in the newborn must recognize keenly.

Clinical issues relating to hydronephrosis in infancy

In the newborn, the relationship between hydronephrosis and obstruction is as complex and enigmatic as is the aetiology of the pelvic dilation and future potential of the dilated kidney. Prior to birth the hydronephrotic kidney may have never been obstructed, its dilation simply related to transient reflux or embryologic malformation, or the kidney may be or no longer be obstructed, or it may become obstructed in the future. Unfortunately, based on 15 years of studies on methods for assessing obstruction in infant hydronephrosis it is now apparent that no extant diagnostic test can diagnose obstruction in this age group, clarify the past history of the kidney, determine whether the kidney is, is not has ever been or will be affected by CUUTPO or predict the fate of the newborn kidney, its response to dilation or its ultimate renal function. At this time of the century the questions, will the hydronephrosis progress, resolve or remain unchanged or will it hurt the kidney remain unanswerable by blood, radiographic or nuclear medicine studies. Faced with these clinical, pathologic and diagnostic dilemmas and a newly recognized near epidemic of ultrasonographically detected hydronephrosis (1 in 500 births), nearly two decades ago it is not surprising that paediatric urologists developed clinical management protocols to try to determine if the dilated kidney was obstructed and to more deliberately approach the problem of managing the infant with hydronephrosis.[1–3,13–19] These protocols were predicated on the concept that since it was not possible to either define or measure obstruction accurately in this age group it was illogical to recommend surgical intervention in the very young child to treat suspicious, but not clearly proven, obstructions. The protocols delayed surgery until sequential testing with ultrasonography, to assess changing degrees of hydronephrosis, and diuretic renography, to measure changes in differential function and isotope washout kinetics, clarified the kidney's response to hydronephrosis. The outcomes of these studies indicated surprisingly that in most cases, 75–80%, hydronephrosis was rather benign and with time spontaneously improved or resolved completely without adversely affecting renal function. The results validated an initial nonoperative approach, demonstrated the feasibility of using serial US and DR testing to determine whether the hydronephrosis and renal function was improving or deteriorating and thereby provide a means for assessing obstruction in newborn hydronephrosis. The protocols ultimately changed the management of this condition. However, in addition to revealing that the initial size of the renal pelvis and the initial level of differential function were unable to accurately determine the presence of obstruction in a given kidney or predict the potential for progression or resolution of hydronephrosis or renal injury, a few studies also demonstrated quite surprisingly that the washout pattern or $T^1/_2$ time on DR was particularly inaccurate in defining obstruction since 40–50% of severely hydronephrotic kidneys, ones whose hydronephrosis improved or resolved spontaneously, had $T^1/_2$ times longer than 20–30 minutes and washout patterns that were clearly in an obstructed range.[3,20,21]

Since DR remains a popular and widely accepted method for assessing obstruction in older patients with hydronephrosis, the nature of this diagnostic fallibility observed in infants required further analysis. In DR, the diagnosis of obstruction has traditionally been based on the rate with which tracer leaves the renal pelvis following diuretic injection. This is reflected in the slope of the drainage curve and often reported as $T^1/_2$ time, the time required for 50% of the isotope to leave the pelvis. It is generally viewed as an accurate reflection of the patency of the UPJ with rapid drainage (low $T^1/_2$ time) indicating no obstruction while impaired drainage, slow or no washout ($T^1/_2$ time > 20 minutes), indicating obstruction. Provided that the testing protocol is standardized and that the conduct and interpretation of the examination follow commonly accepted criteria,[22] DR has been regarded to be an accurate tool for assessing hydronephrosis and suspected obstruction in older children and adults.

The same degree of accuracy probably does not exist in very young children when DR is performed and interpreted using these same protocols and criteria. Technical and physiological error potentials have been well described[22-31] to explain inaccuracy to some degree and these are now well known to nuclear medicine physicians. But there also exist uniquely age-related anatomic variables which have not been well appreciated that can undermine and seriously compromise test accuracy. We have recently shown that the anatomy of the hydronephrotic renal pelvis is so different in very young compared to older children with respect to its ability to expand during diuresis that it can produce excessive dilution of isotope and failure of isotope washout from the renal pelvis.[32] Isotope dilution actually occurs twice during DR. Initially at the time of tracer injection, tracer-free urine already present within the renal pelvis dilutes the concentration of tracer in urine entering the pelvis. The larger the amount of tracer-free urine in the renal pelvis the greater will be the degree of tracer dilution. Dilution occurs again after administration of the diuretic agent, which in most DR proto-

cols is injected typically well after the tracer has been cleared from the blood pool and renal parenchyma. When this diuretic-induced tracer-free urine enters the pelvis it further reduces the concentration of isotope already within the pelvis. As a result of dilution and directly proportional to the size of the hydronephrotic renal pelvis, each cc of urine leaving the renal pelvis will contain progressively less tracer. Consequently, the rate with which tracer washes out from a kidney with a large pelvis will be slower and the $T^1/_2$ time longer than the rate for a kidney with a small pelvis. In addition to this volume effect which hydronephrosis at any age exerts on the behaviour of tracer during diuresis, we noted marked distensibility of the renal pelves in young children during diuresis. By actually measuring with pelvic volume by US during DR, this unique distensibility was observed and served to magnify the effects of dilution and to contribute further to DR inaccuracy. We found that in hydronephrotic kidneys ultimately proven to be nonobstructed, diuresis caused an increase in pelvic volume that averaged 88% and often exceeded by 100% the pre-diuretic hydronephrotic pelvic size. This effect was observed to occur primarily in children under 2 years of age with the greatest potential for volume expansion occurring in the youngest patients. This near doubling of pelvis volume during diuresis, when tracer-free urine is entering the renal pelvis, means that urine containing tracer is accumulating within the pelvis rather than leaving it and this is reflected in a prolonged $T^1/_2$ time. Since urinary tracer concentration is decreased by nearly half it now takes twice as long to empty the large renal pelvis of tracer. Were the urinary outflow rate from the pelvis not to increase at all in response to diuresis it would actually take twice as long to carry tracer out of the pelvis and the $T^1/_2$ time would truly double. In older patients this dilution-induced pelvic enlargement may in fact be mitigated by faster pelvic emptying which accompanies faster inflow during diuresis. However, this does not appear to be the case in very young children whose unique degree of pelvic enlargement during diuresis indicates that these compensating mechanisms are not sufficient to prevent pelvic expansion and that even in the absence of obstruction, urine must be entering the renal pelvis at a rate much faster than it leaves the pelvis. The net effect is one of marked delay in tracer outflow with a prolongation of $T^1/_2$ time. This high compliance anatomic feature of the infant renal pelvis, by allowing the already large pelvis to serve as a ready reservoir for additional volume expansion thus serves to magnify the effect of diuresis on tracer dilution and to compromise the accuracy of DR.

Summary

Hydronephrosis has generally been considered a pathological process, and especially in infancy is widely viewed as caused by obstruction, potentially injurious to the kidney and in need of expeditious surgical treatment. However, a number of clinical and experimental studies suggest exactly the opposite: that hydronephrosis is not pathological but actually a compensating mechanism designed to protect the kidney from high pressures and renal damage. Furthermore, because hydronephrosis in the infant involves an already compliant and distensible renal pelvis its kidney appears to be uniquely protected. In providing the basis for a counter-argument which challenges the pathologic nature of hydronephrosis, these studies also serve as the foundation for evolving clinical management protocols which recognize the limitations and inaccuracies of trying to use adult-based diagnostic tests including DR washout to diagnose obstruction in infants with hydronephrosis. Successful management protocols provide close monitoring of serial changes in pelvic size and differential renal function to identify progressive hydronephrosis or deteriorating differential renal function, to treat correct obstruction with immediate surgery if it occurs, and to reassuringly observe that approximately 80% of patients with affected kidneys managed in this fashion will have their hydronephrosis improve spontaneously or resolve completely without renal impairment.

References

1. Ransley PG, Dhillon HK, Gordon I et al. The postnatal management of hydronephrosis diagnosed by prenatal ultrasound. J Urol 1990; 144: 584.
2. Dhillon HK. Prenatally diagnosed hydronephrosis: The Great Ormand Street experience. Br J Urol 1998; 81: 39.
3. Ulman I, Jayanthi VR, Koff SA. The long-term followup of newborns with severe unilateral hydronephrosis initially treated nonoperatively. J Urol 2000; 164: 1101–5.
4. Djurhuus JC. Dynamics of upper urinary tract. III. The activity of renal pelvis during pressure variations. Invest Urol 1977; 14: 475.
5. Djurhuus JC, Nerstrom B, Gyrd-Hansen N, Rask-Andersen H. Experimental hydronephrosis. Acta Chir Scand 1976; 472: 17.
6. Djurhuus JC, Stage P. Percutaneous and intrapelvic pressure registrations in hydronephrosis during diuresis. Acta Chir Scand 1976; 47: 43.
7. Koff SA. Diagnosis of obstruction in experimental hydroureteronephrosis: mechanisms for progressive urinary tract dilation. Invest Urol 1981; 19: 85–8.
8. Koff SA. Determinants of progression and equilibrium in hydronephrosis. Urology 1983; 21: 496–500.
9. Koff SA. Pressure volume relationships in human hydronephrosis. Urology 1985; 25: 256.
10. Koff SA, Hayden LJ, Cirulli C, Shore R. Pathophysiology of ureteropelvic junction obstruction: experimental and clinical observations. J Urol 1986; 136: 336–8.
11. Koff SA. Editorial: Problematic ureteropelvic junction obstruction. J Urol 1987; 138: 390.
12. Koff SA. Pathophysiology of ureteropelvic junction obstruction. Clinical and experimental observations. Urol Clin North Am 1990; 17: 263–72.
13. Chung YK, Chang PY, Lin CJ et al. Conservative treatment of neonatal hydronephrosis. J Formosan Med Assoc 1992; 91: 75–80.
14. Koff SA, Campbell K. Nonoperative management of unilateral neonatal hydronephrosis. J Urol Aug 1992; 148: 525–31.
15. Freedman ER, Rickwood AMK. Prenatally diagnosed pelvi-ureteric junction obstruction: a benign condition? J Ped Surg 1994; 29: 769–72.
16. Nonomura K, Yamashita T, Kanagawa K et al. Management and outcome of antenatally diagnosed hydronephrosis. Int J Urol J 1994; 1: 121–8.
17. Blachar A, Blachar Y, Livne PM et al. Clinical outcome and follow-up of prenatal hydronephrosis. Pediatr Nephrol 1994; 8: 30–5.
18. Koff SA, Campbell KD. The nonoperative management of unilateral neonatal hydronephrosis: natural history of poorly functioning kidneys. J Urol 1994; 152: 593–5.
19. Josephson S, Dhillon HK, Ransley PG. Post-natal management of antenatally detected, bilateral hydronephrosis. Urol Int 1993; 51: 79–84.
20. Gordon I. Diuretic renography in infants with prenatal unilateral hydronephrosis: an explanation for the controversy about poor drainage. BJU Int'l 2001; 87: 551–5.
21. Amarante J, Anderson PJ, Gordon I. Impaired drainage on diuretic renography using half-time or pelvic excretion efficiency is not a sign of obstruction in children with a prenatal diagnosis of unilateral renal pelvic dilatation. J Urol 2003; 169: 1828–31.
22. Conway JL. 'Well-tempered' diuresis renography: its historical development, physiological and technical pitfalls, and standardized technique protocol. Sem Nucl Med 1992; 22: 74–84.
23. Gungor F, Anderson P, Gordon I. Effect of the size of regions of interest on the estimation of differential renal function in children with congenital hydronephrosis. Nucl Med Commun 2002; 23: 147–51.
24. Connolly LP, Zurakowski D, Peters CA et al. Variability of diuresis renography interpretation due to method of post-diuretic renal pelvic clearance half-time determination. J Urol 2000; 164: 467–71.
25. Wong DC, Rossleigh MA, Farnsworth RH. Diuretic renography with the addition of quantitative gravity-assisted drainage in infants and children. J Nucl Med 2000; 41: 1030–6.
26. Saunders CAB, Choong KKL, Larcos G et al. Assessment of pediatric hydronephrosis using output efficiency. J Nucl Med 1997; 38: 1483–6.
27. Gordon I. Assessment of pediatric hydronephrosis using output efficiency. J Nucl Med 1997; 38: 1487–9.
28. Anderson PJ, Rangarajan V, Gordon I. Assessment of drainage in PUJ dilatation: pelvic excretion efficiency as an index of renal function. Nucl Med Commun 1997; 18: 823–6.
29. Piepsz A, Ham H. Factors influencing the accuracy of renal output efficiency. Nucl Med Commun 2000; 21: 1009–13.
30. Piepsz A, Tondeur M, Ham H. NORA: a simple and reliable

parameter for estimating renal output with or without frusemide challenge. Nucl Med Commun 2000; 21: 317–23.

31. Kuyvenhoven JD, Ham HR, Piepsz A. Optimal time window for measurement of renal output parameters. Nucl Med Rev Cent East Eur 2002; 5: 105–8.

32. Koff SA, Binkovitz I, Coley B, Jayanthi VR. Renal pelvis size during diuresis in children with hydronephrosis: implications for diagnosing obstruction with diuretic renography. J Urology 2005; 174: 303–7.

Renovascular disease

14 Present and future developments of functional and molecular imaging

M Donald Blaufox

This chapter on renovascular hypertension represents an effort to bring together the wide variety of imaging approaches that have been used in studying hypertension and the kidney. The original study that demonstrated a definite relation between the kidney and the regulation of blood pressure was reported in 1898 by Tigerstead and Bergman[1] (see Table 14.1) when they demonstrated that an extract of the kidney injected into experimental animals would cause an elevation of the blood pressure. The substance was named renin because of its origin. A wide variety of experiments were conducted during the following years in an effort to clearly establish that manipulation of the kidney could cause high blood pressure. These studies included partial nephrectomy, infection of the kidney and wrapping the kidney in cellophane among others.[2] The first investigator to show that changes in renal blood flow could affect the blood pressure was Harry Goldblatt, who reported his findings in 1934.[3] Subsequently, the first human case in which it was demonstrated that nephrectomy resulted in a return of blood pressure to normal was published in 1938 by Leadbetter.[4]

Table 14.1 A simplified chronology of developments in renovascular hypertension up to the introduction of the rapid sequence IVP. Although the major developments are shown here, many hundreds of reports appeared in the literature during that time.

Tigerstedt and Bergman	1898
Goldblatt	1934
First human case (Leadbetter)	1938
Howard Test	1954
IVP	1954
Renogram	1956
Rapid sequence IVP	1964

This firmly established a renovascular origin of hypertension in some patients. Following these various observations, the problem arose as to how best to determine which patients with hypertension have renovascular hypertension as their causality and how to cure them.

Table 14.2 This study from London[10] shows the changes that occur in the various physiological parameters in patients with a stenotic kidney causing renovascular hypertension as compared to the contralateral kidney and patients with essential hypertension. These data are obtained by bilateral ureteral catheterization. The difficulty and risk associated with the procedure led to its abandonment as a diagnostic test for renovascular hypertension.

	Essential hypertension		Renovascular hypertension	
	Right kidney (I)	Left kidney (II)	Stenotic kidney (III)	Contralateral kidney (IV)
Cin (ml/min/m^2)	35.2 ± 13.5	33.6 ± 11.6	22.9 ± 9.3*	47.6 ± 12.6‡
CPAH (ml/min/m^2)	160.3 ± 56.9	158.7 ± 45	91.5 ± 47.8*	194.1 ± 63.8‡
EPAH (%)	81.1 ± 10.3	81.4 ± 9.7	84.7 ± 9.7	83.5 ± 11.3
FF (%)	21.8 ± 5.3	21.5 ± 5.0	25.7 ± 7.6†	25.6 ± 6.2†
UV (μl/min)	884 ± 594	836 ± 492	465 ± 372*	1327 ± 692
UNA V (μmol/min)	38.4 ± 24.0	36.7 ± 31	25.1 ± 28.5	77 ± 74‡
UcrR/UcrL	1.08 ± 0.18		2.94 ± 1.7	
PRAR/PRAL	0.90 ± 0.35		2.89 ± 1	
Kidney size (cm)	12.8 ± 0.9	13.0 ± 0.9	10.2 ± 1.6*	13.4 ± 1.3

Values are means ± SD

Abbreviations: UCRR, creatinine concentration in the right or left kidney (or stenotic and contralateral); PRA, plasma renin activity ratio between right or left (or stenotic and contralateral) kidney.

*P<0.001 III v I; II, IV; †P<0.01 III and IV v I and II; ‡P<0.001 IV v I-III; P<0.001 essential AHI v RAM.

Table 14.3 This table from Havey[7] compiles some major studies in patients with suspected renovascular hypertension utilizing radioiosotope renography. The average sensitivity and specificity are not sufficient for a disease of such low prevalence.

Study	Year	Patients with RAS*	Patients without RAS	Sensitivity of renogram (%)	Specificity of renogram (%)
Maxwell et al[3]	1964	42	–	69	–
Burbank et al[10]	1963	37	17	97	82.3
Luke et al[16]	1966	29	66	69	88
Giese et al[19]	1975	38	21	95	90
Kaufman[11]	1979	482	444	70	74
McNeil et al[22]	1975	118	152	85	90
(Data from Cooperative Study)[27]					
Foster et al[12]	1966	44	162	68	69
Hunt et al[20]	1970	85	89	71	70
Buda et al[21]	1976	59	–	78	–
Total	–	934	951	74.4	77

*RAS, renal artery stenosis.

Table 14.4 This table from McNeil[8] shows, in the same patients, a comparison between true-positive and false-positive rates in renography and rapid sequence intravenous urography. It is noteworthy that both tests together improve the true-positive rate to 91% but unfortunately, the very high false-positive rate of 10% is almost doubled. Both tests are done in each patient

	TP (%)	FP (%)
Renogram	85	10
Urogram	78	11
Both	91	18

The search for an ideal test and an ideal therapy has been elusive. Probably one of the most reliable tests was developed by Howard in 1954.[5] It is remarkable that the Howard test was based on only four patients with proven renovascular hypertension. Subsequent data validating the test do not provide us with any information on sensitivity, specificity or any truly scientific way in which the criteria were established. However, they have held up well and in fact characterized the changes in renal function associated with hypertension very nicely (Table 14.2). The IVP came to be used for detection of renovascular hypertension the same year as the Howard test, but provided very nonspecific information. It was not until the introduction of the rapid sequence IVP in 1964[6] that more specific information could be obtained. Patients with renovascular hypertension have delayed concentration of contrast media by the affected kidney and delayed excretion. These changes are exactly analogous to the increased water reabsorption noted in the Howard test. The changes noted in the IVP were paralleled by the changes that were observed in radioisotope renograms as early as

Table 14.5 This table illustrates the effect of prevalence on the false-positive rate for renovascular hypertension studies using tests in which the true-positive rate is 90% and the false-positive rate 10%. In a high prevalence disease, this false-positive rate is very acceptable as shown in the table with the estimated prevalence of 80%. In a relatively low-prevalence disease like renovascular hypertension, this is obviously not a sufficient sensitivity and specificity for screening since the false-positive rate rises to 91.7%

Prevalence 80% RVH	Prevalence 1%
TP – 90%	
FP – 10%	
1000 – 800 RVH	1000 – 10 RVH
200 EH	990 EH
Detect 720 RVH	Detect 9 RVH
$\dfrac{20}{740} = 2.7\%$ FP	$\dfrac{99}{108} = 91.7\%$ FP

1956 (Table 14.3).[7] The true-positive rates and false-positive rates for renography and urography were comparable but far from ideal; each with a false-positive rate of about 10%.[8] The two tests together provided a true-positive rate of about 91% but unfortunately the false-positive rate almost doubled to 18% (Table 14.4). Although one would expect that a test with a 90% true-positive rate and a 10% false-positive rate would be acceptable in many diseases, in the case of renovascular hypertension it is highly unacceptable because of the low prevalence (Table 14.5). If the prevalence of renovascular hypertension in a selected population could be raised to 80%, the test would be superb, but since in a general population it is only about 1% or less, there is an unacceptably high ratio of false positives. Careful selection of the patients for screening can enrich the population to about 30%, which helps but does not resolve completely the false-positive rate.

Another problem that has plagued us with radioisotope renography has been the unbridled early acceptance of the test without any critical review. Winter quotes an investigator whose name is omitted here for obvious reasons as reporting 'X reported in 1961... the renogram as a screening test for renal artery disease....'. He stated '.... there have been no false negative results to date and would be false positive readings had been interpretable or explicable in other ways.' Z... recorded in 1961 'the isotope renogram was distinctly abnormal in 36 of these 37 patients (.... found to have renal artery disease); in the remaining patients the renogram had some abnormal features.'[9] A review of the rapid sequence IVP that had a profound effect on our understanding of the value of the test, was conducted by Havey et al[7] and they found that between the years 1962 and 1983, 2040 patients with renal artery stenosis and 2133 patients with hypertension without renal artery stenosis were reported. The sensitivity in this series was only 74.5% and the specificity only 86.2%. These data and similar studies led to the ultimate demise of the rapid-sequence IVP as a major screening test for renovascular hypertension. We do not have sensitivity or specificity data on the Howard or Howard/Stamey tests. Table 14.2 shows the changes in a series which included 41 patients with renovascular hypertension and 36 with essential hypertension.[10] The differences in the patients with renovascular hypertension are quite impressive, including a reduction in inulin clearance (this abnormality can be seen on a DTPA renogram) and a change in PAH clearance (this can be seen on a MAG3 or hippuran renogram). A marked reduction in urine volume (the reduction that was taken as diagnostic was a 50% decrease in urine volume) and a reduction in urinary sodium excretion of 15% was accepted for diagnostic purposes. Another characteristic is the reduction in renal size that usually occurs ipsilateral to a renal artery stenosis.

Based on numerous studies over the years, we now realize that in renovascular hypertension, renal blood flow and GFR are usually decreased as shown by the Howard test, although this is not an invariable consequence. In some patients, the change in GFR is fully compensated by the renin-angiotensin system. It also became apparent with the introduction of angiotensin-converting enzyme inhibition that the diagnostic accuracy of renography could be improved by showing characteristic haemodynamic changes in which the renal blood flow change is variable and not reliable but in which the GFR is almost invariably decreased after administration of the inhibitor.

Numerous modalities have been introduced to study renovascular disease. Some of these are morphologic and therefore, by their intrinsic nature, cannot be used to diagnose renovascular hypertension but only show us some of the associated morphologic changes. These include colour-coded duplex ultrasound, spiral CT, contrast-

A

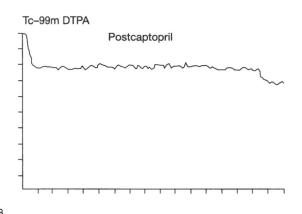

B

Figure 14.1 A: This is a technetium-99m-DTPA renogram obtained in a patient with a renal transplant and renal artery stenosis. Although the patient had renovascular hypertension, the renogram is normal. This renogram shows very nicely the potential for compensatory changes through the renin–angiotensin system to maintain GFR in a patient with renal artery stenosis sufficient to cause renovascular hypertension. B: This renogram was obtained in the same patient after the administration of 25 mg of captopril. The dependence of the kidney function on the renin-angiotensin system is very clearly demonstrated. All renal function is lost as evidenced by a horizontal straight line in a patient who only has one kidney so that there is no source for excretion of the DTPA. This study is diagnostic for renovascular hypertension with a very high sensitivity and specificity and demonstrates clearly the physiology of the disease.

enhanced MR angiography and arteriography. These different modalities of radiology are discussed in detail in Chapter 15.

Colour-coded duplex, another imaging technique, relies on a change in renal artery velocity to greater than 180 cm/s, a change in the renal artery/aorta ratio of greater than 3.5, decreased poststenotic flow velocity, turbulence and a reduction in kidney length to less than 8 cm. The reported sensitivities for colour-coded duplex range from 83% to 87% with a reported specificity of 81–91%. These are really not competitive with the early renograms and IVPs abandoned since. Moreover, the technical failure rate with colour-coded duplex ultrasound has been reported to range from 0–20%.

Although the results are good in highly experienced centres, the generalizability of this is probably poor because of its high user dependence.

Contrast-enhanced spiral CT and MR angiography have progressed to the point where results are almost as good as intra-arterial arteriography, making possible a relatively non-invasive approach to arteriography.

The physiologic diagnostic tests that are available, on the other hand, provide information that is much more specific to the disease. These include colour-coded duplex with angiotensin-converting enzyme inhibition, renal vein renin sampling, peripheral plasma renin and captopril renography. Renal vein renin sampling has been largely abandoned because of its invasive nature, just as the Howard test has been abandoned for the same reason. The peripheral plasma renin has proven too unreliable to use on a routine basis. The present role of nuclear medicine in renovascular hypertension is discussed in Chapter 16.

The changes induced in the radioisotope renogram in patients with renovascular hypertension are very dramatic in many situations. Figure 14.1A shows a technetium-99m-DTPA renogram in a renal transplant recipient. It is for all practical purposes normal; however, Figure 14.1B, shows a renogram in the same patient with technetium-99m-DTPA after receiving captopril. Note the complete absence of renal function after the ACE inhibition that removes the mechanism by which the efferent arteriole maintains GFR. This is a very dramatic in vivo demonstration of the maintenance of GFR in patients with renovascular hypertension through the renin-angiotensin system and its blockade with ACE inhibition.

Besides the radioisotope renogram, numerous other tests have become available over the years in general imaging and methods of analysis. Grunwald[11] reported in 1983 that there is a significant prolongation in parenchymal transit time in renovascular hypertension. However, there is a very large overlap between values in patients who have normal renal function, essential hypertension and renovascular hypertension. A consensus committee of the Society of Nuclear Medicine is currently working on the development of criteria for using parenchymal transit time in renovascular hypertension in an effort to determine its proper use. In our institution, a recent analysis of transit time failed to reveal any advantage over qualitative analysis of the renogram.[12]

Some new approaches are potentially available. It has been demonstrated at Hotel Dieu that labelled atrial natriuretic factor can be shown to concentrate in the monkey kidney. This test, for some reason, although described many years ago, has failed to reach clinical significance in spite of its potential value in determining changes in atrial natriuretic factor in hypertensive patients.[16] Clorius has reported changes in renography associated with exercise for several years but his reports have not been corroborated by other investigators except for a small study from Einstein.[17,18]

Among the new entities that have been introduced are electron beam computed tomography (EBCT), which although still experimental, provides very exciting data. These

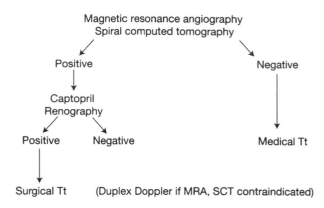

Algorithm for the diagnosis of RVH

Magnetic resonance angiography
Spiral computed tomography

Positive   Negative

Captopril Renography

Positive   Negative   Medical Tt

Surgical Tt   (Duplex Doppler if MRA, SCT contraindicated)

Figure 14.2 The proposed algorithm for the diagnosis of renovascular hypertension aims to diagnose renal artery stenosis in the first step. However, the major question to be resolved at this time is whether captopril renography should be the initial screening test because of its cost efficacy as shown in reference 22 or whether it is more reasonable to initiate diagnosis by first showing whether or not the patient has a renal artery stenosis. It is important to keep in mind that regardless of whether or not renal artery stenosis is present, there is a continuing need for a physiologic test such as captopril renography to demonstrate the functional significance of that stenosis.

data are discussed in detail in Chapter 17. It is possible to generate a time–activity curve for transit using EBCT. This curve is similar to the renogram transit curve. Advantages of the radiographic techniques include their potential to evaluate global kidney, cortical and medullary blood flow[14] and even to discriminate changes in the concentration of contrast media as it transits through the kidney.[15] However, it should be noted that there are disadvantages associated with these techniques as well. These include the partial volume effect of contrast and a radiation dose with EBCT that is about 0.1 Sv/s (10 rads/s) or 0.01 Sv/scan (1 rad/scan). Contrast also causes a diuretic effect and tubular expansion. Associated with this is an increase in renal size. Vasodilatation followed by vasoconstriction may modify the results. These problems are being addressed by the investigators and moving it rapidly toward the potential for clinical utilization. The current state-of-the-art can be found in Chapter 17. In addition, MR contrast also can be used to generate a time–activity curve that can be analysed much like the transit time curves for the renogram.[13] (See Chapter 18.)

Another source for future investigation of renovascular hypertension is the role of positron emission tomography. This is purely experimental at this time, and is discussed in detail in Chapter 19. Although it is possible that the complexity and the high cost of PET for investigation of the kidney may prevent its ultimate clinical application, PET remains one of the few areas in which a significant amount of truly innovative research on kidney function with radioisotopes has been conducted during the past 4 or 5 years.

Finally, in closing these introductory statements, it may be appropriate to introduce a new algorithm for the diagnosis of renovascular hypertension (Figure 14.2) that may provide a template for future diagnostic approaches.

It is my belief that although a great deal of progress has been made in competitive imaging modalities, there still remains a very important role for captopril renography in the diagnosis of renovascular hypertension. It is possible that magnetic resonance angiography may become the initial screening procedure followed by captopril renography only in patients in whom there is a known stenosis. Dr Taylor in Chapter 16 discusses a cost analysis which perhaps puts this in dispute. An earlier cost analysis by our group had similar conclusions.[19]

However, we should keep track of the fact that renal artery stenosis is not synonymous with renovascular hypertension. It is extremely important to keep in mind if patients are going to be subjected to invasive procedures, doing these on the basis of solely the anatomy with an expectation of curing the hypertension is foolhardy. It is essential that some physiologic test be performed that demonstrates that a renal artery stenosis is in fact physiologically significant and the cause of the hypertension. More than 30–40% of patients with hypertension have renal artery stenosis but only a small number of these have renovascular hypertension. Smith showed many years ago that unilateral nephrectomy in patients with a small kidney only cured hypertension in about 50%.[20] We continue to see articles making conclusions about renovascular hypertension used on the presence of renal artery stenosis. The most important message of this introduction is to stress the need to discriminate between these two entities.

References

1. Tigerstedt R, Bergman PG. Niere Und Kreislauf. Skandinav Arch Physiol 1898; 7: 223–71.
2. Blaufox MD. Studies of Renal Function and Experimental Hypertension. (Thesis). Mayo Foundation, University of Minnesota, Rochester Minn. 1963.
3. Goldblatt H, Lynch J, Hanzal RF, Summerville WW. Studies on experimental hypertension. I. The production of persistent elevation of systolic blood pressure by means of renal ischemia. J Exper Med 1934; 59: 347–79.
4. Leadbetter WF, Burkland CE. Hypertension in unilateral artery disease. J Urol 1938; 39: 611–26.
5. Howard JE, Berthrong M, Gould BM, Yend ER. Hypertension resulting from unilateral vascular disease and its relief by nephrectomy. Bulletin, Johns Hopkins Hospital 1954; 94: 51–85.
6. Maxwell MH, Gonick HC, Wilta R, Kaufman JJ. Use of the rapid sequence intravenous pyelogram in the diagnosis of renovascular hypertension. N Engl J Med 1964; 270: 213–20.
7. Havey RJ, Krumlovsky F, del Greco F, Martin HG. Screening for renovascular hypertension. JAMA 1985; 254: 388–93.
8. McNeil BJ, Keeler E, Adelstein SJ. Primer on certain elements of medical decision making. N Engl J Med 1975; 293: 211–15.
9. Winter CC. A kidney function test performed with radioisotope-labeled agents. In: Radioisotope Renography. Baltimore, The Williams and Wilkins Company, 1963.
10. London GM, Safar ME. Renal hemodynamics in patients with sustained essential hypertension and in patients with unilateral stenosis of the renal artery. A J Hyper 1989; 2: 244–52.
11. Gruenewald SM, Collins LT. Renovascular hypertension: quantitative renography as a screening test. Radiol 1983; 149: 287–91.
12. Fine EJ, Li Y, Blaufox MD. Parenchymal mean transit time analysis of ^{99m}Tc-DTPA captopril renography. J Nucl Med 2000; 41: 1627–31.
13. Lee VS, Rofsky NM, Krinsky GA et al. Single-dose breath-hold gadolinium-enhanced three-dimensional MR angiography of the renal arteries. Radiol 1999; 211: 69–78.
14. Lerman LO, Bell MR, Lahera V et al. Quantification of global and regional renal blood flow with electron beam computed tomography. A J Hypert 1994; 7: 829–37.
15. Lerman LL, Rodriquez-Porcel M, Romero JC. The development of X-ray imaging to study renal function. Kidney International 1999; 55: 400 16.
16. Atrial Natriuretic Factor, Hotel Dieu. Personal Communication.
17. Clorius JH, Schmidlin P. The exercise renogram: a new approach documents renal involvement in systemic hypertension. J Nucl Med 1983; 24: 104–9.
18. Fine EJ, Blaufox MD, Blumenfeld JD et al. Exercise renography in untreated subjects with essential hypertension. J Nucl Med 1996; 37: 838–42.
19. Blaufox MD, Middleton ML, Bongiovanni J, Davis B. Cost efficacy of the diagnosis and therapy of renovascular hypertension. J Nucl Med 1996; 37: 171–7.
20. Smith HW. Unilateral nephrectomy in hypertensive disease. J Urol 1956; 76: 685–701.

15 Radiological modalities in renovascular disease

Nicolas Grenier

Introduction

Renovascular disease (RVD) is a complex entity associating atherosclerotic arterial lesions, renal disease and hypertension leading to high renal and cardiovascular risks. The relationships between renal artery stenosis (RAS), hypertension and renal function are variable from patient to patient and difficult to assess, but their severity and their association increase the patient's risks.[1]

As the cardiovascular risk mainly depends on the degree of hypertension, improving the blood pressure control has been a major task. Today, we know that medical treatment can achieve this control without renal revascularization in many cases.[2] Therefore, the management of the patients does not always require, as before, an early diagnosis of RAS, even if recent improvements of radiological techniques allow an accurate diagnosis of RAS noninvasively.

Characterization of the so-called 'atherosclerotic nephropathy' remains difficult and controversial. It is an important cause of end-stage renal failure (ESRF) causing up to 14% of ESRF over the age of 50 years.[3] There are several arguments in favour of nonischaemic factors responsible for atherosclerotic nephropathy:[3] (1) presence of athero-embolic disease and focal segmental glomerulosclerosis at histology; (2) a very variable functional response to revascularization, with evolutive processes independent of a reduction of renal blood flow; (3) the possible observation of either patients with two equally sized kidneys, unilateral RAS and impaired renal function, or patients with severe bilateral RAS and relatively preserved renal function. Atherosclerotic nephropathy is a consequence of the association of multiple factors: decrease of renal blood flow (secondary to bilateral RAS or to unilateral stenosis plus contralateral occlusion or to unilateral stenosis on a solitary kidney), intrarenal atherosclerotic arterial disease, atheroembolism, diabetes, increased oxidative stress, medullary hypoxia, endothelial dysfunction, inflammatory response, proteinuria, etc. This multiplicity of causal factors explains the great heterogeneity of renal damage.

The radiological imaging techniques available today have to reach four objectives:

- to detect and characterize the RAS in terms of anatomical and haemodynamical severity;
- to assess the anatomical consequences of the RAS on the artery itself and on the renal parenchyma;
- to assess the functional and cellular consequences of the RAS on the kidney;
- identify criteria of associated renal impairment related to RVD.

Radiological detection of RAS

Stenoses which reduce the internal diameter by >60% produce a significant decrease in renal blood flow. They can be atheromatous (60% of cases) or dysplastic (fibromuscular dysplasia, 35% of cases),[4] ostial or not, and be located on main, accessory or segmental arteries. Although most of these imaging techniques provide good sensitivity and specificity for diagnosing anatomical RAS, they do not provide information about the relationship between the stenosis (even if haemodynamically significant) and hypertension. These techniques are: Doppler ultrasound (US), helical computerized tomographic angiography (CTA), magnetic resonance angiography (MRA) and intra-arterial (IA) digital subtraction angiography (DSA). Intravenous (IV) urography and IV DSA are no longer recommended.

IADSA

IADSA is considered to be the gold standard for diagnosing RAS,[5] but is limited to confirming stenosis; it can be followed by a transluminal angioplasty during the same procedure. Injection of contrast medium within the aorta is recommended with small catheters (4–5 French) positioned at the level of the renal arteries, to avoid superimposition with the coeliac trunk and superior mesenteric artery. Both posterior oblique and posteroanterior views must be obtained to avoid missed short ostial stenoses, because these stenoses may originate anteriorly or posteriorly from the aortic wall, as shown by two recent CTA-anatomical studies.[6,7] Selective injection in each renal artery is also necessary if a distal stenosis is suspected (e.g. in young patients with fibromuscular dysplasia). If carried out properly, IADSA provides excellent resolution to show the presence, degree, nature and extent of stenosis. However, it has major drawbacks, e.g. invasiveness and cost, justifying the use of other techniques for selection of patients.

Doppler US

With the advent of colour encoding of the Doppler signal, US has gained a major place in the detection of renal artery stenosis. To be of diagnostic use, a complete examination must be undertaken, including B-mode, spectral sampling and colour imaging. The examination should include the measurement of both kidneys; spectral sampling of several interlobar or segmental arteries of each kidney (at lower and upper poles); and spectral sampling of both renal arteries, using colour guidance for angle correction, for velocity profile assessment and peak systolic velocity measurement. This can provide a diagnosis of RAS based on morphological (colour changes in the renal artery) and functional criteria (spectral broadening, velocity increase and distal demodulation).

Proximal criteria

The stenosis may be seen on colour-flow images with focal changes of colour (Figures 15.1A and 15.2A) and/or a perivascular artifact which are related to acceleration and turbulence, respectively. However, the criteria of haemodynamically significant stenosis are essentially based on spectral sampling. At the site of stenosis, there may be spectral broadening and increased velocity (Figures 15.1B and 15.2B). Because the former is difficult to quantify, only the latter is used to separate significant from insignificant stenoses. The main proximal criteria used are: first, a reno-aortic velocity

A

B

Figure 15.1 Fibromuscular dysplasia with stenosis of the right renal artery. A: On the colour flow sonography, acceleration of flow and poststenotic turbulences produce a change of colour on the retrocaval segment of the trunk of renal artery. B: Spectral sampling along renal artery shows progressive spectral broadening and acceleration of flow, with a high peak systolic velocity above 4 m/s at the site of stenosis.

ratio (RAR) higher than 3.5 for a 60% stenosis;[8,9] second, a peak systolic velocity, at the site of stenosis, with an upper limit of either 150 cm/s for a 50% stenosis[10] or 180 cm/s for a 60% stenosis.[11,12] This discrepancy is fairly negligible

Table 15.1 Performance of Doppler US versus angiography for diagnosis of RAS based on proximal criteria

	Arteries (n)	Failures (%)	Stenosis (%)	Criteria	Sensitivity (%)	Specificity (%)
Olin, 1995[13]	102	–	60	200 cm/s	98	98
Miralles, 1996[14]	78	–	60	200 cm/s	89	91
Claudon, 2000[15]	198	35	50	140–200 cm/s	80	84
Hua, 2000[16]	58	–	60	200 cm/s	91	75
Motew, 2000[17]	41	–	60	200 cm/s	91	96
de Cobelli, 2000[18]	45	–	50	200 cm/s	79	93
de Haan, 2002[19]	78%	7	50	180 cm/s	50	91
Napoli, 2002[20]	84	0	60	160 cm/s	93	92
Conkbayir, 2003[21]	50	0	60	180 cm/s	92	88
Nchimi, 2003[22]	91	8.7	60	180 cm/s	91	97

A

B

C

Figure 15.2 Atherosclerotic stenosis of the right renal artery. A: Colour flow sonography, shows typical colour changes at the ostium of right renal artery, extending in the postostial segment. B: Spectral sampling at the site of stenosis shows acceleration of flow and spectral broadening. C: Intrarenal sampling of interlobar arteries shows a decrease of systolic acceleration with an increase of ascension time (0.173 s)

considering the difficulty of separating 50% from 60% stenoses, even at angiography. Using such proximal criteria, the sensitivity and specificity of the technique, compared with angiography, are 89–98% and 90–98%, respectively (Table 15.1).[13-22] In the early experience with colour Doppler imaging, two studies reported 0% sensitivity, which was probably due to difficulty in obtaining a signal in the renal arteries[23,24] with suboptimal US systems.

The percentages of technical success are highly variable in the literature, ranging from 58%[23] to 90%.[12] This probably depends on the experience of the operators and on the type of system used. Although multiple renal arteries can be detected (Figure 15.3), in all series detection of small accessory arteries was reported as very low. The improved sensitivity in depth of the new generation of US systems, a wider use of lateral approaches during examination and wider use of contrast agents (see below) will probably decrease this failure rate.

Intrarenal spectral changes

Because of the difficulties in detecting renal arteries, several authors have proposed sampling intrarenal vessels to detect altered spectral waveforms distally to RAS.[25-30] Severe

Figure 15.3 Multiple right renal arteries with colour flow sonography. Right coronal section shows three right renal arteries emerging from the aorta.

Table 15.2   Performance of Doppler US versus angiography for diagnosis of RAS based on intrarenal distal criteria

	(n)	Stenosis (%)	Criteria	Sensitivity (%)	Specificity (%)
Stavros, 1992[25]	56	60	AT	78	94
		60	ESP	95	97
		60	Acc	89	83
Kliewer, 1993[30]	46	50	AT	82	20
		80	AT	100	23
		50	Acc	71	48
		80	Acc	87	48
Schwerk, 1994[29]		50	RI	82	92
		60	RI	100	94
Halpern, 1995[28]		50	Acc	76	95
Strunk, 1995[32]		50	AT	90	85
Baxter, 1996[33]		70	AT	89	97
Lucas, 1996[34]		60	ΔRI-Acc	68	91
Postma, 1996[35]		50	ESP	63	86
Oliva, 1998[36]		50	AT	81	98
Motew, 2000[17]		60	AT	32	100
Conkbayir, 2003[21]		60	AT	48	93

ESP: early systolic peak; A: acceleration > 3 m/s^2; AT: acceleration time > 0.07 s; ΔRI: resistive index difference >0.05.

stenoses which decrease the diameter by $>75\%$ produce a tardus–parvus phenomenon in the distal intrarenal vessels, with a slowed systolic acceleration and a decreased resistive index (Figure 15.2C).[31] The problems with this approach are that stenoses of 50–75% are not detected. There are many distal criteria proposed in the literature: loss of early systolic peak; acceleration (ascending slope of the systolic peak) lower than 3 m/s^2; acceleration index >4, acceleration time of systolic peak >0.07 s; a difference between kidneys in resistive index of $>5\%$ or in pulsatility index of >0.12. The performances of these correlative studies with angiography are confusing because of the variability in criteria and in corresponding degree of stenosis (Table 15.2).[17,21,25,28,29,30–36] The drawbacks of this transrenal approach are that unsatisfactory results have also been reported with these various criteria,[30,37] interobserver and intraobserver variability is high[38] and intra-arterial Doppler US does not confirm any correlation between distal indices and RAS.[39] Indeed, the factors responsible for changes in the distal waveforms are complex and are probably more dependent on changes of compliance than on pressure decrease.[40,41] Therefore, these criteria are used only when obvious on spectral traces, to quantify the stenosis as severe ($>75\%$) or to identify a downstream pattern of a stenosis on a segmental or an accessory artery that has been missed proximally.

US contrast agents

The development of echo-enhancing agents which affect the Doppler signal has increased the sensitivity of detection of flow when it is too slow or too deep (Figure 15.4).[42] A multi-

centre study performed with the first commercialized agent (Levovist, Schering®, made of microbubbles of air stabilized with galactose and palmitic acid) showed that the feasibility of the US examination was increased, mainly in patients with a high body mass index and in patients with decreased renal function, but neither sensitivity nor specificity were significantly improved.[15] The development of new agents with a stronger and a longer effect in time, together with the improvement in techniques of insonation (e.g. harmonic mode or pulse inversion[43]) will probably improve these results further. However, the easy access to CTA or MRA currently makes the use of US contrast agents quite unusual in clinical practice.

Doppler with captopril

To overcome the lack of sensitivity of distal criteria for detecting proximal RAS, the administration of captopril has been proposed,[36,44] as 'stress test': captopril produces a vasodilation and, when a proximal stenosis is present, increases the pulsus–tardus phenomenon, giving complete sensitivity and specificity for diagnosis of 50% RAS. However, currently it seems more reasonable to seek proximal features of RAS, using contrast agents if necessary, than to give captopril to worsen indirect features.

In summary, US has gained a major place in the detection of RAS because of its advantages of wide availability, low cost, absence of ionizing radiation and lack of harmful effect on renal function. Proximal criteria for diagnosis of RAS are more accurate than intrarenal criteria, as shown by Conkbavir et al[21] who demonstrated that the area under the ROC curve

Figure 15.4   Effect of US contrast agents. A,B: Before injection, the colour flow image does not show the proximal portion of the renal artery (A) and the intensity of spectral waveform is insufficient for diagnosis (B). C,D: After injection of Levovist, the acceleration of flow becomes visible in the proximal portion of the artery (C) and the spectrum displays typical features of stenosis (D).

Table 15.3 Performance of single-slice CT angiography for diagnosis of RAS

	Patients (n)	Stenosis (%)	Rendering technique	Sensitivity (%)	Specificity (%)
Rubin, 1994[47]	31	70	MIP	92	83
			SSD	59	82
Bérégi, 1996[49]	50	50	MIP + SSD	88	98
Kaatee, 1997[50]	71	50	MIP	96	96
Johnson, 1999[48]	25	50	MIP	94	87
			VR	89	99
Wittenberg, 1999[51]	82	50	MIP	96	99

MIP: maximum intensity projection; SSD: shaded surface display; VR: volume rendering.

was greater with the former. However, US has some drawbacks, particularly the possibility of technical failures (the technique is quite difficult and has to be carried out perfectly) and a low detection rate of accessory arteries.

CT angiography

With single-ring CT scanners, optimisation of protocols has led to improvements in the evaluation of renal arteries[45] with the possibility to cover the entire aorta with 3 mm collination.

With single-ring CT scanners, optimization of protocols has led to improvements in the evaluation of renal arteries.[45] With new X-ray tubes capable of greater heat dissipation, it is now possible to cover the entire aorta with 3 mm collimation. For renal artery studies, a 30-second bolus in an antecubital vein is necessary (between 90 ml of contrast material at 3 ml/s and 150 ml at 5 ml/s, depending on the body weight). The delay time between infusion and acquisition ranges from 12 to 25 seconds but automatic control of arrival of the bolus increases the reproducibility of the technique. For image display, Galanski et al[46] reported that axial sections and multiplanar reformatted images were superior to 3D-shaded surface display (SSD) or maximum intensity projection (MIP) algorithm, and Rubin et al[47] showed that MIP projections provided better sensitivity (92%) than SSD (59%). However, Johnson et al[48] reported that the volume rendering technique provided a better specificity (99%) than MIP (87%). If the SSD technique is excluded, the performance of CT angiography in detecting significant stenoses is good with high sensitivity (between 88% and 96%), high specificity (between 83% and 99%) (Table 15.3)[47–52] and close correlation with angiography for grading stenoses.[52] The detection of accessory arteries is much better than with Doppler US (average 90%). CT also shows the exact nature of stenoses, e.g. ostial, truncal or pseudotruncal,[53] and the degree of calcification of lesions before endovascular treatment. Fibromuscular dysplasia stenoses, which are more distal than atherosclerotic stenoses, can also be better characterized using MIP.[54]

With multislice CT, allowing between four and 64 slices per rotation, the axial resolution could be improved forward

with 1 mm slice thickness (Figure 15.5). Compared with single ring CT, the amount of iodinated contrast agent can be reduced. Because of a better spatial resolution, separation of calcification and true lumen is more accurate[55] and distal lesions, as fibromuscular dysplasia, are better delineated (Figure 15.6). Preliminary results of this technique show

A

B

Figure 15.5 Ostial stenosis of the right renal artery shown by contrast-enhanced CT angiography on coronal (A) and axial (B) projections (MIP).

A

B

C

Figure 15.6 Bilateral fibromuscular dysplasia of renal arteries imaged with a 16-ring contrast-enhanced spiral CT angiography on coronal (A) and axial (B) projections (MIP) with DSA correlation (C).

extremely encouraging results but comparative studies with angiography are still not available.

The drawbacks of CT angiography are principally the ionizing radiations and the need to inject large doses of iodinated contrast media, which can be a problem in patients with impaired renal function.

MR angiography

MR angiography has now moved from flow-enhanced (time-of-flight or phase-contrast) sequences to T1-weighted contrast-enhanced acquisitions. With time-of-flight or phase-contrast techniques, MR angiography shows the proximal portion of the renal arteries. Several improvements, e.g. 3D-TONE acquisition, have been necessary to decrease saturation effects and venous overlap. Under the best conditions, only half of the accessory arteries are depicted. Sensitivity and specificity for diagnosis of significant stenosis were between 53% and 100% and between 65% and 97%, respectively, depending on the technique used (Table 15.4).[56–65] This technique has many drawbacks: only the proximal portion (3–3.5 mm) of the renal arteries is visualized because of respiratory movements; only a short segment of the aorta is enhanced because of the saturation effect with time of flight; distal, segmental and accessory artery stenoses are generally not detected; and because of turbulence, stenoses (which are seen as signal loss on MIP images) are often overgraded.

Therefore, with the development of new MR systems with stronger and faster gradients, flow-enhanced sequences have largely been replaced with more reproducible Gd-enhanced sequences. With T1-weighted contrast-enhanced acquisitions, most of the problems are overcome. The vascular contrast is greatly increased by contrast media injected intravenously as a bolus. Images are acquired during one breath-hold with a 3D T1-weighted sequence when the contrast is maximum in the aorta (like CT angiography).[66] New developments, such as fluoroscopic guidance of arrival of the bolus in the aorta, improve the reproducibility of the technique (Figure 15.7).[67] Its performance is excellent with sensitivity and specificity for diagnosis of significant stenosis between 88% and 100% and between 71% and 99%, respectively (Table 15.5).[68–78] This technique shows the entire course of

Table 15.4 Performance of flow-enhanced MR angiography

	Patients (n)	Technique	Sensitivity (%)	Specificity (%)
Debatin, 1991[56]	33	TOF	53	97
		PC	80	91
Richter, 1993[57]	23	PC	100	80
Loubeyre, 1995[58]	46	PC	100	65
Fellner, 1995[59]	46	TOF	100	89
Borrello, 1995[60]	15	TOF	94	94
Gedroyc, 1995[61]	60	PC	84	91
De Cobelli, 1996[62]	50	PC	90	99
De Haan, 1996[63]	38	PC	93	95
Loubeyre, 1996[64]	53	TOF	100	76
Wasser, 1997[65]	16	PC	92	75

PC: phase contrast; TOF: time-of-flight.

Table 15.5 Performance of gadolinium-enhanced MR angiography

	Patients (n)	Renal artery (stenosis/total)	Sensitivity (%)	Specificity (%)
Snidow, 1996[68]	32	5/60	100	89
Rieumont, 1997[69]	30	42/71	100	71
Hany, 1997[70]	39	24/88	93	98
De Cobelli, 1997[71]	55	29/105	94	96
Tello, 1998[72]	20	13/51	100	98
Bakker, 1998[73]	44	40/121	97	92
Thornton, 1999[74]	62	25/138	88	98
Völk, 2000[75]	40	21/78	92.9	83.4
Korst, 2001[76]	38	26/92	100	85
Fain, 2001[77]	25	28/55	97	92
Wilman, 2003[78]	46	73/736 segments	93	99

A

B

Figure 15.7 3D Gd-enhanced MR angiography of the abdominal aorta with coronal (A) and axial (B) projections (MIP), showing bilateral atherosclerotic postostial stenoses of renal arteries, insignificant on the right and high grade on the left.

Figure 15.8 3D Gd-enhanced MR angiography of the abdominal aorta with coronal projection (MIP), showing bilateral truncal stenoses of renal arteries related to fibromuscular dysplasia.

renal arteries up to the renal sinus in most cases, and the complete abdominal aorta including its bifurcation. Most accessory arteries are therefore shown. The evaluation of the degree of stenosis with this method has the same interobserver variability as conventional angiography.[79]

Several improvements are now available. A shorter acquisition time makes it possible to perform a multiphasic angiogram at different phases of vascular filling, as with conventional angiography.[80,81] Also, development of parallel acquisition techniques allows improvement of the spatial resolution without increasing the acquisition time and yielding an isotropic resolution of 1 mm^3 in a single breath-hold. Such a resolution is responsible for an improved grading of stenoses, mainly on the distal part of the trunk for fibromuscular dysplasia (Figure 15.8), and a better detection of accessory arteries.

A recent meta-analysis, from 25 studies, meeting the inclusion criteria, showed that sensitivity and specificity were better for Gd-enhanced MRA (97% (95% CI: 93–98%) and 93% (95% CI: 91–95%), respectively) than for flow-enhanced MRA (94% (95% CI: 90–97%) and 85% (95% CI: 82–87%), respectively); accessory renal arteries were depicted better by Gd-enhanced MRA (82% (95% CI: 75–87%) than for flow-enhanced MRA (49% (95% CI: 42–60%).[82]

Comparison of techniques

Comparison of performance of these noninvasive tests is difficult. A recent meta-analysis[83] tried to compare the validity of CTA, MRA and US for diagnosis of RAS in patients suspected of having RVH. Receiver-operating characteristic (ROC) curves found that CTA and Gd-enhanced 3D MRA performed significantly better than the other diagnostic tests and seemed to be preferred in patients referred for evaluation of RVH. However, because few studies of these tests have been published, further research is recommended.

Figure 15.9 Contrast-enhanced CT of the kidneys showing a cortical atrophy on the left side in a patient presenting with a severe left renal artery stenosis.

Anatomical and haemodynamic consequences of RAS

Detection of a RAS requires further evaluation of the severity of narrowing and its consequences on renal flow, on renal artery, on renal parenchyma and on renal function, in order to improve the interobserver variability and to define predictive factors of improvement after revascularization.

Vascular anatomy

When the stenosis is severe, a *poststenotic dilatation* occurs, as a 'jet-lesion'. This dilatation can be used as a criterion of significant artery stenosis. This morphological change can be assessed with CTA and MRA but not with US. However, this criterion is difficult to quantify; no significant threshold has been defined, even if a 20% dilatation is widely used; it has never been evaluated to our knowledge.

Renal anatomy

When the renal blood flow is significantly decreased, the renal parenchyma shrinks. Several parameters have been proposed to evaluate this effect:

- *Measurement of renal length:* renal length can be measured with any technique: with US, the right renal length is between 98 and 122 mm (median 109 mm) and the left renal length between 101 and 123 mm (median 112 mm).[84] To be significant, a length difference of 1 cm should be considered, attesting to a haemodynamically significant stenosis.[85] If the renal length is less than 8 cm, revascularization is contraindicated because it is less likely to get benefit out of it.

- *Measurement of renal parenchyma thickness* is more difficult because it requires several measurements (upper, mid- and lower poles) due to the irregular inner surface of the renal parenchyma. A thickness of 2–2.5 cm is considered as normal.[86] This parameter, to our knowledge, has never been evaluated in RAS. However, there is a good linear correlation between renal length and renal parenchymal thickness, obviating the need for such a measurement.[86]

- *Measurement of renal volume:* this requires either using the ellipsoid formula[87] or developing a postprocessing software to segment the renal parenchyma from a 3D data set,[88] excluding the fat of renal sinus. None of these has been evaluated in RAS.

- *Measurement of cortical thickness and cortical area:* Mounier-Vehier et al[89] showed that a threshold of 8 mm for cortical thickness and of 800 mm² for cortical area allowed control kidneys to be distinguished from poststenotic kidneys, whereas renal length was still within normal range, suggesting that cortical parameters are more sensitive for early diagnosis of atherosclerotic renal disease than kidney size (Figure 15.9). Cortical atrophy seems to be a useful marker for guidance for revascularization but its prognostic value has still to be evaluated.

Renal haemodynamics

Renal arterial flow below the stenosis

When a significant stenosis occurs (>75% of area narrowing), flow acceleration is associated with a disturbed or destroyed flow profile downstream of the stenosis. Only two techniques allow assessment of the intravascular flow profile: Doppler US and MR imaging using the cine-phase contrast method.

Diagnosis of RAS with Doppler US is based on the detection of spectral broadening on the Doppler waveforms.

A

B

Figure 15.10 Phase-contrast acquisition on renal arteries in a patient with left renal artery stenosis. A: Example of MR angiography showing left renal artery stenosis with a small kidney. B: The flow velocity–time curves, obtained on each renal artery, show a normal curve on the right with early systolic peak, and an altered flow within left renal artery without early systolic peak. (Courtesy of Dr Stephan Schoenberg, Muenchen, Germany.)

However, no quantification of such a broadening is possible. This is the reason why measurement of peak systolic velocity is used to separate significant from nonsignificant stenoses.

With Gd-enhanced MRA, no haemodynamical information is available and this separation is based on morphological analysis of the artery only (as for CTA). However, by using 3D phase contrast sequences, with flow encoding in the three directions, signal intensity within the artery becomes sensitive to flow velocity. The flow profile alteration is responsible for a

severe dephasing of MR signal with these sequences. It has been shown, in vitro, that the degree of spin dephasing was directly correlated with the trans-stenotic pressure gradient (Figure 15.10).[90] Velocity–time curves can also be obtained: the imaging plane has to be perpendicular to the artery for accurate measurements of velocity changes during the cardiac cycle (results similar to Doppler sampling). A normal velocity–time curve is characterized by an early systolic peak (ESP), a subsequent incision and a lower second midsystolic peak. Schoenberg et al[91,92] showed in animals and patients that either a normal curve or partial loss of the ESP were consistent with low-grade stenosis; complete loss of the ESP and decrease of the midsystolic peak indicated moderate stenosis (50%); flattened flow profile with no systolic velocity components was representative of high-grade stenosis.[93] Using this classification, the combined approach of 3D Gd-enhanced MRA and phase-contrast flow sequence revealed the best interobserver variability and almost perfect intermodality agreement with DSA. Administration of angiotensin converting enzyme inhibitors does not significantly change the renal velocities in renal artery stenoses.[37]

This method also allows the measurement of renal blood flow in the renal artery below the stenosis as the product of the mean velocity within the artery and the cross-sectional area of renal artery. Binkert et al[94] reported a renal flow index (renal flow (ml/min) divided by renal volume (cm³)) less than 1.5 ml/min/cm³ as predictive of successful outcome of revascularization.

Intrarenal haemodynamics

By sampling the distal intrarenal vessels (as segmental or interlobar arteries), essentially with Doppler US, two types of flow curve changes can be observed:

Figure 15.11 Intrarenal colour Doppler examination in a patient with severe renal artery stenosis showing an increased ascension time (0.17 s) related to stenosis associated with an increased resistivity index (0.86).

- A decreased resistive index (RI, defined as the ratio: systolic velocity – diastolic velocity/systolic velocity), related to a compensatory vasodilatation because of the presence of a severe RAS proximally; usually, this feature is associated with an increase in the ascension time (see above) because of a slower systolic acceleration.

- An increased RI, which is not specific but compatible, in this context, with the diagnosis of atherosclerotic nephropathy (Figure 15.11). The RI increases when small intrarenal arteries are diseased, as in chronic nephropathies, or constricted or compressed, as in acute nephropathies. Therefore, spectral waveforms from these vessels can give us information about the intensity of renal consequences of RAS. Radermacher et al[95] demonstrated that an increased RI > 0.8 was associated with a poor prognosis in patients with RAS shown by an absence of improvement of hypertension, renal function or kidney survival after revascularization.

Renal function

Glomerular filtration

Baseline semiquantitative evaluation or quantification of glomerular filtration is neither sensitive enough nor specific enough to detect a renal dysfunction due to RAS. Blockade of the renin-angiotensin system is mandatory for this purpose.

Captopril-enhanced filtration studies

ACE inhibitors, such as captopril, decrease the synthesis of angiotensin II, and block its vasoconstrictor-stimulating effect, mostly on the efferent arterioles. This block produces a decrease in hydrostatic pressure within the glomerulus and a decrease in filtration on the side of the stenosis. The principle of the test is to image the renal elimination of a tracer before

A

B

C

Figure 15.12 Dynamic Gd-enhanced MR imaging of the kidneys before (A) and after (B) captopril administration in a patient with stenosis of the left renal artery (from top-to-bottom then left-to-right). A: Before captopril, the tubular phase with a low signal intensity within medulla and excretion of contrast medium within renal collecting system are symmetrical. B: After captopril, the tubular phase is delayed in the left kidney compared to the right, but enhances with time, extending within the cortex; this effect is related to a severe retention of the contrast agent within the entire left kidney induced by captopril. C: Positive captopril ^{99m}Tc-MAG3 scintigraphy obtained in the same patient: the baseline study shows symmetrical elimination of the tracer (right of the image). After captopril (left of the image), there is an accumulation of the tracer within the left kidney (red line) whereas it remains unchanged in the right (yellow line). (Reprinted with permission, from reference 96.)

and after administration of captopril to detect captopril-induced functional changes. A positive test demonstrates the diagnosis of 'functional stenoses' producing renovascular hypertension. This test has been coupled with scintigraphy (see Chapter 16) and, more recently, with dynamic MR.

Gadolinium chelates behave as glomerular tracers in the same manner as iodine contrast media. After infusion of a bolus of 0.1 mmol/kg, it is possible to follow the intrarenal transit of this chelate with a series of coronal gradient-echo images obtained during breath holding (Figure 15.8). This transit begins with a vasculo-interstitial phase producing a cortical, then a medullary, enhancement of signal intensity (T1-shortening effect), a tubular phase characterized by a drop of signal intensity (T2-shortening effect) within the external medulla that extends centripetally towards the papilla, and finally a ductal phase characterized by a late low signal intensity within the internal medulla and the renal collecting system (Figure 15.12). In RVH, the normal contrast kinetics is altered by captopril on the side of the stenosis, thus inducing a delay or disappearance of the tubular and ductal phases or a late T2 effect extending across the whole kidney.[96] In that preliminary study, the MR results were concordant with scintigraphy but need to be studied more extensively.

Renal perfusion

Absolute quantification of parenchymal perfusion can be assessed with diffusible (as Gd-chelates)[97] or purely intravascular contrast agents (as iron oxide particles) (see Chapter 18).[98] A 50% decrease in cortical perfusion (from 400 ml/min/100 g to 200 ml/min/100 g) has been observed below a tight (80%) stenosis; however, atherosclerotic nephropathy, because of its vascular components, can also be responsible for a decrease of perfusion to 180 ml/min/100 g.[98] Distinction between these two types of cortical perfusion changes, and their potential role in prognosis has not yet been demonstrated.

Other functional parameters

MR imaging is able to provide other new functional parameters as a diffusion coefficient or a BOLD (Blood Oxygen Level Dependent) effect. Principles of these techniques are detailed in Chapter 18. In RAS, their results are preliminary and their significance and role in strategy still under debate. They showed a decrease of renal diffusion coefficients in patients with RAS[99] and a decreased intrarenal oxygenation during acute experimental occlusion of the renal artery in pigs.[100]

Strategy

The best strategy to explore RVD remains a matter of debate. The choice of the best noninvasive test at present depends on the experience of each group in every technique and the availability of these techniques, knowing that US is cheaper and more available than CT or MR but requires training. In good hands, using proximal criteria of RAS, US remains the most useful tool as a first line study. Based on haemodynamic features, it provides criteria of significant (>60%) RAS (if peak systolic velocity is > 160 cm/s) or severe (>75%) RAS (if intrarenal acceleration time is increased) and prognosis information about the possibility of improvement of hypertension, renal function or kidney survival after revascularization. If accurate US examination is not available, or if the US is inconclusive, MRA or CTA should be performed. Their comparative performances have not been compared in a blind trial, but, in practice, CTA is preferred because of its wider availability, its higher spatial resolution with multislice systems and its lower cost. MRA is performed in most centres if the patient has an impaired renal function or intolerance to iodinated contrast agents. However, 'downstream damage', so-called atherosclerotic nephropathy, remains difficult to characterize whereas it represents the essential prognostic factor.

References

1. Safian RD, Textor SC. Renal artery stenosis. N Engl J Med 2001; 344: 431–42.
2. Plouin PF, Rossignol P, Bobrie G. Atherosclerotic renal artery stenosis: to treat conservatively, to dilate, to stent, or to operate? J Am Soc Nephrol 2001; 12: 2190–6.
3. Scoble JE. Atherosclerotic nephropathy. Kidney Int 1999; 56: S106–9.
4. Maxwell MH, Bleifer KH, Franklin SS, Varady PO. Cooperative study of renovascular hypertension. Demographic analysis of the study. J Am Med Assoc 1972; 220: 1195–204.
5. Hillman BJ. Imaging advances in the diagnosis of renovascular hypertension. AJR 1989; 153: 5–14.
6. Verschuyl EJ, Kaatee R, Beek FJA et al. Renal artery origins: location and distribution in the transverse plane at CT. Radiology 1997; 203: 71–5.
7. Beregi JP, Mauroy B, Willoteaux S et al. Anatomic variation in the origin of the main renal arteries: spiral CTA evaluation. Eur Radiol 1999; 9: 1330–4.
8. Kohler TR, Zierler RE, Martin RL et al. Noninvasive diagnosis of renal artery stenosis by ultrasonic duplex scanning. J Vasc Surg 1986; 4: 450–6.
9. Taylor DC, Kettler MD, Moneta GL et al. Duplex ultrasound scanning in the diagnosis of renal artery stenosis: A prospective evaluation. J Vasc Surg 1988; 7: 363–9.
10. Hélénon O, El Rody F, Correas JM et al. Color Doppler US

of renovascular disease in native kidneys. RadioGraphics 1995; 15: 833–54.

11. Hoffmann U, Edwards JM, Carter S et al. Role of duplex scanning for the detection of atherosclerotic renal artery disease. Kidney Int 1991; 39: 1232–9.

12. Strandness DE. Duplex imaging for the detection of renal artery stenosis. Am J Kidney Dis 1994; 24: 674–8.

13. Olin JW, Piedmonte MR, Young JR et al. The utility of duplex ultrasound scanning of the renal arteries for diagnosing significant renal artery stenosis. Ann Intern Med 1995; 122: 833–8.

14. Miralles M, Cairols M, Cotillas J et al. Value of Doppler parameters in the diagnosis of renal artery stenosis. J Vasc Surg 1996; 23: 428–35.

15. Claudon M, Plouin PF, Baxter G et al. Renal arteries in patients at risk of renal artery stenosis: multicenter evaluation of the echo enhancer SH508A at color and spectral Doppler US. Radiology 2000; 214: 739–46.

16. Hua HT, Hood DB, Jensen CC et al. The use of colorflow duplex scanning to detect significant renal artery stenosis. Ann Vasc Surg 2000; 14: 118–24.

17. Motew SJ, Cherr GS, Craven TE et al. Renal duplex sonography: main renal artery versus hilar analysis. J Vasc Surg 2000; 32: 462–9; 469–71.

18. De Cobelli F, Venturini M, Vanzulli A et al. Renal arterial stenosis: prospective comparison of color Doppler US and breath-hold, three-dimensional, dynamic, gadolinium-enhanced MR angiography. Radiology 2000; 214: 373–80.

19. de Haan MW, Kroon AA, Flobbe K et al. Renovascular disease in patients with hypertension: detection with duplex ultrasound. J Hum Hypertens 2002; 16: 501–7.

20. Napoli V, Pinto S, Bargellini I et al. Duplex ultrasonographic study of the renal arteries before and after renal artery stenting. Eur Radiol 2002; 12: 796–803.

21. Conkbayir I, Yucesoy C, Edguer T et al. Doppler sonography in renal artery stenosis. An evaluation of intrarenal and extrarenal imaging parameters. Clin Imaging 2003; 27: 256–60.

22. Nchimi A, Biquet JF, Brisbois D et al. Duplex ultrasound as first-line screening test for patients suspected of renal artery stenosis: prospective evaluation in high-risk group. Eur Radiol 2003; 13: 1413–19.

23. Berland LL, Koslin DB, Routh WD, Keller FS. Renal artery stenosis: Prospective evaluation of diagnosis with color duplex US compared with angiography. Radiology 1990; 174: 421–3.

24. Desberg AL, Paushter DM, Lammert GK et al. Renal artery stenosis: Evaluation with color Doppler flow imaging. Radiology 1990; 177: 749–53.

25. Stavros AT, Parker SH, Yakes WF et al. Segmental stenosis of the renal artery: Pattern recognition of tardus and parvus abnormalities with duplex sonography. Radiology 1992; 184: 487–92.

26. Patriquin HB, Lafortune M, Jequier JC et al. Stenosis of the renal artery: assessment of slowed systole in the downstream circulation with Doppler sonography. Radiology 1992; 184: 479–85.

27. Ozbek SS, Aytac SK, Erden MI, Sanlidilek NU. Intrarenal Doppler findings of upstream renal artery stenosis: A preliminary report. Ultrasound Med Biol 1993; 19: 3–12.

28. Halpern EJ, Needleman L, Nack TL, East SA. Renal artery stenosis: should we study the main renal artery or segmental vessels? Radiology 1995; 195: 799–804.

29. Schwerk WB, Restrepo IK, Stellwaag M et al. Renal artery stenosis: Grading with image-directed Doppler US evaluation of renal resistive index. Radiology 1994; 190: 785–90.

30. Kliewer MA, Tupler RH, Carroll BA et al. Renal artery stenosis: analysis of Doppler waveform parameters and tardus-parvus pattern. Radiology 1993; 189: 779–87.

31. Lafortune M, Patriquin HB, Demeule E et al. Renal arterial stenosis: slowed systole in the downstream circulation – experimental study in dogs. Radiology 1992; 184: 475–8.

32. Strunk H, Jaeger U. Duplex ultrasonographic diagnosis of renal artery stenosis by intrarenal acceleration determination and recognition of the tardus-parvus phenomenon with special regard to multiple renal arteries. Rofo Fortschr Geb Rontgenstr Neuen Bildgeb Verfahr 1995; 162: 420–8.

33. Baxter GM, Aitchison F, Sheppard D et al. Colour Doppler ultrasound in renal artery stenosis: intrarenal waveform analysis. Br J Radiol 1996; 69: 810–5.

34. Lucas P, Blome S, Roche J. Intra-renal Doppler wave-form analysis as a screening test for renal artery stenosis. Australas Radiol 1996; 40: 276–82.

35. Postma CT, Bijlstra PJ, Rosenbusch G, Thien T. Pattern recognition of loss of early systolic peak by Doppler ultrasound has a low sensitivity for the detection of renal artery stenosis. J Hum Hypertens 1996; 10: 181–4.

36. Oliva VL, Soulez G, Lesage D et al. Detection of renal artery stenosis with Doppler sonography before and after administration of captopril: Value of early systolic rise. AJR 1998; 170: 169–75.

37. Kliewer MA, Tupler RH, Hertzberg BS et al. Doppler evaluation of renal artery stenosis: interobserver agreement in the interpretation of waveform morphology. AJR 1994; 162: 1371–6.

38. Gottlieb RH, Snitzer EL, Hartley DF et al. Interobserver and intraobserver variation in determining intrarenal parameters by Doppler sonography. AJR 1997; 168: 627–31.

39. Van der Hulst VPM, Van Baalen J, Schultze Kool L et al. Renal artery stenosis: Endovascular flow wire study for validation of Doppler US. Radiology 1996; 200: 165–8.

40. Bude RO, Rubin JM, Platt JF et al. Pulsus tardus: its cause and potential limitations in detection of arterial stenosis. Radiology 1994; 190: 779–84.

41. Bude RO, Rubin JM. Detection of renal artery stenosis with Doppler sonography: It is more complicated than originally thought. Radiology 1995; 196: 612–13.

42. Goldberg BB, Liu JB, Forsberg F. Ultrasound contrast agents: A review. Ultrasound Med Biol 1994; 20: 319–33.

43. Burns PN, Powers JE, Simpson DH et al. Harmonic imaging principles and preliminary results. Angiology 1996; 47: S63–74.

44. René PC, Oliva VL, Bui BT et al. Renal artery stenosis: Evaluation of Doppler US after inhibition of angiotensin-converting enzyme with captopril. Radiology 1995; 196: 675–9.

45. Brink JA, Lim JT, Wang Ge et al. Technical optimization of spiral CT for depiction of renal artery stenosis: in vitro analysis. Radiology 1995; 194: 157–63.

46. Galanski M, Prokop M, Chavan A et al. Renal artery stenoses: spiral CT angiography. Radiology 1993; 189: 185–92.

47. Rubin GD, Dake MD, Napel S et al. Spiral CT of renal artery stenosis: comparison of three-dimensional rendering techniques. Radiology 1994; 190: 181–9.

48. Johnson PT, Halpern EJ, Kuszyk BS et al. Renal artery stenosis: CT angiography – comparison of real-time volume-rendering and maximum intensity projection algorithms. Radiology 1999; 211: 337–43.

49. Beregi JP, Elkohen M, Deklunder G et al. Helical CT angiography compared with arteriography in the detection of renal artery stenosis. AJR 1996; 167: 495–501.

50. Kaatee R, Beek FJA, de Lange EE et al. Renal artery stenosis: Detection and quantification with spiral CT angiography versus optimized digital subtraction angiography. Radiology 1997; 205: 121–7.

51. Wittenberg G, Kenn W, Tschammler A et al. Spiral CT angiography of renal arteries: comparison with angiography. Eur Radiol 1999; 9: 546–51.

52. Van Hoe L, Vandermeulen D, Gryspeerdt S et al. Assessment of accuracy of renal artery stenosis grading in helical CT angiography using maximum intensity projections. Eur Radiol 1996; 6: 658–64.

53. Kaatee R, Beek FJA, Verschuyl EJ et al. Renal artery stenosis: Detection and quantification with spiral CT angiography versus optimized digital subtraction angiography. Radiology 1996; 199: 637–640.

54. Beregi JP, Louvegny S, Gautier C et al. Fibromuscular dysplasia of the renal arteries: Comparison of helical CT angiography and arteriography. AJR 1999; 172: 27–34.

55. Fleischmann D. Multiple detector-row CT angiography of the renal and mesenteric vessels. Eur J Radiol 2003; 45: S79–S87.

56. Debatin JF, Spritzer CE, Grist TM et al. Imaging of the renal arteries: value of MR angiography. AJR 1991; 157: 981–90.

57. Richter CS, Krestin GP, Eichenberger AC et al. Assessment of renal artery stenosis by phase-contrast magnetic resonance angiography. Eur Radiol 1993; 3: 493–8.

58. Loubeyre P, Revel D, Garcia P et al. Screening patients for renal artery stenosis: value of three-dimensional time-of-flight MR angiography. AJR 1995; 162: 847–52.

59. Fellner C, Strotzer M, Geissler A et al. Renal arteries: evaluation with optimized 2D and 3D time-of-flight MR angiography. Radiology 1995; 196: 681–7.

60. Borrello JA, Li D, Vesely TM et al. Renal arteries: Clinical comparison of three-dimensional time of flight MR angiographic sequences and radiographic angiography. Radiology 1995; 197: 793–9.

61. Gedroyc WMW, Neerhut P, Negus R et al. Magnetic resonance angiography of renal artery stenosis. Clin Radiol 1995; 50: 436–9.

62. De Cobelli F, Mellone R, Salvioni M et al. Renal artery stenosis: Value of screening with three-dimensional phase-contrast MR angiography with a phased-array multicoil. Radiology 1996; 201: 697–703.

63. De Haan MW, Kouwenhoven M, Thelissen GRP et al. Renovascular disease in patients with hypertension: detection with systolic and diastolic gating in three-dimensional, phase-contrast MR angiography. Radiology 1996; 198: 449–56.

64. Loubeyre P, Trolliet P, Cahen R et al. MR angiography of renal artery stenosis: Value of the combination of three-dimensional time-of-flight and three-dimensional phase-contrast MR angiography sequences. AJR 1996; 167: 489–94.

65. Wasser MN, Westenberg J, Van der Hulst VPM et al. Hemodynamic significance of renal artery stenosis: Digital subtraction angiography versus systolically gated three-dimensional phase-contrast MR angiography. Radiology 1997; 202: 333–8.

66. Prince MR, Narasimhan DL, Stanley JC et al. Breath-hold Gadolinium-enhanced MR angiography of the abdominal aorta and its major branches. Radiology 1995; 197: 785–92.

67. Wilman AH, Riederer SJ, King BF et al. Fluoroscopically triggered contrast-enhanced three-dimensional MR angiography with elliptical centric view order: Application to the renal arteries. Radiology 1997; 205: 137–46.

68. Snidow JJ, Johnson MS, Harris VJ et al. Three-dimensional Gadolinium-enhanced MR angiography for aortoiliac inflow assessment plus renal artery screening in a single breath hold. Radiology 1996; 198: 725–32.

69. Rieumont MJ, Kaufman JA, Geller SC et al. Evaluation of renal artery stenosis with dynamic gadolinium-enhanced MR angiography. AJR 1997; 169: 39–44.

70. Hany TF, Debatin JF, Leung DA, Pfammatter T. Evaluation of the aortoiliac and renal arteries: Comparison of breath-hold, contrast-enhanced, three-dimensional MR angiography with conventional catheter angiography. Radiology 1997; 204: 357–62.

71. De Cobelli F, Vanzulli A, Sironi S et al. Renal artery stenosis: evaluation with breath-hold, three-dimensional, dynamic, gadolinium-enhanced versus three-dimensional, phase-contrast MR angiography. Radiology 1997; 205: 689–95.

72. Tello R, Thomson KR, Witte D et al. Standard dose Gd-DTPA dynamic MR of renal arteries. JMRI 1998; 8: 421–6.

73. Bakker J, Beek FJA, Beutler JJ et al. Renal artery stenosis and accessory renal arteries: accuracy of detection and visualization with gadolinium-enhanced breath-hold MR angiography. Radiology 1998; 207: 497–504.

74. Thornton J, O'Callaghan J, Walshe J et al. Comparison of digital subtraction angiography with gadolinium-enhanced magnetic resonance angiography in the diagnosis of renal artery stenosis. Eur Radiol 1999; 9: 930–4.

75. Völk M, Strotzer M, Lenhart M et al. Time-resolved contrast-enhanced MR angiography of renal artery stenosis: diagnostic accuracy and interobserver variability, AJR 2000; 174: 1583–8.

76. Korst MB, Joosten FB, Postma CT et al. Accuracy of normal-dose contrast-enhanced MR angiography in assessing renal artery stenosis and accessory renal arteries. AJR 2000; 174: 629–34.

77. Fain SB, King BF, Breen JF et al. High-spatial resolution contrast enhanced MR angiography of the renal arteries: a prospective comparison with digital subtraction angiography, Radiology 2001; 218: 481–90.

78. Wilman AH, Riederer SJ, King BF et al. Fluoroscopically triggered contrast-enhanced three-dimensional MR angiography with elliptical centric view order: application to the renal arteries. Radiology 1997; 205: 137–46.

79. Gilfeather M, Yoon HC, Siegelman ES et al. Renal artery stenosis: Evaluation with conventional angiography versus gadolinium-enhanced MR angiography. Radiology 1999; 210: 367–72.

80. Masunaga H, Takehara Y, Isoda H et al. Assessment of gadolinium-enhanced time-resolved three-dimensional MR angiography for evaluating renal artery stenosis, AJR 2001; 176: 1213–19.

81. Van Hoe L, De Jaegere T, Bosmans H et al. Breath-hold contrast-enhanced three-dimensional MR angiography of the abdomen: time-resolved imaging versus single-phase imaging, Radiology 2000; 214: 149–56.

82. Tan KT, Van Beek EJR, Brown PWG et al. Magnetic resonance angiography for the diagnosis of renal artery stenosis: a meta-analysis, Clin Radiol 2002; 57: 617–24.

83. Vasbinder GB, Nelemans PJ, Kessels AG et al. Diagnostic tests for renal artery stenosis in patients suspected of having renovascular hypertension: a meta-analysis. Ann Intern Med 2001 18; 135: 401–11.

84. Emamian SA, Bachmann Nielsen M, Pedersen JF, Ytte L. Kidney dimensions at sonography: Correlation with age, sex, and habitus in 665 adult volunteers, AJR 1993; 160: 83–6.

85. Zhang HL, Schoenberg SO, Resnick LM, Prince MR. Diagnosis of renal artery stenosis: combining gadolinium-enhanced three-dimensional magnetic resonance angiography with functional magnetic resonance pulse sequences. Am J Hypertens 2003; 16: 1079–82.

86. Roger SD, Beale AM, Cattell WR, Webb JAW. What is the value of measuring renal parenchymal thickness before renal biopsy? Clin Radiol 1994; 49: 45–9.

87. Bakker J, Olree M, Kaatee R et al. Renal volume measurements: accuracy and repeatability of US compared with that of MR imaging. Radiology 1999; 211: 623–8.

88. Coulam CH, Bouley DM, Graham Sommer F. Measurement of renal volumes with contrast-enhanced MRI. JMRI 2000; 15: 174–9.

89. Mounier-Vehier C, Lions C, Devos P et al. Cortical thickness: an early morphological marker of atherosclerotic renal disease, Kidney Int 2002; 61: 591–8.

90. Mustert BR, Williams DM, Prince MR. In vitro model of arterial stenosis: correlation of MR signal dephasing and trans-stenotic pressure gradients. Magn Reson Imaging 1998; 16: 301–10.

91. Schoenberg SO, Knopp MV, Bock M et al. Combined morphologic and functional assessment of renal artery stenosis using gadolinium enhanced magnetic resonance imaging.

92. Schoenberg SO, Bock M, Kallinowski F, Just A. Correlation of hemodynamic impact and morphologic degree of renal artery stenosis in a canine model. J Am Soc Nephrol 2000; 11: 2190–8.

93. Schoenberg SO, Knopp MV, Londy F et al. Morphologic and functional magnetic resonance imaging of renal artery stenosis: a multireader tricenter study. J Am Soc Nephrol 2002; 13: 158–69.

94. Binkert CA, Debatin JF, Schneider E et al. Can MR measurement of renal artery flow and renal volume predict the outcome of percutaneous transluminal renal angioplasty? Cardiovasc Intervent Radiol 2001; 24: 233–9.

95. Radermacher J, Chavan A, Bleck J et al. Use of Doppler ultrasonography to predict the outcome of therapy for renal-artery stenosis. N Engl J Med 2001; 344: 410–417.

96. Grenier N, Trillaud H, Combe C et al. Diagnosis of renovascular hypertension with captopril-sensitized dynamic MR of the kidney: feasability and comparison with scintigraphy. AJR 1996; 166: 835–43.

97. Vallee JP, Lazeyras F, Khan HG, Terrier F. Absolute renal blood flow quantification by dynamic MRI and Gd-DTPA. Eur Radiol 2000; 10: 1245–52.

98. Schoenberg SO, Aumann S, Just A et al. Quantification of renal perfusion abnormalities using an intravascular contrast agent (part 2): results in animals and humans with renal artery stenosis. Magn Reson Med 2003; 49: 288–98.

99. Namimoto T, Yamashita Y, Mitsuzaki K et al. Measurement of the apparent diffusion coefficient in diffuse renal disease by diffusion-weighted echo-planar MR imaging. J Magn Reson Imaging 1999; 9: 832–7.

100. Juillard L, Lerman LO, Kruger DG et al. Blood oxygen level dependent measurement of acute intra-renal ischemia. Kidney Int 2004; 65: 944–50.

16 ACE inhibition renography in the evaluation of suspected renovascular hypertension

Andrew Taylor

Introduction

Goldblatt first demonstrated the link between renal artery stenosis (RAS) and persistent hypertension in 1934.[1] In this experimental work, he showed that hypertension could be induced by placement of a clip on the renal artery and he subsequently showed that the hypertension would subside after the clip was removed. While the presence of such curable hypertension has been proven in humans, the cause-and-effect relationship between renal artery stenosis and hypertension is more complex than originally suspected. Renal artery stenosis does not always result in hypertension; in fact, it is common in the ageing normotensive population and it is far more common than renovascular hypertension (RVH), whose classical definition is based on cure or amelioration of the hypertension after revascularization. Indeed, based on autopsy and arteriographic studies, up to 30–50% of normotensive patients can have moderate or even severe RAS with the prevalence increasing with age.[2-4] Moreover, RAS is often present as an incidental or secondary finding in hypertensive patients and does not represent the aetiology of the hypertension.[4] Consequently, even though renovascular disease is the most common cause of secondary hypertension,[5] it comes as no surprise that revascularization of an atherosclerotic renal artery stenosis (the commonest cause of renovascular disease) does not always result in amelioration or cure of the hypertension. Consequently, the clinical question still remains: Which hypertensive patients have a renal artery stenosis that, if corrected, will lead to cure or amelioration of the hypertension?

Renovascular hypertension (RVH) occurs in only 0.5–3% of the unselected hypertensive population but a careful clinical screening can significantly increase the prevalence of RVH to as high as 5–40%.[6-8] RAS correction is readily available as a result of the widespread use of percutaneous transluminal renal angioplasty (PTRA) and stenting, but correction of renal artery stenosis in unselected patients will ameliorate blood pressure in only 55–80% of hypertensive patients with an anatomical renal artery stenosis.[8-10] Moreover, angioplasty with or without stent placement has a complication rate of 10–20%; these complications include haematoma, pseudo-aneurysm, dissection, thrombosis, bleeding, atheroembolism, myocardial infarction, acute renal failure and infection and the incidence of a major complication has been reported to be as high as 10%.[11] This *complication rate* further underscores the need for optimized patient selection before revascularization.

Angiography is still considered to be the gold standard for diagnosing renal artery stenosis but it does not adequately assess the functional importance of the stenotic lesion. Moreover, angiography may also cause atheromatous embolization of the kidneys or renal impairment due to contrast nephrotoxicity.[13] Spiral computed tomography (CTA) and magnetic resonance angiography (MRA) are noninvasive imaging techniques that have high sensitivity and specificity for detecting renal artery stenosis[5,12] but these techniques are associated with higher costs than scintigraphy and spiral CT requires the use of potentially nephrotoxic contrast agents. MRA is not suitable for patients with claustrophobia, certain types of metallic implants and is relatively expensive. Duplex sonography has achieved excellent results in some centres but others have found it to be too time consuming, too operator dependent and too unreliable in obese individuals to be an efficient tool to screen hypertensive patients for RVH.

This introduction underscores the need for diagnostic procedures that can accurately select those hypertensive patients with RAS most likely to be cured or improved after revascularization. Angiotensin converting enzyme (ACE) inhibition renography in an appropriately screened hypertensive patient with preserved renal function can detect renovascular disease with a sensitivity and specificity in excess of 90%.[14] Several detailed reviews present the radionuclide approaches to the evaluation of the patient with suspected RVH and discuss the technical features of this diagnostic procedure.[15-18] The goal of this chapter is not to recapitulate those reviews but to address areas of controversy, focus on selected issues and suggest directions for future research.

Detection of a functionally significant renal artery stenosis

A functionally significant RAS decreases the perfusion pressure to the afferent arteriole resulting in a decrease in GFR and a decrease in sodium delivery to the distal tubule.[18] The decrease in pressure and reduction in distal tubule sodium delivery stimulate the juxtaglomerular apparatus to release renin which cleaves angiotensin I from angiotensinogen; angiotensin I is then converted to angiotensin II by angiotensin-converting enzyme. Angiotensin II is a potent vasoconstrictor and acts preferentially on the efferent glomerular arteriole. Constriction of the efferent arteriole raises the transglomerular pressure gradient and can maintain GFR even in the face of a moderate reduction in perfusion pressure resulting from a functionally significant renal artery stenosis.

ACE inhibitors have two important mechanisms of action. (1) ACE inhibitors block the conversion of angiotensin I to angiotensin II and thereby interfere with the angiotensin II constriction of the efferent arteriole. The reduction in GFR induced by ACE inhibition can be detected by renography. For ^{99m}Tc-diethyltriaminepenta-acetic acid (DTPA), the primary effect is a reduction in renal uptake secondary to the reduction in GFR. For tubular secreted tracers such as ^{99m}Tc-mercaptoacetyltriglycine (MAG3), the primary effect is retention of the tracer in the parenchyma due to the reduction in GFR and the resulting reduction in primitive urine flow in the proximal tubules. (2) ACE inhibitors also inhibit kininase II, a dipeptidylcarboxy-peptidase that inactivates bradykinin; bradykinin, a potent vasodilator, accumulates following ACE inhibition and causes selective efferent arteriolar dilation.[19-21] The vasodilatory effects of bradykinin on the efferent arteriole also contribute to the reduction in GFR and the development of an abnormal renogram curve in patients with RVH following ACE inhibition. This second mechanism is probably quite important since only 60% of angiotensin II is produced by ACE-dependent pathways in the human renal cortex and neither acute nor chronic ACE inhibition completely eliminates angiotensin II from the plasma.[22,23]

Should renovascular hypertension be treated medically?

In a recent study of the effect of angioplasty on hypertension in atherosclerotic RAS, van Jaarsveld et al. concluded that, 'angioplasty has little advantage over anti-hypertensive drug therapy'.[24] In an accompanying editorial, Ritz and Mann concluded, 'We are left with the question of whether renal angioplasty should be considered at all for the treatment of patients with atherosclerotic renal-artery stenosis. Clearly, the screening of all hypertensive patients for atherosclerotic renal-artery stenosis is no longer justified'.[25]

If these conclusions are valid, then the use of ACE inhibition renography to detect RVH is rarely justified. Similarly, the use of other noninvasive tests (CTA, MRA, duplex US) is seldom justified and angioplasty with or without stent placement is rarely appropriate. Since this interpretation is primarily based on the Scottish, French and Dutch studies,[24-27] it is useful to re-examine these studies with an emphasis on ACE inhibition renography.

The Scottish study

The Scottish study identified 135 eligible patients of whom 55 (44%) were randomized.[26] Entry criteria included atheromatous disease, a 50% stenosis in the affected vessel and a serum creatinine less or equal to 500 μmol/l (5.8 mg/dl). The randomization group included 28 with bilateral disease and 27 with unilateral disease. Mean serum creatinine in the six subgroups ranged from 138 μmol/l (1.6 mg/dl) to 182 μmol/l (2.1 mg/dl). These investigators concluded that, compared with medical therapy alone, *percutaneous renal angioplasty resulted in a modest improvement in systolic BP only in patients with bilateral disease*. Furthermore, 'No patient was "cured", renal function did not improve and intervention was accompanied by a significant complication rate.'[26] The authors concluded, 'Our data support the use of angioplasty in hypertensive renovascular disease as a reserve procedure for patients whose blood pressure cannot be controlled by medical therapy or for those whose renal function is deteriorating despite medical therapy rather than as a primary form of intervention'.[26]

These data could be interpreted differently. The entry criterion of a 50% or greater stenosis undoubtedly allowed some patients into the study who did not have a functionally significant stenosis and who did not have RVH. Moreover, many patients, even with unilateral stenosis, had an elevated serum creatinine; these patients, therefore, had bilateral renal disease and may well have had hypertension that was no longer renin dependent or essential hypertension with associated atheromatous renal artery stenosis rather than renal artery stenosis causing the hypertension. In conclusion, the randomization group almost certainly included a number of patients without RVH; consequently, the results were likely diluted and the effect of PTCA in RVH could not be appropriately assessed. The authors concluded, 'The selection of patients for intervention will continue to tax the skills of all clinicians involved'.[26] Perhaps if a distinction had been made between patients with and without azotemia (see below) and ACE inhibition renography had been used to guide intervention, the results would have been different (and the skills of clinicians not so severely taxed).

The French study

Entry criteria for the French study required a unilateral renal artery stenosis > 75% or > 60% if there was a lateralizing test (renal scintigraphy, IVP or renal vein renin). In addition to unilateral atherosclerotic RAS, the creatinine clearance was required to be greater than 0.83 ml/s (50 ml/min).[27] A total of 49 patients with a mean serum creatinine of 100 μmol/l (1.16 mg/dl) entered the study and were randomized to receive angioplasty or medical therapy. At 6 months, there was no significant difference in the mean blood pressures of the medically treated group and the angioplasty group. Analysed differently, angioplasty reduced by 60% the probability of requiring two or more drugs to control blood pressure at 6 months; however, it is important to note that the complication rate from angioplasty was 26% with one patient having a branch dissection that resulted in infarction of 30% of the kidney. The authors did not issue general recommendations but stated that the reduction in drug therapy resulting from angioplasty should be weighed against the risks of complications and restenosis for each individual patient.

The French study made an effort to select patients with RVH by selecting patients with unilateral RAS and a tighter stenosis than those selected for the Scottish study.[26,27] In contrast to the Scottish study, angioplasty reduced the likelihood of requiring two or more drugs to control hypertension in patients with unilateral disease and 26% (6/23) of patients achieved a normal blood pressure without drugs at the 6 month follow-up period versus 0% (0/25) in the Scottish study.[26,27] However, the fact that the entry criteria accepted patients with a creatinine clearance as low as 50 ml/min indicates that some of the patients in the study had bilateral disease and may have had essential hypertension with associated renal artery stenosis or nonrenin-dependent hypertension. Moreover, the authors of the French study also concluded, 'It is difficult to differentiate patients with primary hypertension associated with RAS from those having hypertension secondary to RAS, that is, renovascular hypertension.'[27] Nevertheless, the French study shows that as the selection criteria for detecting patients with RVH improve, the outcome (response to revascularization) also improves.

The Dutch study

The Dutch study, as indicated in the title of their paper, 'The effect of balloon angioplasty on hypertension in atherosclerotic renal-artery stenosis', only claims to evaluate patients with RAS but the results have been interpreted as applying to patients with RVH.[24,25] Hypertensive patients were selected for the study if the diastolic BP was greater than 95 mmHg despite treatment with two antihypertensive drugs or if the creatinine increased in patients receiving an ACE inhibitor. In addition, at least one renal artery was required to have a stenosis of 50% and the patient's serum creatinine had to be <200 μmol/l (2.3 mg/dl). Based on the selection criteria, it would be expected that a substantial number of patients would have essential hypertension with associated RAS and not RVH. This interpretation is confirmed by the results of renal scintigraphy where one third of patients had a normal captopril scan. It is not surprising that these patients would not show BP improvement since they were unlikely to have RVH. Second, intermediate probability scans were given equal treatment as positive scans. Intermediate probability scans do not have a high predictive value for angioplasty success and combining these scans with high-probability scans reduces the specificity.[15,17,28] In spite of this bias, abnormal renal scans decreased from 65% in the preangioplasty group to 36% at 3 months following angioplasty compared to a change of 65% to 70% in the drug therapy group suggesting that a subset of angioplasty patients may have received substantial benefit; it would be interesting to know the BP response in this selected group of patients.

In conclusion, RAS increases in frequency in the ageing population[1] and RAS may occur in the nonhypertensive patients or be a nonaetiologic finding in a patient with hypertension. The clinical question is not whether or not a patient has RAS but whether or not the patient has RVH that will improve with revascularization. These three major studies illustrate the difficulty of selecting hypertensive patients with RVH using clinical data and anatomic screening and point to the need of a functional test such as ACE inhibition renography to determine the physiological significance of the stenosis.

Factors affecting the performance and/or the perceived performance of ACE inhibition renography

Several factors affecting the performance and/or the perceived performance of ACE inhibition renography need to be emphasized. They are listed below and then individually addressed.

1. Use of the anatomic presence of a renal artery stenosis, often as low as 50%, as a surrogate for renovascular hypertension.
2. Inconsistent use of recommended criteria for interpreting ACE inhibition renograms.
3. Failure to recognize the differences in the performance of ACE inhibition in azotemic and nonazotemic populations and to distinguish between results obtained in these different population.
4. The 'intermediate probability' or indeterminate scan.
5. Performance of the examination.

Use of the anatomic presence of a renal artery stenosis, often as low as 50%, as a surrogate for renovascular hypertension

In the evaluation of ACE inhibition renography, it is essential to keep in mind that *ACE inhibition renography is a test to detect a functionally significant renal artery stenosis, not a test to detect the presence of a renal artery stenosis.*[12,15] Nevertheless, as summarized in several reviews, many investigators have used the angiographic presence of a renal artery stenosis >50% RAS as the gold standard to make the diagnosis of RVH in spite of the fact that many of these stenotic lesions will not be haemodynamically significant.[7,18,29,30] In an attempt to circumvent this problem, other investigators have used the more stringent standard of >70% stenosis. Not surprisingly, however, the sensitivity and specificity of ACEI renography is improved when the gold standard is the response to revascularization rather than the anatomic presence of RAS.[31,32] Although consensus panels have recommended that the gold standard be response to revascularization, the presence of RAS continues to be used as a gold standard.[15,17,25,33] In view of the fact that RAS is not equivalent to RVH, the failure to use an appropriate gold standard adds to the difficulty of objectively appraising the literature.

Inconsistent use of recommended criteria for interpreting ACE inhibition renograms

In a recent meta-analysis evaluating the use of ACE inhibition renography to detect RVH, Boudewijn et a.l note a wide variation in results reported by different centres and attribute part of this variability to 'the lack of standard criteria to define a positive test result.'[34] Although most of the studies in the meta-analysis were published prior to 1996,[34] it is important to note that interpretative criteria for ACE inhibition renography have been developed and were published as an international consensus report in 1996.[15] These consensus RVH guidelines and interpretative criteria have been subsequently updated by the Society of Nuclear Medicine, published on the Society's website[17] and are summarized below. While it may be possible to improve on these criteria, future studies of ACE inhibition for the detection of RVH should include an analysis using these criteria to allow better comparisons between centres.

Low probability

A normal ACE inhibition renogram with normal indices (relative function, time to peak height of the renogram curve, 20 min/max count ratios) or Grade 2 renogram which is

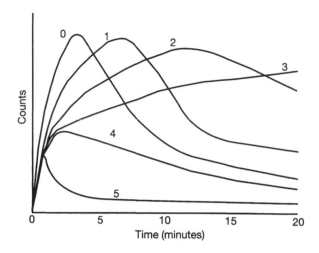

Figure 16.1 Common renogram patterns used for the visual interpretation of ACEI renography. Type 0: Normal. Type 1: Time to peak (T_{max}) is > 5 minutes and 20 min/max count ratio is > 0.3 for background subtracted OIH and MAG3 curves. Type 2: There are more exaggerated delays in time to peak and in parenchymal washout. Type 3: Progressive parenchymal accumulation (no washout detected). Type 4: Renal failure pattern, but with measurable renal uptake. Type 5: Renal failure pattern, representing blood background activity only.

unchanged or improves following ACE inhibition (Figures 16.1 and 16.2).

Intermediate (indeterminate) probability

Small or poorly functioning kidney (kidney with less than 30% of the relative function) or kidneys with abnormal baseline renograms (Grades 3–5) which are unchanged following ACE inhibition (Figures 16.1 and 16.3).

High probability

Unilateral deterioration of the renogram curve and/or of the relative function following ACE inhibition compared to the baseline study (Figure 16.4).

Tc-99m DTPA

The principal diagnostic criterion for the GFR tracer, DTPA, is a change in the relative uptake. A reduction in the relative uptake greater than 10 percentage points (50/50 to 60/40) is a highly significant change and 5–9 percentage points is considered to be an intermediate response although studies performed under carefully controlled conditions suggest that smaller changes in relative uptake may be significant. Parenchymal retention following ACE inhibition can also be

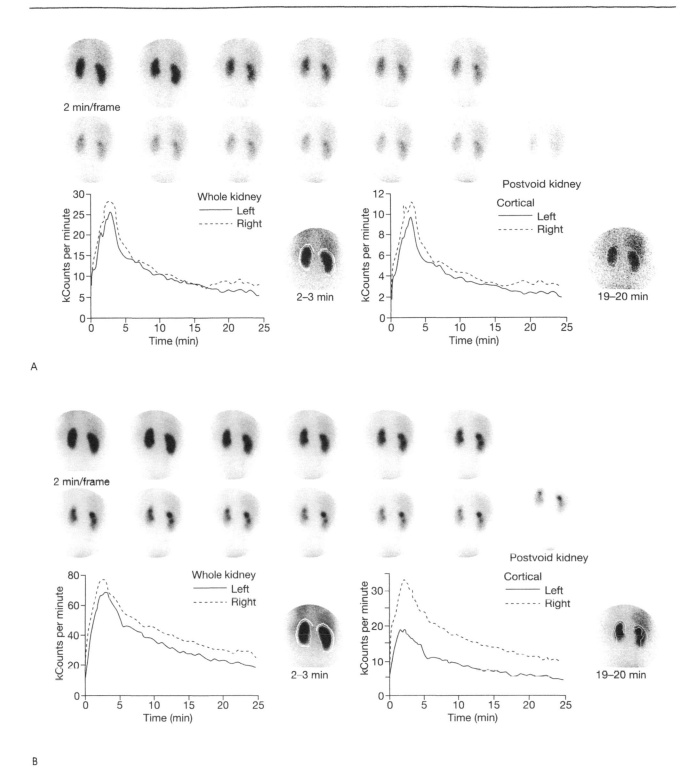

Figure 16.2 A 53-year-old male with poorly controlled hypertension was referred for ACE inhibition renography. A: The baseline study was performed following the intravenous injection of 1.53 mCi (57 MBq). The 2-minute sequential images and whole kidney and cortical renogram curves are normal with the time to peak counts less than 5 minutes and the 20 minute to maximum count ratio <0.3. The relative uptake was 54% in the right kidney and 46% in the left kidney. The MAG3 clearance (not shown) was also normal. B: Following the intravenous administration of 2.5 mg of enalaprilat, the study was repeated with 10.3 mCi (381 MBq) of MAG3. The relative uptake and configuration of the renogram curves were essentially unchanged. A normal study that remains normal following ACE inhibition is low probability for renovascular hypertension.

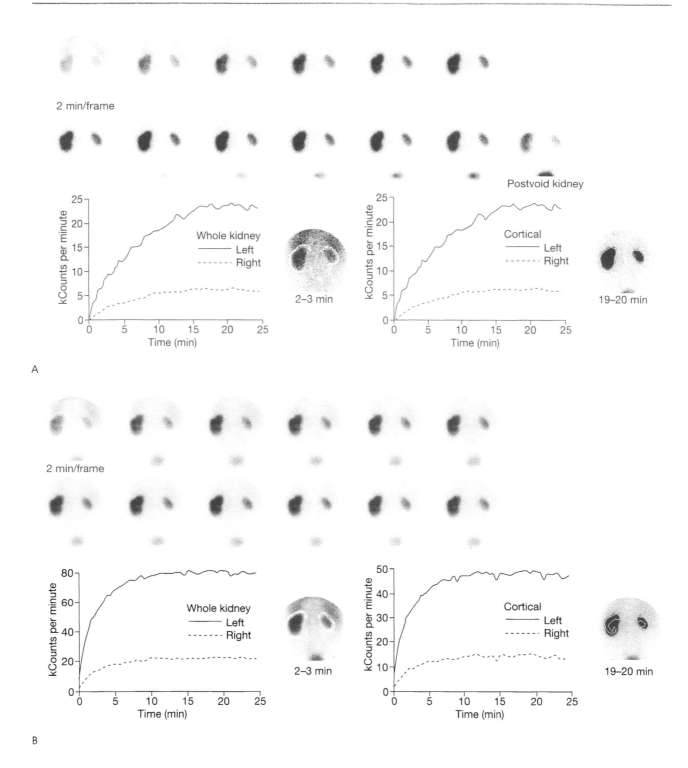

Figure 16.3 A 73-year-old hypertensive male with biventricular heart failure and an elevated serum creatinine was referred for ACE inhibition renography. A: The baseline study was performed following the intravenous injection of 1.54 mCi (57 MBq). The 2-minute sequential images and whole kidney and cortical renogram curves show bilateral type 3 rising renogram curves (Figure 16.1). The relative uptake was 80% in the right kidney and 20% in the left kidney. The MAG3 clearance (not shown) was reduced. B: Following the intravenous administration of 2.5 mg of enalaprilat, the study was repeated with 9.81 mCi (363 MBq) of MAG3. The relative uptake and configuration of the renogram curves were essentially unchanged. This pattern is an intermediate (indeterminate) probability of renovascular hypertension and occurs in as many as 50% of patients with renal failure.

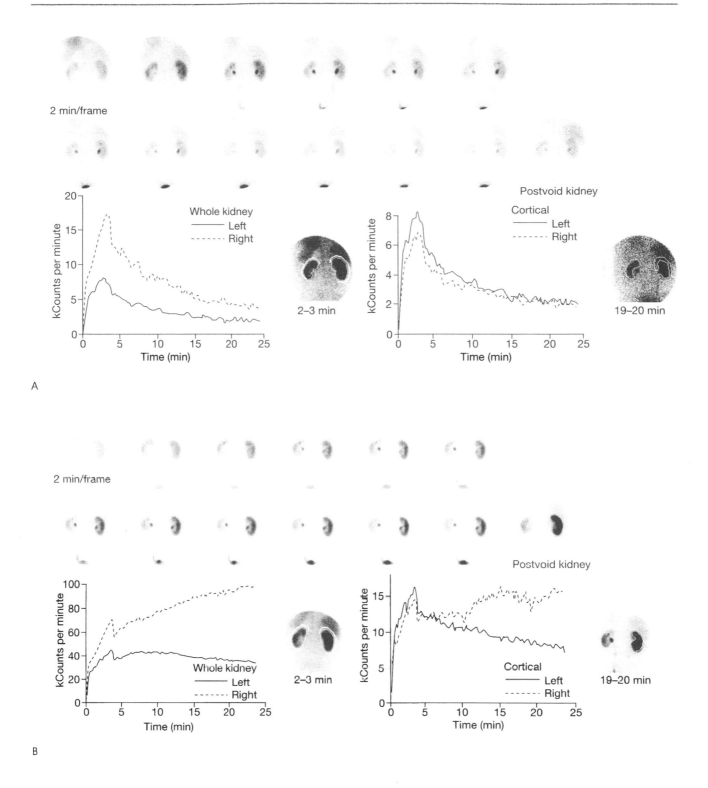

Figure 16.4 A 66-year-old hypertensive male with coronary artery disease, peripheral vascular disease and renal insufficiency was referred for ACEI renography. A: The patient received 2.2 mCi (81 MBq) of MAG3 and data were acquired for 24 minutes. The MAG3 clearance (not shown) was reduced; relative uptake was 65% in the right kidney and 35% in the left kidney. Two minute sequential images and the whole kidney and cortical renogram curves show normal time to peak counts and normal 20 minute to maximum count ratios. B: Following the intravenous administration of 2.5 mg of enalaprilat, the study was repeated with 7.2 mCi (252 MBq) of MAG3. The MAG3 clearance and relative uptake were unchanged but the time to peak counts for the left kidney has increased to 7.2 minutes and the 20 minute to maximum count ratio has increased to 0.79. The renogram curve for the right kidney has become markedly abnormal with a persistent rising renogram curve (Grade 3, Figure 16.1). The unilateral pattern shift from Grade 1 to Grade 3 is characteristic of renovascular hypertension and is highly specific even in patients with impaired renal function.

an important diagnostic finding and can be quantitated by a delay in the time to peak or an increase in the 20–30 min/max ratios although, in general, changes have to be much more pronounced than with ^{99m}Tc MAG3 and I-131 or I-123 orthoiodohippurate (OIH) to be significant due to the slower clearance of DTPA compared with the tubular agents.

MAG3/OIH

An increase in the 20 min/max ratio of 0.15 or greater for parenchymal ROIs represents the 90% confidence limit for a significant change. A prolongation of the time to peak of 120 seconds for a cortical ROI is significant at the 90–95% confidence limit. It is important to note, however, that a change from 5 to 7 minutes is much more significant that a change from 15 to 17 minutes and, for this reason, consensus panels recommend an increase of 2 minutes or 40% of the baseline value before the change is considered to be significant. Renograms derived from the cortical ROIs (parenchymal ROIs that avoid activity in the collecting system) may help avoid error or the diagnostic difficulty that can be introduced when there is retention of the tracer in the collecting system. A change in the relative uptake of MAG3 or OIH by 10 percentage points (50/50 to 40/60) is uncommon even in a patient with RVH but it is highly significant when it occurs. Smaller changes may have diagnostic significance but they should be accompanied by confirmatory changes in the shape of the renogram curve or increases in the T_{max} or 20–30 min/max ratio. In regard to qualitative criteria, most experts accept a change in one grade as a positive response (Figure 16.1).

Failure to recognize the differences in the performance of ACE inhibition renography in azotemic and nonazotemic populations and to distinguish between results obtained in these different populations

Excellent results have been obtained in patients with normal or near normal renal function with sensitivities around 90% and specificity ranging from 90–100%,[28,35–37] Although good results have been reported in azotemic patients,[38–40] most investigators have found ACE inhibition renography to be less accurate in patients with azotemic renovascular disease.[15,17,18,28,16,35,36] While a positive test result in a patient with azotemia or in a patient with a small, poorly functioning kidney indicates a high likelihood that the hypertension will be ameliorated by revascularization, as many as 50% of patients in this population may have an intermediate probability test result.[28] In a recent prospective study using simultaneous DTPA and OIH renography in 60 patients with a high prevalence of a renal artery stenosis greater than 50%, Blaufox et al observed that about

50% of baseline renograms were abnormal and were unchanged after ACEI challenge (i.e., nondiagnostic or intermediate probability).[28] Twenty-seven of these 29 nondiagnostic tests were associated with a GFR lower than 50 ml/min ($n = 17$), one small kidney ($n = 17$) and/or bilateral RAS ($n = 16$). The authors concluded that, in the azotemic population, a high probability scan indicates that hypertension is very likely to improve after revascularization. However, the sensitivity of ACE inhibition renography is diminished to about 80% in the azotemic population even when nondiagnostic/intermediate probability scans are combined with high probability scans. False negative results appear to be more likely in azotemic patients with bilateral disease, probably due to suppression of the renin-angiotensin system.[18,28,41]

The 'intermediate probability' or indeterminate scan

The recommendation that the studies be interpreted as high, intermediate and low probability for renovascular disease has resulted in a problem in reporting sensitivities and specificities determined from a 2×2 table. Intermediate probability scans have to be reclassified to be incorporated into a binary scoring system since an intermediate or indeterminate result is neither positive nor negative. If intermediate probability results are included with the positive studies, sensitivity will be increased at the expense of specificity; if intermediate probability studies are considered negative, specificity will be improved at the expense of sensitivity. Alternatively, intermediate probability studies can simply be counted as incorrect or they can be omitted from the data analysis. The reported values for sensitivity and specificity will vary depending on the frequency of intermediate probability studies in the study population and how these results are handled in the data analysis. As emphasized above, intermediate probability scans are uncommon in patients with normal or near normal renal function but they occur in patients with a unilateral small kidney and/or azotemia.[17,28,35]

Performance of the examination

Recommended protocols for performance of ACE inhibition renography as well as recommended methods for calculating the quantitative variables have been well described[17,18,42] but several points should be emphasized.

Blood pressure must be monitored

Asymptomatic hypotension secondary to ACE inhibition can result in bilateral symmetrical abnormalities in the renogram curves (Figure 16.5).[43–45] This phenomenon is relatively

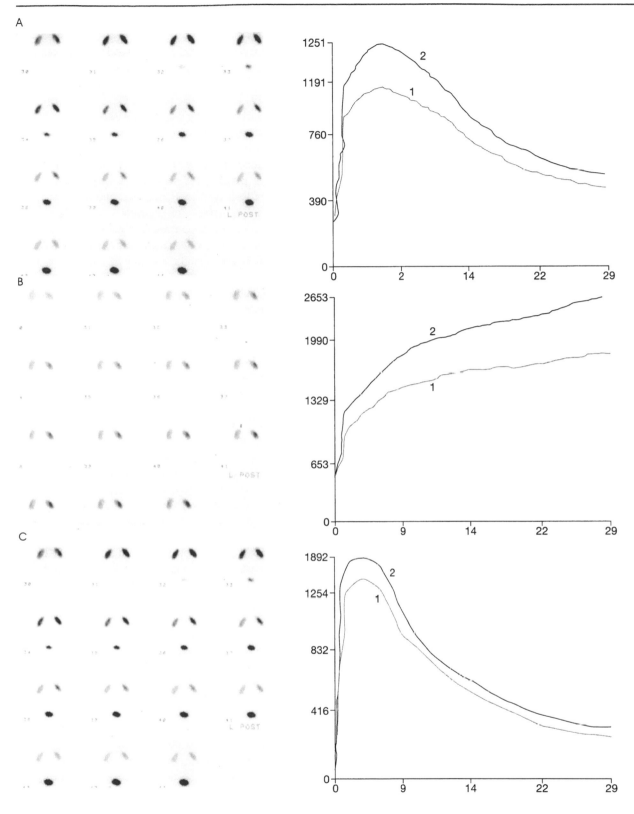

Figure 16.5 A middle-age male with refractory hypertension was referred for ACE inhibition renography. A: Sequential 2-minute images and whole-kidney renogram curves were obtained following a baseline injection of approximately 1.0 (37 MBq) of MAG3. B: The patient received 50 mg of captopril and 10 mCi (370 MBq) were injected an hour later. The 2-minute images demonstrate parenchymal retention with bilateral rising whole-kidney renogram curves. Usually, renovascular hypertension produces asymmetrical abnormalities. On further review, the patient's precaptopril blood pressure was 165/71 but it fell to 102/41 during the study even though the patient remained asymptomatic. C: Several days later the study was repeated with 50 mg of captopril and intravenous hydration to maintain blood pressure. The 2-minute sequential images and renogram curves are normal. Bilateral symmetrical abnormalities following ACE inhibition are a nonspecific finding and are often due to volume depletion and hypotension.[43–45]

uncommon but may occur in as many as 3% of patients referred for ACEI renography, usually in patients who are volume or salt depleted.[43] ACE inhibitors can also cause a major hypotensive episode, although the prevalence appears to be quite low in a well-hydrated patient. Some centres establish an intravenous line before scintigraphy; this precaution is important for high-risk patients, who include patients with angina, recent myocardial infarction, a history of transient ischaemic attacks, recent stroke and patients receiving enalaprilat or furosemide.

ACE inhibitors and angiotensin II receptor blockers (ARBs)

The majority of ACE inhibition studies have been performed with captopril but enalaprilat is an acceptable alternative.[17,29,38] Limited data suggest that chronic ACE inhibition may reduce the sensitivity of the test[40,46] and the consensus recommendation is to discontinue captopril for 4 days prior to the study and discontinue the longer half-life ACE inhibitors for 7 days.[17] Because ARBs also block the vasoconstrictive effect of angiotensin II on the efferent vessels in patients with RVH, it was thought that the sensitivity of the ACE inhibition renography might be reduced in patients receiving angiotensin receptor blockers but it is probably not necessary to discontinue this class of drugs. Captopril renograms were obtained in 26 patients with normal or near normal renal function who were receiving angiotensin II receptor blockers; in this patient population, the sensitivity of ACE inhibition renography for renovascular hypertension was 92% and specificity was 100%, values comparable to those obtained in patients not taking angiotensin II receptor blockers.[47] Finally, a recent study showed that ARB renography is considerably less sensitive than captopril renography for detecting RAS in hypertensive patients or for detecting RVH.[20] The superiority of ACE inhibitors over the ARBs in detecting renovascular hypertension probably derives from the action of ACE inhibitors on kininase II (see above).

Sensitivity/specificity of ACE inhibition renography and diagnostic strategy

ACE inhibition renography has recently been criticized for having sensitivities and specificities that are too low compared to other diagnostic options;[33,34] however, the study by Huot et al and the meta-analysis of Boudewijn et al base their conclusions on data using RAS, not RVH, as the end point.[33,34] In spite of the problems of inconsistent interpretative criteria and the problem of the indeterminate scan, *ACE inhibition renography has performed reasonably well even when the gold standard is RAS.* Most of the studies evaluating the performance of ACE inhibition renography in either the detection of RAS and/or RVH (i.e., prediction of blood pressure outcome after revascularization) have been summarized in comprehensive reviews.[7,17,18,29,30] In a recent review of 12 studies including 2291 hypertensive patients, the overall mean sensitivity and specificity for the detection of RAS were 92.5% and 92.2%, respectively, although the sensitivity may have been artifactually elevated since not all patients underwent angiography.[29] In another review of 17 studies involving about 3000 hypertensive patients, the sensitivity and specificity for the detection of RAS (with only two exceptions) ranged from 83–100% and 62–100%, respectively.[18] Using the criterion of ACEI-induced changes between baseline and ACEI renography to define a positive test, most studies show that the test has a specificity ≥90% and consequently the test has a high positive predictive value.[18,29,30] Finally, in a separate analysis of ten studies published between 1987 and 1998, the mean positive predictive value of ACEI-induced changes between baseline and ACEI renography for predicting improvement or cure of hypertension in 291 patients undergoing revascularization was 92%.[29]

It is important to note that in the two reviews published in 2000,[29,30] in a population where RAS prevalence varies between 20–65%, the positive and negative predictive values of ACEI-renography in the detection of RAS were the same, 90% and 95%, respectively. In these series, the average prevalence of RAS was about 50%; however, even when RAS prevalence is only about 5%, as reported in two large studies containing 667 and 450 hypertensive patients respectively, the sensitivity and specificity remain high, i.e., 90–100% for sensitivity and 94–95% for specificity,[48,49] Helin et al reported a clinically relevant prevalence of RVH of 12% in 173 patients with no obvious renal parenchymal disease and unresponsive to two antihypertensive drugs and showed that ACEI renography was cost effective in this population.[49]

Technologies are evolving and multiple diagnostic imaging strategies have been proposed; four recent reviews[8,29,30,50] recommended strategies incorporating renal scintigraphy but, to date, there is no generally accepted approach. Costs need to be considered in determining the clinical approach but a cost analysis is a moving target. Costs are often hard to ascertain and costs and technologies continue to evolve. Nevertheless, a recent study showed that the diagnostic strategy of first evaluating patients with CTA or MRA is less cost-effective than the use of ACEI renography as the first test in patients with normal or near normal serum creatinine and without a small poorly functioning kidney.[51] Nelemans et al subsequently assessed eight strategies for the diagnosis of RVH followed by treatment with percutaneous transluminal angioplasty with or without stent placement and concluded that computed tomography angiography followed by angiography was less cost-effective (although more effective) than ACEI renography followed by angiography.[52]

A common clinical approach in some areas of the United States is to perform MRA or CTA followed by angioplasty with stent placement. Based on current Medicare reimburse-

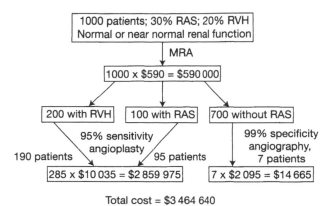

Total cost = $3 464 640

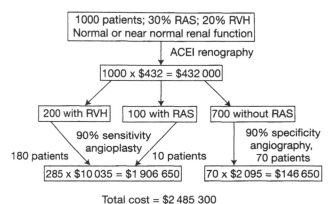

Total cost = $2 485 300

Figure 16.6 Based on Medicare Part B and DRG reimbursement rates (see text), the strategy of MRA followed by angioplasty and stent placement to diagnose and treat 1000 patients with a 30% prevalence of RAS (20% prevalence of RVH) will miss ten patients with RVH and cost $3 464 640.

Figure 16.7 Based on Medicare Part B and DRG reimbursement rates (see text), the strategy of ^{99m}Tc MAG3 renography followed by angioplasty and stent placement to diagnose and treat 1000 patients with a 30% prevalence of RAS (20% prevalence of RVH) will miss 20 patients with RVH and cost $2 485 300.

ment rates, this approach is not cost effective in hypertensive patients suspected of having RVH who have normal to near normal renal function (Figures 16.6 and 16.7). For example, assuming an extra $50 to cover the cost of the contrast media and $180 to cover the cost of ^{99m}Tc MAG3 for the baseline and ACE inhibition studies, the 2005 Medicare Part B reimbursement rates (RVU or relative value units) unadjusted for geography are $2095 for renal angiography, $590 for MRA, $619 for CTA and $432 for ACE inhibition renography. It is important to note that the cost estimate for ACE inhibition renography is actually conservative since many institutions begin with the ACE inhibition renogram; if it is negative, the baseline study is not performed and cost of the MAG3 can be reduced. Moreover, if ^{99m}Tc DTPA were used, the cost estimates for the ACE inhibition renogram would be further reduced. The cost for renal angioplasty with or without stent placement can best be estimated from the DRG (diagnostic related grouping) payment. The DRG payment is all-inclusive and is the average payment for the entire hospital stay for a particular procedure. Assuming no complications, the DRG reimbursement for a renal angioplasty with stent placement is $10 035. These procedure reimbursements from Medicare were used for the simplified cost analysis supplied in Figures 16.6 and 16.7.

The prevalence of RAS in the unselected hypertensive population varies from 0.5–3%; but ranges from 20–50% in selected populations.[12,30] If a population of 1000 patients with normal to near normal renal function has a 30% prevalence of RAS and a 20% prevalence of RVH and they are first screened with MRA, assuming 95% sensitivity and 99% specificity,[13] then 285 patients with RAS will be identified (Figure 16.6). If angioplasty and stent placement is then performed in these patients, the total cost (MRA, angiography and angioplasty with stent placement), will be $3 464 640 (Figure 16.6). Since the reimbursement for CTA is higher

than that for MRA, a strategy of CTA followed by angioplasty would result in an even higher cost than that of MRA followed by angioplasty. This analysis underestimates the actual cost since the DRG reimbursement assumes no complications while the actual complication rate may be as high as 20%.[11]

In contrast, the cost will be $2 485 300 if these 1000 patients are first screened with ACE inhibition renography, assuming a sensitivity and specificity of only 90% (Figure 16.7). Seventy patients without RAS would have false-positive studies and would be sent for angiography. Ten of the 100 patients with RAS who did not have RVH would have false-positive studies and would be sent for revascularization and 180 patients with RVH would be sent for angioplasty and stent placement (Figure 16.7). This figure translates into a saving of about $4500 per patient with RVH; moreover, the approach is conservative since the specificity for ACE inhibition renography in this patient population is probably higher than 90%. This strategy would miss 20 patients with RVH compared to ten patients with MRA but these patients would be managed with medical therapy. If the hypertension could not be controlled, CTA, MRA, Doppler ultrasound or ACE inhibition renography would likely be obtained depending on circumstances. Depending on the prevalence of disease and the value used for the specificity of ACE inhibition renography, obtaining a MRA in patients with a positive ACE inhibition scan would reduce the number of angioplasties but would slightly increase the total cost.

Based on these considerations, a cost-effective approach would be to classify hypertensive patients at moderate to high risk for RVH into those with a normal or near normal serum creatinine and those with significant azotemia. Patients with a normal to near normal creatinine should first be evaluated with ACE inhibition renography (Figure 16.8). Those with impaired function may best be initially evaluated by MRA or Duplex sonography (Figure 16.8).

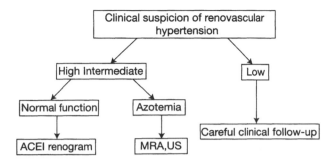

Figure 16.8   Flow chart outlining the initial management of hypertensive patients with suspected renovascular hypertension.

Future directions

Aspirin renography (alone or in combination with ACE inhibition renography) for the detection of RVH

Preliminary data suggest that aspirin renography may provide a sensitive test for renovascular hypertension comparable to that obtained with ACE inhibitors.[53,54] Administration of nonsteroidal anti-inflammatory agents such as aspirin inhibits prostaglandin synthesis and lead to a preglomerular vaso-contriction with a reduction in renal blood flow and GFR.[55] The reduction in renal blood flow and GFR caused by prostaglandin inhibitors appears to accentuate the effect of a functionally significant renal artery stenosis and allows detection by renography. Since the mechanisms of action differ, the combination of aspirin and an ACE inhibitor may result in a higher sensitivity and even further improve the predictive value of a negative test for excluding renovascular hypertension.

Use of ACE inhibition induced changes in total and individual kidney clearance measurements as additional diagnostic factors

In a recent study, the mean ^{99m}Tc MAG3 clearance increased from 221 to 239 ml/min in 20 patients with a low probability of RAS whereas in 22 patients with a RAS greater than or equal to 50%, the MAG3 clearance decreased from a mean of 233 to 186 ml/min.[56] If this observation is corroborated by future studies, it could provide an additional diagnostic aid for distinguishing between RAS and RVH.

Modification of the Santa Fe criteria for patients with a small unilateral kidney and azotemia

Fernandez et al studied 38 hypertensive patients with a mean baseline GFR of 35 ml/min with captopril renography.[39] The authors suggest modifying the Santa Fe consensus criteria so that a small unilateral kidney with a rising curve on baseline and captopril is considered a positive study and interpreting bilateral symmetrical rising curves before and after ACE inhibition as a negative study. Using these modified criteria, the test showed good performance for detection of RAS in renal failure patients with a sensitivity of 100%, specificity of 83%, positive predictive value of 64% and negative predictive value of 100%. There was also 100% sensitivity for predicting response to revascularization but the number of patients was low. Future studies should evaluate both the standard and modified criteria in patients with azotemia to determine if the modified criteria improve results.

Automated processing and interpretation of ACE inhibition renography

Criteria for the interpretation of ACE inhibition renography include time to peak height of the renogram curve, relative uptake and the 20 min/max count ratio. Measurement of DTPA and MAG3 clearances before and after ACE inhibition may also be useful in determining the presence or absence of RVH. Prigent et al have developed guidelines for extracting quantitative data from a radionuclide renal scan, camera-based techniques are available to estimate the MAG3 and DTPA (GFR) clearances and approaches are being developed to automatically assign kidney and background regions of interest.[42,57–60] Use of validated software to extract the relevant quantitative variables and apply the diagnostic criteria should minimize interobserver variability, facilitate the comparison of results between centres and provide a decision support system for physicians who are not expert in interpreting these studies.

Summary

Cost-effective patient management requires that the functional significance of the stenosis be determined before intervention.[12,61] ACEI renography is a sensitive, specific and cost-effective test for renovascular hypertension in patients with normal or near normal renal function; it is not a test for the detection of the presence or absence of renal artery stenosis. For this reason, it is essential to recognize that many of the conclusions drawn from the literature (1) do not distinguish between RVH and RAS and (2) do not distinguish between azotemic patients and those with a normal or near normal serum creatinine. When ACE inhibition renography is performed in patients with ischaemic nephropathy or a small poorly functioning kidney, as many as 50% of the studies may be indeterminate or intermediate probability. Finally, future studies may refine the test and lead to even higher values for sensitivity and specificity, particularly in patients with impaired renal function.

References

1. Goldblatt H, Lynch J, Hanzal RF, Summerville WW. Studies on experimental hypertension, 1, the production of persistent elevation of systolic blood pressure by means of renal ischemia. J Exp Med 1934; 59: 347–78.

2. Chen CC, Hoffer PB, Vahjen G et al. Patients at high risk for renal artery stenosis: a simple method of renal scintigraphic analysis with Tc-99m DTPA and captopril, Radiology 1990; 176: 365–70.

3. Dustan HP, Humphries AW, Dewolfe VG, Page IH. Normal arterial pressure in patients with renal arterial stenosis. JAMA 1964; 187: 1028–9.

4. Holley KE, Hunt JC, Brown AL Jr et al. Renal artery stenosis: a clinical-pathologic study in normotensive and hypertensive patients. Am J Med 1964; 37: 14–22.

5. Dawson DL. Noninvasive assessment of renal artery stenosis. Semin Vasc Surg 1996; 9: 172–81.

6. Working Group on Renovascular Hypertension. Detection, evaluation, and treatment of renovascular hypertension. Arch Intern Med 1987; 147: 820–9.

7. Prigent A. The diagnosis of renovascular hypertension: the role of captopril renal scintigraphy and related issues. Eur J Nucl Med 1993; 20: 625–44.

8. Bloch MJ, Basile J. The diagnosis and management of renovascular disease: a primary care perspective. J Clin Hypertens 2003; 5: 210–18.

9. Radermacher J, Haller H. The right diagnostic work-up: investigating renal and renovascular disorders. J Hypertens 2003; 21: S19–S24.

10. Meier GH, Sumpio B, Setaro JF et al. Captopril renal scintigraphy: a new standard for predicting outcome after renal revascularization. J Vasc Surg 1993; 17: 280–5; discussion 285–7.

11. Slonim SM, Dake MD. Radiographic evaluation and treatment of renovascular disease. In: Rutherford RB, ed. Vascular Surgery. Philadelphia, PA: WB Saunders Company; 2000; 1611–39.

12. Bloch MJ, Basile J. The diagnosis and management of renovascular disease: a primary care perspective. Part II. Issues in management. J Clin Hypertens 2003; 5: 261–8.

13. Willmann JK, Wildermuth S, Pfammatter T et al. Aortoiliac and renal arteries: prospective intraindividual comparison of contrast-enhanced three-dimensional MR angiography and multi-detector row CT angiography. Radiology 2003; 226: 798–811.

14. Barton D, Nally JV Jr. Provocative captopril testing in renovascular hypertension. Urol Clin N Am 2001; 28: 781–91.

15. Taylor A, Nally J, Aurell M et al. Consensus report on ACE inhibitor renography for detecting renovascular hypertension. Radionuclides in Nephrourology Group. Consensus Group on ACEI Renography. J Nucl Med 1996; 37: 1876–82.

16. Taylor A. Renovascular hypertension: nuclear medicine techniques. Q J Nucl Med 2002; 46: 268–82.

17. Taylor A, Blaufox MD, Dubovsky EV et al. Society of Nuclear Medicine procedure guideline for diagnosis of renovascular hypertension 3.0. Procedure guidelines, Policy and Practice, www.snm.org, 2003.

18. Prigent A, Taylor A. The role of ACE inhibitor renography in the diagnosis of renovascular hypertension, In: Henkin RE, Bova D, Dillehay GL et al, eds, Nuclear Medicine, 2nd edn. Elsiever, Philadelphia, PA 2005. In press.

19. Gainer JV, Morrow JD, Loveland A et al. Effect of bradykinin-receptor blockade on the response to angiotensin-converting-enzyme inhibitor in normotensive and hypertensive subjects. N Eng J Med 1998; 339: 1285–92.

20. Karanikas G, Becherer A, Wiesner K et al. ACE inhibition is superior to angiotensin receptor blockade for renography in renal artery stenosis, Eur J Nucl Med 2002; 29: 312–18.

21. Kon V, Fogo A, Ichikawa I et al. Bradykinin causes selective efferent arteriolar dilation during angiotensin I converting enzyme inhibition. Kidney International 1993; 44: 545–50.

22. Nussberger J, Brunner DB, Waeber B, Brunner HR. Plasma angiotensin under sustained converting enzyme inhibition with enalapril in normal humans. J Hypertension 1985; 3: S269–70.

23. Sandberg K, Hong J. Kidney angiotensin receptors and their role in renal pathophysiology. Semin Nephrol 2000; 20: 402–16.

24. van Jaarsveld BC, Krijnen P, Pieterman H et al. The effect of balloon angioplasty on hypertension in atherosclerotic renal-artery stenosis. Dutch Renal Artery Stenosis Intervention Cooperative Study Group. N Engl J Med 2000; 342: 1007–14.

25. Ritz E, Mann JFE. Renal angioplasty for lowering blood pressure. N Engl J Med 2000; 342: 1042–3.

26. Webster J, Marshall F, Abdalla M et al. Randomised comparison of percutaneous angioplasty vs continued medical therapy for hypertensive patients with atheromatous renal artery stenosis. Scottish and Newcastle Renal Artery Stenosis Collaborative Group. J Hum Hypertens 1998; 12: 329–35.

27. Plouin PF, Chatellier G, Darne B, Raynaud A. Blood pressure outcome of angioplasty in atherosclerotic renal artery stenosis: a randomized trial. Essai Multicentrique Medicaments vs Angioplastie (EMMA; Study Group. Hypertension 1998; 31: 823–9.

28. Blaufox MD, Fine EJ, Heller S et al. Prospective study of simultaneous orthoiodohippurate and diethylenetriaminepentaacetic acid captopril renography. The Einstein/Cornell Collaborative Hypertension Group. J Nucl Med 1998; 39: 522–8.

29. Taylor A. Functional testing: ACEI renography. Semin Nephrol 2000; 20: 437–44.

30. Pedersen EB. New tools in diagnosing renal artery stenosis. Kidney Int 2000; 57: 2657–77.

31. Kahn D, Ben-Haim S, Bushnell DL et al. Captopril-enhanced 99Tcm-MAG3 renal scintigraphy in subjects with suspected renovascular hypertension. Nucl Med Commun 1994; 15: 515–28.

32. Mittal BR, Kumar P, Arora P et al. Role of captopril renography in the diagnosis of renovascular hypertension. Am J Kidney Dis 1996; 28: 209–13.

33. Huot SJ, Hansson JH, Dey H, Concato J. Utility of captopril renal scans for detecting renal artery stenosis. Arch Intern Med 2002; 162: 1981–4.

34. Boudewijn C, Vasbinder C, Nelemans PJ et al. Diagnostic tests for renal artery stenosis in patients suspected of having renovascular hypertension: A meta-analysis. Ann Intern Med 2001; 135: 401–11.

35. Fommei E, Ghione S, Hilson AJ et al. Captopril radionuclide test in renovascular hypertension: a European multicentre study. European Multicentre Study Group. Eur J Nucl Med 1993; 20: 617–23.

36. Fommei E, Ghione S, Hilson AJW et al. Captopril radionuclide test in renovascular hypertension: European Multicentre Study. In: O'Reilly PH, Taylor A, Nally JV, eds. Radionuclides in Nephrourology. Blue Bell, Pennsylvania, USA: Field & Wood, Medical Periodicals, Inc. 1994; 33–7.

37. Fommei E, Mezzasalma L, Multicentre Study Group. Detection of renovascular hypertension by captopril renography with MAG3: a multicentre study. Eur J Nucl Med 1997; 24: 941(abstract).

38. Erbslöh-Möller B, Dumas A, Roth D et al. Furosemide-131I-hippuran renography after angiotensin-converting enzyme inhibition for the diagnosis of renovascular hypertension. Am J Med 1991; 90: 23–9.

39. Fernandez P, Morel D, Jeandot R et al. Value of captopril renal scintigraphy in hypertensive patients with renal failure. J Nucl Med 1999; 40: 412–17.

40. Setaro JF, Saddler MC, Chen CC et al. Simplified captopril renography in diagnosis and treatment of renal artery stenosis. Hypertension 1991; 18: 289–298.

41. Rossi GP, Pavan E, Chiesura-Corona M et al. Renovascular hypertension with low to normal plasma renin: Clinical and angiographic features. Clin Sci 1997; 93: 435–43.

42. Prigent A, Cosgriff P, Gates GF et al. Consensus report on quality control of quantitative measurements of renal function obtained from renogram. Semin Nucl Med 1999; 29: 146–59.

43. Fanti S, Dondi M, Guidalotti PL et al. Bilateral symmetrical induced changes in captopril scintigraphy. J Nucl Med 1998; 39: 86P.

44. Taylor A. Radionuclide scintigraphy: a personal approach. Sem Nucl Med 1999; 29: 102–27

45. Stavropoulos SW, Sevigny SA, Ende JF, Drane WE. Hypotensive response to captopril: a potential pitfall of scinti-graphic assessment for renal artery stenosis. J Nucl Med 1999; 40: 406–11.

46. Visscher CA, de Zeeuw D, Huisman RM. Effect of chronic ACE inhibition on the diagnostic value of renography for renovascular hypertension: a preliminary report. Nephrol Dial Transplant 1995; 10: 263–5.

47. Picciotto G, Sargiotto A, Petrarulo M et al. Reliability of captopril renography in patients under chronic therapy with angiotensin II (AT1; receptor antagonists. J Nucl Med 2003; 44: 1574–81.

48. Roccatello D, Picciotto G, Rabbia C et al. Prospective study on captopril renography in hypertensive patients. Am J Nephrol 1992; 12: 406–11.

49. Helin KH, Tikkanen I, von Knorring JE et al. Screening for renovascular hypertension in a population with relatively low prevalence. J Hypertens 1998; 16: 1523–9.

50. Safian RD, Textor SC. Renal-artery stenosis. N Engl J Med 2001; 344: 431–42.

51. Blaufox MD, Middleton ML, Bongiovanni J, Davis BR. Cost efficacy of the diagnosis and therapy of renovascular hypertension. J Nucl Med 1996; 37: 171–7.

52. Nelemans PJ, Kessels AG, De Leeuw P et al. The cost-effectiveness of the diagnosis of renal artery stenosis. Eur J Radiol 1998; 27: 95–107.

53. Imanishi M, Kawamura M, Akabane S et al. Aspirin lowers blood pressure in patients with renovascular hypertension. Hypertension 1989; 14: 461–8.

54. van de Ven PJG, de Klerk JMH, Mertens IJR et al. Aspirin renography and captopril renography in the diagnosis of renal artery stenosis. J Nucl Med 2000; 41: 1337–42.

55. Milot A, Lambert R, Lebel M et al. Prostaglandins and renal function in hypertensive patients with unilateral renal artery stenosis and patients with essential hypertension. J Hypertension 1996; 14: 765–71.

56. Müller-Suur R, Tidgren B, Fehrm A, Lundberg HJ. Captopril-induced changes in MAG3 clearance in patients with renal artery stenosis and the effect of renal angioplasty. J Nucl Med 2000; 41: 1203–8.

57. Taylor A, Corrigan PL, Galt J et al. Measuring technetium-99m-MAG3 clearance with an improved camera-based method. J Nucl Med, 1995; 36: 1689–95.

58. Gates GF. Glomerular filtration rate: estimation from fractional renal accumulation of Tc-99m DTPA (stannous). AJR 1982; 138: 565–70

59. Inoue Y, Yoshikawa K, Yoshioka N et al. Evaluation of renal function with Tc-99m MAG3 using semiautomated regions of interest. J Nucl Med 2000; 41: 1947–54.

60. Bergmann H, Dworak E, Konig B et al. Improved automatic separation of renal parenchyma and pelvis in dynamic renal scintigraphy using fuzzy regions of interest. Eur J Nucl Med 1999; 26: 837–43.

61. Radermacher J. Ultrasonography in the diagnosis of renovascular disease. Imaging Decisions 2002; 2: 15–22.

Functional and molecular imaging

17 Functional imaging of the kidney with electron beam CT

Lilach O Lerman

Introduction

The kidney is involved in regulation of homeostasis and controls a variety of physiological processes including electrolyte balance, blood volume and arterial pressure, and has various endocrine functions. It is also a vulnerable target organ to drugs, toxins and other risk factors. Renal dysfunction and maladjusted responses may well have grave repercussions on the wide spectrum of functions of the kidney, and may contribute to progression of renal and cardiovascular disease. Because of the potential ramifications of renal impairment, diverse techniques have been developed and utilized for measurement of renal haemodynamic function, including renal perfusion and renal blood flow (RBF), glomerular filtration rate (GFR), and the dynamics of the tubular reabsorption process. However, the complexity and spatial heterogeneity of intrarenal structure and function have made it difficult to reliably quantify these characteristics noninvasively in the intact single kidney under a wide spectrum of physiologic conditions.

Development of X-ray techniques for functional imaging of the kidney

Since their discovery, X-rays have been widely applied to identification of anatomic and physiologic processes. One of the first applications of X-rays to the kidney was in the 1920s in the advent of excretory urography, in which sequential X-ray images were acquired during injection of contrast media to explore renal excretory function.[1] The first functional imaging of the kidney using X-rays was then introduced in 1923 as the important technique of intravenous pyelography.[2] In the 1940s Trueta et al,[3] who assessed and timed the transit of intravascular contrast media through the renal vasculature using angiography, pioneered dynamic studies of the renal circulation and intrarenal distribution of blood flow. Subsequently, Erikson et al used videodensitometry to study total and regional renal blood flow[4] as well as function.[5] Using

injection of a glomerular filterable (urographic) contrast medium, they were able to evaluate the amount of filterable contrast that was filtered from the glomerular to the tubular compartment and estimate filtration fraction. However, the use of projection imaging, and low spatial and temporal resolution, limited the accuracy of these approaches to quantify renal function.

Mathematical development of 3D reconstruction[6] and its application in the late 1950s and 1960s to transaxial image reconstruction[7-9] enabled development of computed tomography (CT). Tomographic imaging techniques in conjunction with intravenous injections of contrast media may be clinically useful, because their cross-sectional capability allows assessment of the circulation of the single-kidneys noninvasively, bilaterally and simultaneously. Cross-sectional CT imaging also overcomes superimposition observed in projection images and allows anatomically discerning intrarenal regions (e.g. cortex and medulla) and external detection of the transit of a bolus of X-ray filterable contrast media. Since the cortex receives about 90% of renal blood flow, vascular transit of contrast media opacifies the cortex more than the medulla and marks the cortico-medullary junction.

One of the advantages of CT for quantitative assessment of renal functional imaging is that because of the linear relationship between X-ray contrast media concentration and CT-derived tissue attenuation, measurements of tissue density reflect and can provide absolute quantifications of tissue concentration of the contrast media contained in the renal vasculature, interstitium or tubular fluid. Much progress has been made towards development of concepts for exploration and interpretation of renal transit of contrast media.[10,11] However, the first generations of CT scanners, introduced in the 1980s, were limited by long data acquisition times and low sampling rate that hampered their ability to accurately record subsecond changes in contrast concentration.

The dynamic spatial reconstructor (DSR) developed in the late 1970s[12] was the first three-dimensional volume-scanning CT scanner, and exhibited stop-action (to minimize motion artifacts) and very high temporal resolution (up to 60 frames/s), which enabled assessment of functional movements (e.g. of the heart or lung) and distribution of X-ray contrast media in blood and tissue. It provided the opportunity to assess renal structure and function,[13-15] measurement of renal perfusion, blood flow distribution,[16]

Figure 17.1 Schematic demonstrating the configuration of the EBCT. An electron gun located behind the patient produces an electron beam, which is magnetically deflected sequentially onto four tungsten target rings located underneath the patient. Fan beams of X-rays subsequently pass through the patient (up to 17 frames/s at the cine mode), and their attenuation is detected by a semicircular detector array located on the opposite side of the patient.

Figure 17.2 Representative EBCT image of a pig kidney obtained after intravenous injection of a bolus of a contrast medium, showing the cortex manually traced. Similar images were used to generate the time–density curves demonstrated in Figure 17.3.

and dynamic changes in the renal circulation.[17] However, despite the sophistication and potential of the DSR, its limited availability, high operating costs, and unavailability of adequate computing power to facilitate data handling at that time restricted its use.

Electron beam computerized tomography (EBCT)

EBCT was introduced in the 1980s. Its configuration is such (Figure 17.1) that the absence of moving mechanical parts (i.e. X-ray tubes and/or TV cameras revolving around the subject) other than the patient table, decreases heat production compared to conventional CT, and enables ultrafast scanning. Using the multislice mode, this configuration allows studying eight parallel 8-mm-thick tomographic slices almost simultaneously at around 50 ms/image. Using the single-slice stop-action mode, which resembles conventional CT acquisition, thinner slices (1–10 mm) can be obtained at 100 ms/image and above. Its spatial and temporal resolution is therefore suitable to quantify renal function, which can be obtained from any region of interest within the kidney. Figure 17.2 shows an example of a cortical region of interest traced on an EBCT image.

Jaschke et al were the first to show the potential of the EBCT for measuring renal blood flow.[18–20] We have subsequently validated the accuracy of EBCT-derived measure-

ments of renal, cortical and medullary volumes,[21,22] perfusion and blood flow distribution within a wide range of renal blood flow values.[17,23] These measurements also proved to be feasible and highly reproducible in humans[24–26] and animals.[27,28]

Renal perfusion and blood flow

CT measurements of parenchymal perfusion are usually based on repetitive scanning of tomographic slices during the transit (first pass) of a bolus of contrast media. Distribution of X-ray contrast media follows blood distribution patterns, and the degree of change in tissue density (CT numbers, Hounsfield Units) reflects the amount of blood that perfuses the tissue. After depicting the change in tissue attenuation as a time–density curve (TDC) (Figure 17.3), regional perfusion (e.g. cortical or medullary, depending on the region of interest from which the data was sampled) can be assessed following the principles of the indicator-dilution theory.[29] Regional perfusion (ml blood/min/cc tissue) multiplied by the corresponding regional volume then yields regional (cortical or medullary) or total (the sum of cortical and medullary) renal blood flow (in units of ml blood/min).

Renal function

Measurement of renal perfusion relies on the presence of contrast media within the renal vascular compartment. The mathematical basis for calculations of tissue perfusion and vascular volume, the classical indicator-dilution theory, is

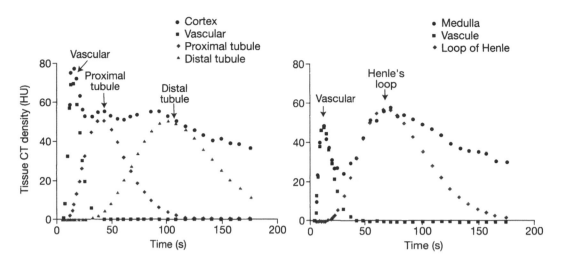

Figure 17.3 Time–density curves obtained with EBCT from the renal cortex (left panel) and medulla (right panel) of a pig after an intravenous bolus injection of iopamidol. The raw data of each curve have been modelled, and display the vascular and tubular location of the bolus during its transit along the nephron.

based on several assumptions regarding the haemodynamic, physical and physiological characteristics of the contrast bolus, as well as the microvascular branching structure. Implicit to this theory is the requirement that the indicator (i.e. contrast medium) should essentially remain intravascular during its first pass through the tissue.[29] The curves can be then fitted with standard gamma-variate curve-fitting algorithms:[30]

$$C(t) = C\ t^a\ \{\exp(-t/b)\} \qquad (1)$$

where $C(t)$ is the contrast concentration as a function of time t (s), and the remaining are curve-fitting parameters describing the magnitude and spread of the curve. The curve-fitting parameters are utilized to calculate the area under the curve ($c\Gamma(a + 1)\ b^{a+1}$), blood volume, mean transit time ($MTT = (a + 1)\ b$), and tissue perfusion as $Perfusion = 60 \times$ blood volume/MTT/$(1 - $ blood volume).[28] The input function for the kidney is typically obtained from the abdominal aorta, and is modelled as a simple gamma-variate curve (equation 1).

Blood volume (microvascular volume fraction) is determined from the ratio of the regional vascular and input TDC.[31] The input curve depicts the concentration of the contrast medium in pure blood, whereas tissue density measured during the vascular phase is in fact a weighted mean between the density of intravascular contrast media and that of the surrounding parenchyma. The ratio between contrast concentration in the tissue vascular curve and that of pure blood is hence directly related to the relative blood (vascular) volume fraction of the tissue.

However, due to their small molecular size, the soluble iodinated contrast media commonly used for cardiovascular X-ray imaging are extravascular markers[32] and leak from microvessels. In the myocardium, under physiological condi-

tions 15–30% of the indicator may be extracted into the extravascular compartment during its first pass through the vasculature,[33,34] and this fraction may increase during myocardial ischaemia. Consequently, rather than return to baseline levels, tissue density exhibits residual opacity,[35] whose magnitude depends on the fraction of the contrast remaining in the extravascular space, and to a lesser degree on recirculation.[31] A similar phenomenon takes place in the kidney as a result of glomerular filtration. Because of their chemical and physical properties, urographic contrast media are cleared from the body primarily via renal glomerular filtration in a manner similar to inulin. Using EBCT we have previously shown that although the majority of a contrast bolus washes out through the renal vein during its first pass, around 20% undergoes filtration in the glomerular capillaries and accumulates in the proximal tubule.[36] Since they are neither secreted nor reabsorbed in the renal tubules, their fate resembles that of inulin, and the determination of their elimination rate can be used to estimate tubular transit as well as the rate of glomerular filtration.

Therefore, residual tissue density that remains in the kidney following the vascular phase and venous washout of the contrast media[16] can be utilized to assess renal function. As mentioned earlier, Erikson et al took advantage of this phenomenon to assess filtration fraction using videodensitometry by comparing transit of two different types of contrast media: intravascular versus filterable.[5] More recently, the residual opacity in the kidney after a first pass of a single injection of contrast was used to assess filtration fraction,[16,37] and changes in density of the whole kidney during a first pass of contrast was used in an attempt to calculate renal permeability[38] and filtration.[39,40]

Subsequent tubular flow of the contrast along the nephron segments contained in the cortex or medulla leads to distinct changes in their X-ray densities (Figure 17.4). Changes in fluid

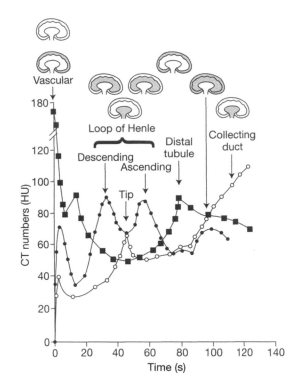

Figure 17.4 Time–density curves obtained with EBCT from the renal cortex and medulla of a normal dog. Because the canine kidney is unipapillary, the medullary region of interest is relatively well-defined, and enables outlining and depiction of contrast transit in the outer (descending and ascending limbs of the loops of Henle) and inner medulla. The corresponding anatomic location of the contrast in the renal cross-sectional regions is illustrated at the top panel. Reproduced with permission from reference 56.

concentration due to intratubular fluid reabsorption or secretion along the nephron also contribute to intratubular contrast concentration (ITC) and to the ultimate characteristics of these TDC.

Furthermore, because of bolus dispersion and the heterogeneous lengths of the tubular segments, these TDC overlap and require mathematical stripping. Therefore, we have recently developed mathematical models, which extend the standard gamma-variate curve-fitting algorithms. This modelling approach breaks the TDC into their individual components to delineate renal vascular and tubular fluid flow in individual nephron segments,[27,28] and permits calculation of curve parameters for each segment for assessment of regional perfusion, ITC, tubular transit times (the first moment of the curve) and GFR. These algorithms have been designed to model the TDC raw data in accordance with the region of interest from which the data were originally obtained (e.g. cortex, medulla or papilla, see Figure 17.4).

Distribution of contrast in the renal cortex is observed mainly in the vascular, proximal tubular, and distal tubular compartments (Figure 17.3, left panel), and the TDC can therefore be fitted with a tricompartmental curve-fitting algorithm:

$$C(t) = ct^a \{\exp^{(-t/b)} + d \exp^{(-t/h)}\} + it^j \exp^{(-t/k)} \qquad (2)$$

Distribution of contrast in the renal medulla corresponds to transit of the contrast medium in the vascular compartment and then the loop of Henle (Figure 17.3, right panel), and the model applied to the medullary TDC is therefore bicompartmental:[27,28]

$$C(t) = ct^a \exp^{(-t/b)} + it^j \exp^{(-t/k)} \qquad (3)$$

The vascular gamma-variate curve in each region is used to calculate regional perfusion, whereas data obtained from all subsequent peaks are used to calculate tubular dynamics (ITC and transit times), reflecting the degree of tubular fluid reabsorption (i.e. concentration or dilution) along the nephron. ITC is calculated for each nephron segment as the ratio of the area under each curve to that of the cortical vascular curve and GFR (to render ITC independent of concurrent contrast delivery via the vascular circulation or glomerular filtration).

Furthermore, the maximal slope of the ascending arm of the proximal tubular curve, which represents the rate of contrast accumulation secondary to glomerular filtration, is used to calculate unit GFR (ml/min/cc tissue).[27,28] It is calculated for each kidney from the right and left cortical time–density curves as:

$$GFR = \left\{ \frac{slope \times cortical\ vascular\ MTT}{area\ under\ aortic\ curve} \right\} \times 60$$

EBCT measurements of renal blood flow correlate well with those obtained with an electromagnetic flow probe[23] and with an intravascular Doppler wire,[28] which measure blood velocity in the main renal artery. EBCT-derived GFR correlated well with the clearance of the reference standard inulin.[27,28] This suggests that this model (e.g. equation 2) provided faithful depiction of the accumulation of contrast media in the proximal tubule.

Functional imaging of renal physiology and pathophysiology (Figure 17.5)

Analysis of renal TDC allows derivation of unique measures of intrarenal regional haemodynamics and function. EBCT detected physiological changes in renal perfusion and function during a number of challenges, such as administration of diuretics and renal vasodilators, Figure 17.5.[21,27,36,41–43] Acute changes in renal perfusion pressure within the range of RBF autoregulation disclosed changes of ITC (i.e., fluid reabsorption) that paralleled and were concordant with altered

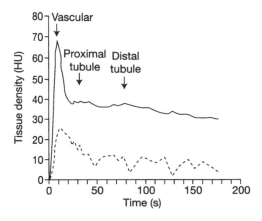

Figure 17.5 Inner medullary time-density curves obtained in the canine kidney before (solid squares) and after (circles) systemic furosemide injection. This loop-diuretic induced a marked dilution (and hence a decrease in tissue densities) in the nephron segments from the loop of Henle and distally. Reproduced with permission from reference 56.

Figure 17.6 Time–density curves obtained with EBCT from the renal cortex of a pig with left renal artery stenosis. The vascular and tubular curves of the stenotic cortex (dashed line) are considerably flatter that that from the contralateral (solid line) cortex, indicating lower perfusion and tubular content of contrast. Reproduced with permission from reference 45.

pressure natriuresis.[17,36,42] Moreover, similar changes were observed under chronic conditions in animals with renovascular hypertension, which showed diluted intratubular fluid,[44] while the stenotic kidney exposed to low renal perfusion pressure showed contrarily an increase in ITC (Figure 17.6).[45]

The significance of measurements of tubular function is underscored by the observation that superimposition of atherosclerosis (simulated by a high-cholesterol diet) markedly accentuated impairment in tubular fluid reabsorption in the stenotic kidney (Figure 17.7).[46] These findings of tubular injury *in vivo* were supported by morphological examination of the stenotic kidney, which revealed a marked increase in tubulo-interstitial injury *in vitro*.[46,47] The renal tubules, and particularly the S3 segment of the proximal tubule, are distinctly vulnerable to renal circulatory compromise and hypoxic injury. Renal susceptibility to hypoperfusion is further aggravated by insults that increase medullary vulnerability to hypoxia, especially models combining multiple insults.[48] Indeed, decreased filtrate-concentration capacity is a measure of intrinsic renal damage, suggesting a potential role for ITC as an index of tubular integrity and function.

The success of therapeutic intervention has also been evaluated using EBCT. For example, chronic endothelin-1[49] or angiotensin II AT1 receptor[50] blockade improves renal perfusion, function and structural integrity in hypercholesterolaemia. HMG-CoA-reductase inhibitors (simvastatin) also

Figure 17.7 Profiles of contrast media concentration in the renal tubules assessed in pigs that were either normal or hypercholesterolaemic (HC), had renal artery stenosis (RAS), or both HC and RAS (*P <0.05 vs normal and HC, † P <0.05 vs RAS). Intratubular concentration was similar in normal and HC, but significantly higher in the proximal tubule and Henle's loop of RAS, suggesting increased fluid reabsorption. However, in HC+RAS intratubular contrast media concentration was significantly lower along the nephron, suggesting impaired tubular fluid reabsorption and tubular injury. Reproduced with permission from reference 46.

attenuated the inflammatory and pro-oxidative environment as well as fibrosis in kidneys in pigs with diet-induced hypercholesterolaemia, in association with enhanced renal perfusion.[51] Chronic supplementation of antioxidant vitamins preserved renal vascular responses to endothelium-dependent vasodilators[52] and improved renal haemodynamics in the ischaemic kidney.[53-55] Therefore, these imaging techniques appear to be sufficiently sensitive to detect and monitor both acute and chronic subtle changes in renal function during physiology, pathophysiology and in response to treatment.

Tubular dynamics have not been extended to humans yet, but EBCT estimates of the renal perfusion and volume have been shown to be feasible and highly reproducible in normal humans under controlled conditions.[24] Cortical perfusion was decreased in normotensive humans predisposed to essential hypertension compared to humans without a family history of this syndrome.[26] In the ischaemic kidney of renovascular hypertensive patients, cortical and medullary perfusion were further decreased compared to essential hypertension.[25]

Limitation of EBCT techniques

Tomographic X-ray methods may be limited by imaging artifacts such as partial volume effects, beam hardening (an artificial increase in the average energy of the transmitted beam), or photon scatter (detection of X-ray information originating outside the X-ray source and detector plane).[56]

They are also associated with exposure to radiation and contrast media, which bear the risk for nephrotoxicity and may present a limitation in patients with greatly compromised renal function. However, serum creatinine of up to 2 mg/dl does not usually increase the risk for contrast nephropathy, which is under 2% in nondiabetic subjects.[57] Therefore, use of small doses of nonionic, low-osmolar contrast media during functional imaging as well as adequate hydration decrease this risk for adverse effects.

Conclusion

In conclusion, X-ray techniques offer a unique insight into the synchronous intrarenal haemodynamics and function. The high spatial and temporal resolution of EBCT, and the linear relationship between CT image density and iodine concentration, allow illustration of contrast transit in the renal vascular and tubular compartments, and thus simultaneous and reproducible measurements of regional renal perfusion, tubular dynamics and GFR in the intact bilateral kidneys. This technique can provide an opportunity to elucidate mechanisms underlying renal regulation of homeostatic and other processes, and monitor renal disease progression and regression, in a manner potentially applicable to humans.

References

1. Carelli HH, Sordelli E. A new procedure for examining the kidney. Rev Assoc Med Argent 1921; 34: 18-9.

2. Osborne EA, Sutherland CG, Scholl J et al. Roentgenography of urinary tract during excretion of sodium iodide. J Am Med Assoc 1923; 80: 368-73.

3. Trueta J, Barclay AE, Daniel PM et al. Studies of the renal circulation. Springfield: Thomas, C.C.; 1947.

4. Erikson U, Lidgren PG, Lofroth PO et al. Measurement of total and regional renal blood flow. Acta Radiol Diagn 1973; 18: 225-34.

5. Erikson U, Lorelius LE, Ruhn G, Wolfgast M. Regional renal function measured by videodensitometry. Scand J Urol Nephrol 1981; 15: 131-5.

6. Radon J. Über die Bie Bestimmung von Funktionen durch ihre Integralwerte längs gewisser Mannigfaltigkeiten. Ber Sachs Akad Wiss Math Phys Kl 1917; 69: 262-77.

7. Oldendorf WH. Isolated flying spot detection of radiodensity discontinuities – displaying the internal structural pattern of a complex object. IRE Trans Biomed Electron 1961; 8: 68-72.

8. Cormack AM. Representation of a function by its time integrals, with some radiological applications. J Appl Physiol 1964; 35: 2908-13.

9. Hounsfield GN. Computed transverse axial scanning (tomography): Part I. Description of system. Br J Radiol 1973; 46: 1016-22.

10. Jaschke W, Lipton MJ, Boyd DP et al. Attenuation changes of the normal and ischemic canine kidney. Dynamic CT scanning after intravenous contrast medium bolus. Acta Radiol (Diagn) (Stockh) 1985; 26: 321-30.

11. Heinz ER, Dubois PJ, Drayer BP, Hill R. A preliminary investigation of the role of dynamic computed tomography in renovascular hypertension. J Comput Assist Tomogr 1980; 4: 63-6.

12. Ritman EL, Kinsey JH, Robb RA et al. Three-dimensional imaging of heart, lungs, and circulation. Science 1980; 210: 273-80.

13. Iwasaki T, Ritman EL, Fiksen-Olsen MJ et al. Renal cortical perfusion – preliminary experience with the Dynamic Spatial Reconstructor (DSR). Ann Biomed Eng 1985; 13: 259-71.

14. Bentley MD, Fiksen-Olsen MJ, Knox FG et al. The use of the Dynamic Spatial Reconstructor to study renal function. In: Kaufman W, ed. Primary Hypertension. Berlin Heidelberg: Springer-Verlag; 1986: 126-41.

15. Bentley MD, Hoffman EA, Fiksen-Olsen MJ et al. Three dimensional canine renovascular structure and circulation visualized in situ with the Dynamic Spatial Reconstructor. Am J Anat 1988; 181: 77-88.

16. Bentley MD, Lerman LO, Hoffman EA et al. Measurement of renal perfusion and blood flow with fast computed tomography. Circ Res 1994; 74: 945-51.

17. Lerman LO, Bentley MD, Fiksen-Olsen MJ et al. Pressure dependency of canine intrarenal blood flow within the range of autoregulation. Am J Physiol 1995; 268: F404-F9.

18. Jaschke W, Gould R, Assimakopoulos PA, Lipton MJ. Flow measurements with a high-speed computed tomography scanner. Med Phys 1987; 14: 238–43.

19. Jaschke W, Gould R, Cogan MG et al. Cine-CT measurement of cortical renal blood flow. J Comput Assist Tomogr 1987; 11: 779–84.

20. Jaschke W, Sievers RS, Lipton MJ, Cogan MG. Cine-computed tomographic assessment of regional renal blood flow. Acta Radiol 1989; 31: 77–81.

21. Lerman LO, Bentley MD, Bell MR et al. Quantitation of the in vivo kidney volume with cine computed tomography. Invest Radiol 1990; 25: 1206–11.

22. Lerman LO, Bentley MD, Bell MR et al. The effect of a low-osmolar radiographic contrast medium on in vivo and postmortem renal size. Invest Radiol 1991; 26: 992–7.

23. Lerman LO, Bell MR, Lahera V et al. Quantification of global and regional renal blood flow with Electron Beam Computed Tomography. Am J Hypertens 1994; 7: 829–37.

24. Lerman LO, Flickinger AL, Sheedy PF, Turner ST. Reproducibility of human kidney perfusion and volume determinations with electron beam computed tomography. Invest Radiol 1996; 31: 204–10.

25. Lerman LO, Taler SJ, Textor S et al. CT-derived intra-renal blood flow in renovascular and essential hypertension. Kidney Int 1996; 49: 846–54.

26. Flickinger AL, Lerman LO, Sheedy PF, Turner ST. The relationship between renal cortical volume and predisposition to hypertension. Am J Hypertens 1996; 9: 779–86.

27. Lerman LO, Krier JD, Ritman EL et al. Quantification of single-kidney glomerular filtration rate with electron-beam computed tomography. SPIE Proc 2000; 3978: 539–46.

28. Krier JD, Ritman EL, Bajzer Z et al. Noninvasive measurement of concurrent, single-kidney perfusion, glomerular filtration, and tubular function. Am J Physiol Renal Physiol 2001; 281: F630–8.

29. Rumberger JA, Bell MR, Feiring AJ et al. Measurement of myocardial perfusion using fast computed tomography. In: Marcus M, Schelbert H, Skorton D, Wolf G, eds. Cardiac imaging: a companion to Braunwald's Heart disease. Philadelphia, PA: W. B. Saunders; 1991: 688–702.

30. Thompson HK, Starmer F, Whalen RE, McIntosh HD. Indicator transit time considered as a gamma variate. Circ Res 1964; 14: 502–15.

31. Lerman LO, Siripornpitak S, Luna Muffei N et al. Measurement of in vivo myocardial microcirculatory function with electron beam CT. J Comput Assist Tomogr 1999; 23: 390–8.

32. Morris TW, Fischer HW. The pharmacology of intravascular radiocontrast media. Ann Rev Pharmacol Toxicol 1986; 26: 143–60.

33. Canty JM Jr, Judd RM, Brody AS, Klocke FJ. First-pass entry of nonionic contrast agent into the myocardial extravascular space. Effects on radiographic estimates of transit time and blood volume. Circulation 1991; 84: 2071–8.

34. Wu X, Ewert DL, Liu YH, Ritman EL. In vivo relation of intramyocardial blood volume to myocardial perfusion. Circulation 1992; 85: 730–7.

35. Sako M, Sugimoto K, Matsumoto S et al. CT evaluation of extravascular perfusion of contrast medium and its potential to a new method of diagnosis: an experimental study using macro, micro-molecular contrast media. Nippon Igaku Hoshasen Gakkai Zasshi 1994; 54: 289–91.

36. Lerman LO, Rodriguez-Porcel M, Sheedy PFI, Romero JC. Renal tubular dynamics in the intact canine kidney. Kidney Int 1996; 50: 1358–62.

37. Lumsden CJ, Silverman M, Zielinski A et al. Vascular exchange in the kidney. Regional characterization by multiple indicator tomography. Circ Res 1993; 72: 1172–80.

38. Miles KA, Kelley BB. CT measurements of capillary permeability within nodal masses: a potential technique for assessing the activity of lymphoma. Br J Radiol 1997; 70: 74–9.

39. Ishikawa I, Masuzaki S, Saito T et al. Dynamic computed tomography in acute renal failure: Analysis of time-density curves. J Comput Assist Tomogr 1985; 9: 1097–102.

40. Dawson P, Peters M. Dynamic contrast bolus computed tomography for the assessment of renal function. Invest Radiol 1993; 28: 1039–42.

41. Lerman LO, Rodriguez-Porcel M. Functional assessment of the circulation of the single kidney. Hypertension 2001; 38: 625–9.

42. Rodriguez Porcel M, Lerman LO, Sheedy PF II, Romero JC. Pressure dependency of renal tubular flow. Am J Physiol 1997; 273: F667–F73.

43. Feldstein A, Krier JD, Hershman Sarafov M et al. In vivo renal vascular and tubular function in experimental hypercholesterolemia. Hypertension 1999; 31: 859–61.

44. Rodriguez-Porcel M, Krier JD, Lerman A et al. Combination of hypercholesterolemia and hypertension augments renal function abnormalities. Hypertension 2001; 37: 774–80.

45. Lerman LO, Schwartz RS, Grande JP et al. Noninvasive evaluation of a novel swine model of renal artery stenosis. J Am Soc Nephrol 1999; 10: 1455–65.

46. Chade AR, Rodriguez-Porcel M, Grande JP et al. Distinct renal injury in early atherosclerosis and renovascular disease. Circulation 2002; 106: 1165–71.

47. Chade AR, Rodriguez-Porcel M, Grande JP et al. Mechanisms of renal structural alterations in combined hypercholesterolemia and renal artery stenosis. Arterioscler Thromb Vasc Biol 2003; 23: 1295–301.

48. Brezis M, Rosen S. Mechanisms of disease: Hypoxia of the renal medulla – its implications for disease. N Engl J Med 1995; 332: 647–55.

49. Chade AR, Best PJ, Rodriguez-Porcel M et al. Endothelin-1 receptor blockade prevents renal injury in experimental hypercholesterolemia. Kidney Int 2003; 64: 962–9.

50. Chade A, Rodriguez-Porcel M, Rippentrop SJ et al. Angiotensin II AT1 receptor blockade improves renal perfusion in hypercholesterolemia. Am J Hypertens 2003; 16: 111–5.

51. Wilson SH, Chade AR, Feldstein A et al. Lipid-lowering-independent effects of simvastatin on the kidney in experimental hypercholesterolaemia. Nephrol Dial Transplant 2003; 18: 703–9.

52. Stulak JM, Lerman A, Rodriguez Porcel M et al. Renal vascular function in experimental hypercholesterolemia is preserved by chronic antioxidant vitamin supplementation. J Am Soc Nephrol 2001; 12: 1882–91.

53. Chade AR, Rodriguez-Porcel M, Herrmann J et al. Beneficial Effects of Antioxidant Vitamins on the Stenotic Kidney. Hypertension 2003; 42: 605–12.

54. Chade AR, Rodriguez-Porcel M, Herrmann J et al. Antioxidant Intervention Blunts Renal Injury in Experimental Renovascular Disease. J Am Soc Nephrol 2004; 15: 958–66.

55. Zhu XY, Chade AR, Rodriguez-Porcel M et al. Cortical Microvascular Remodeling in the Stenotic Kidney. Role of Increased Oxidative Stress. Arterioscler Thromb Vasc Biol 2004.

56. Lerman LO, Rodriguez Porcel M, Romero JC. The development of x-ray imaging to study renal function. Kidney Int 1999; 55: 400–16.

57. Rihal CS, Textor SC, Grill DE et al. Incidence and prognostic importance of acute renal failure after percutaneous coronary intervention. Circulation 2002; 105: 2259–64.

18 Functional and cellular imaging of the kidney by MRI

Nicolas Grenier, Michael Pedersen, Olivier Hauger

Introduction

Imaging of parenchymal renal diseases has for long been restricted to renal length, cortico-medullary differentiation, evaluated by various radiological techniques, and functional information, evaluated by nuclear medicine technique. Today, the new developments of both magnetic resonance imaging (MRI) systems, providing higher signal-to-noise ratio and higher spatial and/or temporal resolution, and MR contrast agents have the potential to drive new opportunities for obtaining reliable and quantitative functional data, as well as information on tissue characteristics relevant to various renal diseases.

Functional MR imaging

Although the physiology of the kidney is quite complex, some functional parameters become available from MRI, based on qualitative, semiquantitative or quantitative analyses. Such functional approaches have received attention for many years[1] but the clinical applications are nowadays limited to semiquantitative evaluation of a few useful parameters for several reasons. First, it is difficult to obtain accurate and reproducible information in a mobile organ, subject to respiratory movements and to magnetic susceptibility artifacts arising from the surrounding bowel; second, the complexity of the relationship between the observed signal changes and the concentration of the contrast agent makes quantitative analysis difficult. Therefore, nuclear medicine remains at present the reference method for quantification of most renal functional parameters, but MRI is now able to compete in many fields. Functional parameters that can be evaluated noninvasively with MRI and will be covered in this chapter include blood flow and perfusion, glomerular filtration, tubular concentration, renal transit time, molecular diffusion of water and tissue oxygenation. These parameters are calculated from MRI measurements using either exogenous contrast agents such as gadolinium (Gd) chelates or iron oxide particles or endogenous contrast agents such as water protons or blood deoxyhaemoglobin.

Technical issues for studies requiring exogenous contrast agents

Most of these approaches are based on dynamic contrast-enhanced acquisitions, either with T1 weighting (R1 relaxation-enhanced) using paramagnetic Gd chelates, or with T2* weighting (R2* susceptibility-enhanced) using superparamagnetic iron oxide particles, and the fundamental differences between these two methods will be emphasized. Because both types of agents have a concomitant effect on all components of relaxivity, Gd chelates may produce T2 and T2* effects at high concentration and, conversely, iron oxide particles may produce T1 effects at low concentration. Therefore, depending on the type of agent used, specific optimization of the injected dose and of the imaging sequence is necessary.

Quantification of physiological parameters using dynamic contrast-enhanced MRI requires a conversion of signal intensity (SI) values into concentrations. Use of relative SI only precludes quantification of these parameters but allows instead calculation of parameters that, to some extent, reflect blood flow or filtration without being in absolute units. These parameters can only be used in the same individual to compare different renal areas or one kidney from the other.

Dynamic relaxivity contrast-enhanced MRI (T1 weighting)

Optimization of sequences

When Gd chelates are used, a reasonable T1 weighting can be accomplished using spoiled gradient-echo (type FLASH – Fast Low Angle SHot). Here, an RF-flip angle of 90° has been preferred by several authors to obtain a relative linear relationship between SI and Gd concentration.[2] If very short acquisition times are required, a nonselective magnetization preparation is convenient combined with very short TR and TE values to obtain a heavy T1 weighting. The preparation pulse is either realized as a saturation pulse (90°) or as an inversion pulse (180°), or alternatively, a more complex pulse scheme (90–180°) to eliminate arrhythmia.[3] Interestingly, Ivancevic et al[4] proposed, for a quantitative analysis of perfusion, coupling a 90–180° magnetization preparation with a large acquisition RF-flip angle to obtain a large contrast dynamic range which seemed more relevant, even if the temporal resolution was decreased. Therefore, according to selected geometric parameters and the performance of the MRI system used, a compromise may often be necessary.

Measurement of renal perfusion and filtration requires accurate sampling of the vascular phase of the kidney in order to measure the arterial input function (AIF). The AIF is usually the SI–time curve observed in the suprarenal abdominal aorta or in a renal artery and is used for different kinetic models in order to compensate for the noninstantaneous bolus injection into the blood. This need for a high temporal resolution explains why most studies have been performed using a single-slice acquisition scheme and not multislice or 3D techniques. However, the required extrapolation of functional data from one slice to the whole kidney is not always valid if the renal disease is irregularly or focally distributed. Recent advances in MR instrumentation and hardware facilitate coverage of the entire kidneys with several slices using 3D sequences while maintaining a temporal resolution around 1.5 s.[5] The acquisition plane (coronal or axial) has to include both kidneys for renal sampling and the suprarenal abdominal aorta for AIF. Moreover, the dynamic procedure has to be prolonged for minutes after injection of contrast for measurements of renal blood perfusion (1–2 min) and measurements of renal filtration (up to 3 min).

Optimization of the dose of contrast agent

The concentration of Gd within the kidney has to be decreased (to decrease the T2* contribution occurring at high concentration within the aorta and renal medulla), by decreasing the injected dose and by hydrating the patient. There is no consensus about the optimal dose to be used for MR renography, but it is generally accepted that MR renographic studies should be performed with a lower dose than that usually accepted clinically (0.1–0.2 mmol/kg). The standard dose must be avoided because of the high concentrations reached in the abdominal aorta during the bolus and within the renal medulla after water reabsorption. The choice between 0.025 mmol/kg and 0.05 mmol/kg depends on the level of signal-to-noise ratio obtained with the sequence and the system used.

Conversion of SI into Gd concentration

Absolute quantification of the tissue concentration of contrast agent C can usually be estimated using the equation (C) = (R1 − R1$_0$)/r, where R1 is th relaxation rate in the tissue

(R1 = 1/T1), R1$_0$ is the bulk R1 in the tissue without contrast agent, and r is the specific relaxivity of the contrast agent. In principle, this means that a precontrast measurement of R1 should be performed before injection of the contrast agent.

To convert changes in SI into changes in R1, different approaches can be used. A commonly used method is based on a phantom of tubes filled with Gd solutions at various concentrations, which is then imaged with the sequence used for the dynamic study. The acquired SI values are plotted against measured R1 values, and a polynomial fit is made to obtain a calibration curve. However, this approach has some drawbacks, including the assumption that the relaxivity is equivalent in solution and in tissues. Another method of conversion is to use the relationship between SI and R1 given by the equation driven by the sequence used,[6] which unfortunately is not straightforward. In addition, some sequences may not even have an analytical formula that can be used for this method.[7]

One important factor contributing to erroneous measurements of T1 of blood is subjected to the inflow effect, because the coherent movement of flowing fluid can alter T1 of the signal arising from spins therein.[8] The value of T1 for blood is therefore difficult to measure in vivo. Consequently, the T1 of the arterial blood has in many studies not actually been measured, but has been assumed from previously measured T1 values in humans[9] or has been assumed to be the same as the value measured ex vivo.[10]

This mathematically complex conversion from SI to R1 can be avoided using direct dynamic measurement of R1 (instead of SI). Very fast dynamic measurements of R1, based on the Look–Locker sequence,[11] providing dynamic T1 mapping of kidneys and aorta, is one possibility to eliminate this problem.[12,13] Preliminary renal studies appear extremely encouraging[14] but their accuracy in dynamic quantification has yet to be investigated.

Dynamic susceptibility contrast enhanced MRI (T2* weighting)

The passage of magnetopharmaceuticals leads to differences in the local magnetic susceptibility between vessels and the surrounding tissue. Although the fraction of the vascular space is generally a small fraction of the total tissue blood volume, this compartmentalization of contrast agent leads to a disruption of the local magnetic field homogeneity extending beyond the immediate confines of the vascular compartment, within which the contrast agent is retained. With iron oxide particles, the increased magnetic susceptibility caused by the ferromagnetic atom causes a relatively large spin dephasing, and thus T2*-weighted sequences can conveniently be used to detect the passage of the agent through a tissue of interest. Since these compounds are currently restricted to experimental studies in animals, T2*-weighted perfusion with these agents has received little clinical attentions. However, recent advances in developments of iron-containing magneto-pharmaceuticals have presented some prospective results, potentially attractive for evaluation of perfusion in the kidney.

Optimization of the sequence

These studies have predominantly been performed using snapshot FLASH-type sequences, with small TR and TE values together with a relatively small flip angle in order to facilitate T2* weighting. The T1 contribution to the signal expression of FLASH sequences is generally considered to be negligible in situations where iron particles are administered. Nevertheless, Bjørnerud et al[15] demonstrated that, using iron-oxide particles, the T1 effect in FLASH sequences was responsible for a significant distortion of the first-pass curves, leading to a significant underestimation of blood flow in the renal tissue. This effect decreases with increasing TE and agent dose, but is completely eliminated using a double-echo gradient-echo sequence that is inherently insensitive to changes in T1.

Gradient echo based echo-planar imaging is another type of sequence that can be used because the relatively large acquisition time is sensitive to changes in the magnetic susceptibility. Since those sequences are extremely suscepti-ble to image artifacts and distortions, their use for renal perfu-sion has been limited.

Optimization of the dose of contrast agent

For iron oxide-enhanced sequences using ultra-small particles of iron oxide (USPIO), the standard doses are between 20–40 μmol Fe/kg employing magnetization-prepared sequences. Among these agents, in humans only Clariscan® (GE Healthcare) can be injected as a bolus, whereas others such as ferumoxtran 10 (Sinerem®, Guerbet Group) must be slowly infused.

Conversion of SI into contrast agent concentration

Dynamic susceptibility contrast imaging (T2* weighted) does not make quantification of SI into concentration units possible. However, a relative measure of the concentration for iron oxide particles can be estimated using the linear proportion-ality between the concentration of the contrast agent and R2* changes given by the equation:

$$\Delta R2^*(t) = C(t)/K$$

where K is the proportionality constant, which depends on the properties of the tissue, the type of microvasculature, the

contrast agent and the sequence used. Measured SI is then converted into changes in R2* by the following relationship:

$$\Delta R2^*(t) = -\ln(S(t)/S_0)/TE$$

where TE is the echo time of the sequence and S_0 the baseline signal before arrival of the tracer.

Renal flow rate and perfusion

Renal blood flow (RBF), or flow rate, refers to the global amount of blood reaching the kidney per unit of time, normally expressed in ml/min. This parameter is usually measured on a renal artery or a renal vein or, alternatively, measured in the abdominal aorta as the difference of flow above and below the renal arteries. In contrast, renal perfu-sion refers to the blood flow that passes through a unit mass of renal tissue (ml/min/g) in order to vascularize it and exchange with the extravascular space. The degree of perfu-sion depends on both the arterial flow rate and local factors such as regional blood volume and vasoreactivity. In clinical practice, measurement of renal blood flow or perfusion may become important for the evaluation of renal artery stenosis or nephropathies with microvascular involvement[16] and help in monitoring intravascular interventions.

Renal flow rate

In a similar way to Doppler sonography, the cine-phase-contrast MR method is useful to evaluate the intra-arterial velocity profile and to quantify the renal blood flow in each renal vessel without injection of contrast agent. This technique is well described in the literature[17] and is based on the measurement of phase shifts of flowing spins along one direction (usually perpendicular to the vessel of interest). By using heart-triggered 3D phase contrast sequences, used with flow encoding in all three directions, it is possible to measure a vector-map of all flow components that may potentially elucidate wall shear stress patterns circumferen-tially and longitudinally in renal arteries. For accurate flow measurements in human arteries the imaging plane is usually positioned 10–15 mm downstream from the ostium, where respiratory movements are minimal, and perpendicular to the renal artery, often requiring a double obliquity.

It has been shown, in vitro, that the degree of spin dephas-ing is directly correlated with the trans-stenotic pressure gradient.[18] With a time resolution of 32 ms per timeframe, Schœnberg et al[19–21] described a gradation of velocity profile alteration (Figure 18.1): a normal curve or a partial loss of the early systolic peak (ESP) was consistent with low grade steno-sis; complete loss of the ESP and decrease of the midsystolic

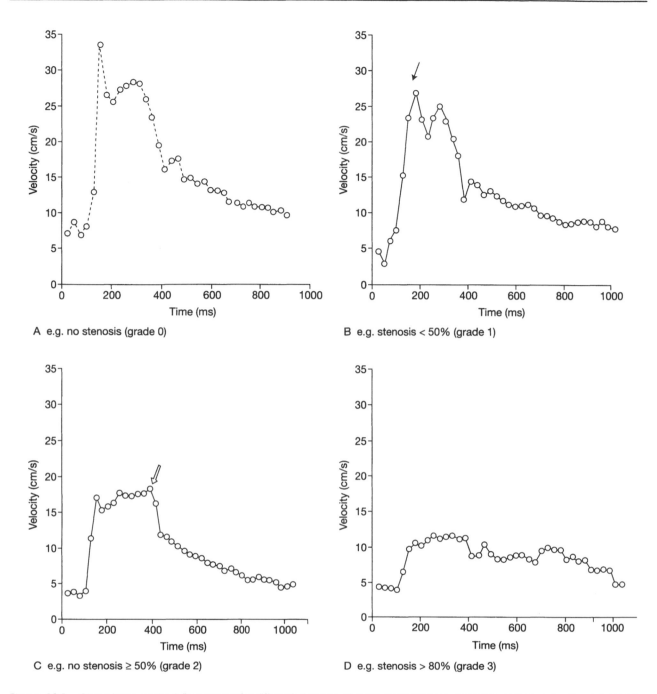

Figure 18.1 Cine phase-contrast flow curves for different degrees of renal artery stenosis. A semiquantitative grading scheme is applied on the basis of distinct changes in the waveform pattern. This scheme is shown as a guideline for the grading of haemodynamic changes. Note that the absolute scaling is the same for all four flow curves. Normal flow profiles (A) reveal a characteristic early systolic peak and a midsystolic maximum. Low-grade stenoses (B) typically reveal only a partial loss of the early systolic peak (solid arrow). Moderate stenoses (C) demonstrate an almost complete loss of the early systolic peak and a decrease of the midsystolic maximum (open arrow). High-grade stenoses (D) have a featureless flattened flow profile. Reprinted with permission from reference 21.

peak indicated moderate stenosis (50%); a flattened flow profile with no systolic velocity components was representative of high-grade stenosis. Using this classification, the combined approach of 3D Gd-enhanced MRA and phase-contrast flow sequence revealed the best interobserver and intermodality agreement. Sensitivity and specificity of detection of significant renal artery stenosis (>50%) were 100% and 93%, respectively. Therefore, this technique has been considered to be a useful complement to MR angiography of renal arteries. This method is also capable of measuring the renal blood flow in the renal artery below a stenosis as the product of the mean velocity within the artery and the cross-sectional area of renal artery. Although this technique is useful for measuring aortic flow rate, renal arteries are more difficult to evaluate because of their small size and because of respiratory movements.

Renal perfusion

Renal perfusion parameters, such as renal blood volume (RBV) and renal blood flow (RBF), can be assessed using different approaches: contrast-enhanced dynamic studies, contrast-enhanced steady-state studies, oxygen-enhanced acquisitions and water spin-labelling techniques.

Renal perfusion with contrast-enhanced dynamic studies

The theory of perfusion calculation as well as imaging methods depends on the type of contrast agent used. Within the brain, regular Gd chelates and iodine compounds are considered as nondiffusible tracers, because of the blood–brain barrier, and thus can be used to measure cerebral perfusion using MRI or CT.[22] Within the kidney, only agents that show neither interstitial diffusion nor glomerular filtration can be considered to be completely intravascularly confined. Two categories of such agents have been proposed: iron oxide particles and blood-pool Gd chelates (macromolecular or albumin-bound). First-pass intensity–time curves, in conjunction with these compounds, have been used for renal perfusion.[23,24]

Semiquantitative parameters such as maximal signal change (MSC), time to MSC (T_{MSC}) or wash-in and wash-out slopes can be measured for comparison from right to left kidney, from cortex to medulla or from one region to another. However, absolute quantification of regional perfusion is not straightforward and requires several signal processing steps together with several assumptions. Therefore, most studies have been conducted using either qualitative or semiquantitative indices.

For absolute blood flow calculations, the acquired SI–time curves of the aorta and the renal parenchyma must be converted into concentration–time curves as explained earlier. The former serves as an arterial input function (AIF), and the calculated concentration–time curves must then be processed using specific mathematical models. If the effect of a noninstantaneous bolus administration is not taken into account (i.e. absence of deconvolution), the calculated RBV, and RBF, will appear as representative parameters that may not give absolute measures but may instead be useful for qualitative diagnosis, such as the identification of abnormal regions or comparison of left and right kidneys.

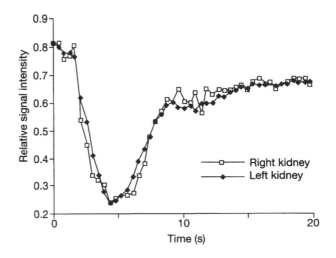

Figure 18.2   Plots of relative signal intensity changes versus time during iron-oxide particle transit within normal rabbit kidneys. The decrease of signal intensity is related to a T2* effect.

First-pass dynamic studies using intravascular agents with a T2* effect

Once injected intravenously as a bolus, iron oxide particles produce dynamic signal-intensity changes based on a T2* effect caused by alterations in the local magnetic susceptibility, as after Gd chelates for studies of brain perfusion (Figure 18.2). As these agents are considered as having a unicompartmental distribution within the kidney, regional renal blood flow can be calculated (in ml/min/g) according to Stewart and Hamilton's central volume theorem:

$$rRBF = rRBV \times MTT$$

where rRBF is the regional renal blood flow, rRBV is the regional renal blood volume and MTT is the mean transit time. Calculation of rRBV (in ml/g of renal tissue) can be estimated using the equation:

$$rRBF = k_h/\rho . \int C(t)dt / \int Ca(t)dt$$

where $\int C(t)dt$ is the area under the fitted first-pass concentration–time curve; $\int Ca(t)dt$ is the area under the AIF curve; ρ is the mean renal density ($\rho = 1.04$ g/ml) and k_h, a correction factor taking into account the difference between arterial and capillary haematocrits[25] (k_h is occasionally estimated at about 0.73):

The real MTT is difficult to measure because it would require a better understanding of the range of microvasculature structure within the tissues. However, it has been shown that the first moment of the renal fitted concentration–time curve is a

A

B

reasonable estimation of the relative MTT (rMTT), subsequently allowing a calculation of the renal perfusion that is fairly independent of a vasculature model.[26] Calculation of the real MTT is possible by mathematical deconvolution using the equation:

$$MTT = \int R(t)dt/R(t_0)$$

where R(t) is the residue function found from the deconvolution of C(t) with AIF(t).[27]

Because of the marked reduction in T2*, a bolus injection of iron-oxide particles produces an initial drop of signal intensity in the cortex that is secondarily followed by a decreased signal intensity in the medulla. Experimental applications with Endorem® (Guerbet Group) in rabbits subjected to hydronephrosis[23] or renal artery stenosis,[28] showed that the concentration–time curves of the ischaemic kidneys had a lower slope and a higher area under the curve than the normal contralateral kidney. In animals having unilateral renal artery stenosis, rRBF was decreased and rRBV was increased in the ipsilateral kidney.[28]

In a dog study, perfusion measurements based on the described indicator dilution theory and deconvolution demonstrated that rRBF values measured by MR correlated

C

Figure 18.3 Perfusion study with iron oxide particles: 62-year-old patient with left-sided high-grade renal artery stenosis at MRA (A). Phase-contrast MR-flow measurements (B) reveal a significantly flattened flow profile on the left side and normal profile on the right side. Colour-coded mapping of the regional perfusion (C) shows clearly reduced cortical perfusion on the left side with mean values of 229 ml/100 g/min and normal perfusion values on the right side with 350 ml/100 g/min. Scintigraphy (D) confirms the differences in renal perfusion of both kidneys at a right-to-left ratio of 77% over 23%. The diagnosis is a haemodynamically and functionally significant renal artery stenosis on the left side with consecutive ischaemic parenchymal damage. (Courtesy of Dr Stefan O. Schoenberg and Dr Henrik Michaely, Department of Clinical Radiology, Ludwig-Maximilians-University Munich, Germany.)

D

with those measured by implanted flow probe, but with a tendency to overestimate in the order of 20% in the renal parenchyma and about 100% in the medulla.[25] Mean values of rRBF, rRBV and MTT were 524 ml/min/100 g, 28 ml/100 g and 3.4 s, respectively. According to the authors, the overestimation of RBF measured by MRI was thought to be related to an overestimation of RBV, due to an inappropriate representation of the AIF observed in a renal artery. However, determination of AIF in the suprarenal abdominal artery appeared much more robust, but in cases of renal artery stenosis (RAS), dispersion of the bolus could not be taken into account. Other possible sources of error were ascribed to T1 contribution at low dosages, an improper choice of the constant K used for estimating R2*(t) an erroneous k_h value due to the fact that knowledge about haematocrit value within renal capillaries is limited, especially within the medulla where haematocrit changes may be complex.

Application of this quantitative technique to experimental models of RAS in dogs and a series of RAS in humans has been reported recently.[29] In these studies, the acquisition was performed in the sagittal plane to sample both the renal artery (for AIF) and the kidney. In the dog study, with four degrees of stenosis, an increase of MTT and a decreased rRBF occurred only for severe stenosis above 90%. In patients, a decreased rRBF was noted only for severe stenosis (Figure 18.3) or in kidney suffering from chronic damage related to other renal diseases, illustrating the complementary role of morphological information provided by MR angiography and haemodynamic data.

First-pass dynamic studies using intravascular agents with a T1 effect

Macromolecular Gd chelates have also been applied to renal perfusion evaluation, based on the same mathematical models. In a model of RAS in pigs, dynamic contrast-enhanced MRI using a new Gd chelate which targets albumin within the blood (MS-325, Epix Medical Inc.) demonstrated that the measured rRBF appeared comparable to microsphere measurements, but with a slight overestimation (258 ± 19.8 vs 198 ± 12.2 ml/min/100 g). However, RBF did not appear significantly altered, even when the diameter reduction exceeded 75%, which may well be explained by an intrarenal vascular regulation.[24]

First-pass dynamic studies using diffusible Gd chelates

Renal perfusion can also be evaluated with standard Gd chelates that are freely diffusible within the interstitial space and excreted exclusively by glomerular filtration. Although first-pass studies with these agents allow measurement of both renal perfusion and glomerular filtration during the same acquisition protocol, different assumptions and restrictions are put to the imaging scheme in order to calculate either renal perfusion or renal filtration. In general, renal perfusion is calculated from the first-pass renal curve following an instan-

taneous bolus of the contrast agent, which requires both a high temporal resolution and absence of recirculation of blood.

The most widely used perfusion model is derived from Peters' model,[30] developed for nuclear medicine with ^{99m}Tc-DTPA as the radiopharmaceutical.[31] Since ^{99m}Tc and Gd chelates have similar pharmacokinetic properties (around 10% is diffused into the interstitial space and around 20% is extracted by the glomeruli during the first pass), the dynamic uptake curves obtained by MRI are comparable with those obtained with a gamma camera. Peters et al[31] hypothesized that before leaving the kidney, the contrast agent behaves like microspheres that are trapped in the capillary system during a short time interval, inferior to the minimal vascular transit time. Therefore, the simple kinetic description of microspheres can be applied to the initial wash-in of the renal MR signal–time curve. Accordingly, renal perfusion is related to the amount of contrast medium trapped in the kidney using the following equation:

$$RBF/CO = M_{kidney}/M_{total}$$

where CO is the cardiac output, M_{kidney} is the amount of contrast agent trapped in the kidney at a time shorter than minimum vascular transit time and M_{total} is the total amount of contrast agent injected. As the extravascular leakage of Gd chelate is considered to be negligible during the initial first-pass, the amount of contrast trapped in the kidney vasculature is derived from the initial slopes of the renal and aortic wash-in curves and the arterial residue function (i.e. the integral of the AIF fitted to a gamma variate function). Moreover, introducing the arterial changes of RI ($\Delta(RI)_{art}$) allows the calculation of renal perfusion per unit of volume using the mathematical expression:

$$RBF/vol = max\ slope_{renal}/max\ \Delta(RI)_{art}$$

where $\Delta(RI)_{art}$ is calculated from the changes in aortic SI using a priori knowledge of the SI-vs-RI relationship that can be determined in vitro. Using this method, with a small bolus of contrast (0.025 mmol/kg) and a T1-weighted gradient-echo sequence, Vallée et al[30] were able to measure cortical BF in 16 normal kidney patients (254 ± 116 ml/min/100 g), decreasing to 109 ± 75 ml/min/100 g in cases of RAS and to 51 ± 34 ml/min/100 g in cases of renal failure. Unfortunately, reference measurements with radiopharmaceutical techniques were not used to reveal the inflow detected in aorta and the effects of the saturation observed at high Gd concentrations. Note, however, that the anticipated inflow effect was accounted for by introducing a flow-sensitive calibration model.[4] Such flow-corrected MR measurements of renal perfusion have been applied to a model of reversible RAS in rabbits (Figure 18.4), demonstrating values of cortical RBF that correlated linearly with reference values observed with a transit-timed ultrasound flow probe around the renal artery. These cortical RBF values were nonetheless

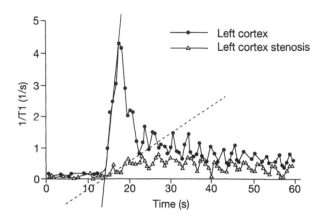

Figure 18.4 Arterial and cortical transit curves obtained after injection of GD-DTPA in a rabbit with left renal artery stenosis. SI is converted into 1/T1. An important decrease of the maximal slope of the cortical transit curve between the normal right kidney and the stenosed left kidney is observed. The calculated cortical perfusion was 26 ml/min before the stenosis was turned on and 19.7 ml/min after the stenosis was turned on. Reprinted with permission from reference 3.

systematically underestimated,[3] which could be related to a limitation of the upslope model at high flow.

Dujardin et al[32] generalized the tracer kinetic theory from intravascular to diffusible tracers and provided intrarenal maps of rRBF and rMTT with sufficient quality to allow accurate cortical delineation using deconvolution (Figure 18.5).

A

B

Figure 18.5 Comparison of relative renal blood flow mapping obtained in normal kidneys with dynamic Gd-enhanced sequences without (A) and with deconvolution (B). Quality of cortical delineation is better with deconvolution. (Reprinted with permission from Dujardin et al. MRM 2005, in press.)

Renal perfusion with contrast-enhanced steady-state studies using intravascular agents

Once intravascularly confined nondiffusible contrast agents are injected into the vasculature, they reach an equilibrium phase and the observed SI is then related to rRBV. In a rabbit study, iron oxide particles were administered during acquisition with T2- or T2*-weighted sequences leading to a decrease of SI in all renal compartments, which was greatest in the outer medulla.[33] This intrarenal distribution is in accordance with several studies demonstrating that the proportion of capillaries to tubular structures and interstitial tissue is greater in the medulla than in the cortex, with the largest percentage in the outer medulla (30% in the inner stripe). In addition, the interlobar arteries and veins restricted to the cortico-medullary junction are responsible for producing large susceptibility effects (Figure 18.6).

In a model of medullary ischaemia induced by glycerol, the signal change produced by either iron-oxide particles[34] or macromolecular blood pool Gd chelate[35] was lower in the outer medulla, where histological criteria of ischaemia predominated.[35]

Vascular ischaemia is also considered to be a major contributor to contrast media-induced acute renal failure (ARF). In an experimental model of radiocontrast nephropathy, the decreased SI following iron oxide injection seemed to be correlated with the reversibility of induced lesions.[36,37]

Renal perfusion with steady-state studies using inhalation of pure oxygen

Molecular dissolved oxygen is a weakly paramagnetic agent reducing the T1 of the blood without affecting the transverse relaxation. Functional imaging of the lung based on these changes in T1 induced by inhaling pure oxygen has been

A

B

Figure 18.6 T2*-weighted sequence obtained on a kidney transplant, before (A) and 15 minutes after (B) IV injection of iron-oxide particles, showing the maximum drop of signal intensity within the outer medulla. Interlobar arteries and veins restricted to the cortico-medullary junction are responsible for producing large susceptibility effects.

Figure 18.7 Image from one volunteer obtained using the dynamic, inversion prepared TSE sequence. O_2-enhanced: images are obtained by subtracting mean signal while breathing air from mean signal while breathing oxygen. The cross-correlation image is superimposed on one of the dynamic images. (Reprinted with permission from Jones et al. MRM 2002; 47: 728–35.)

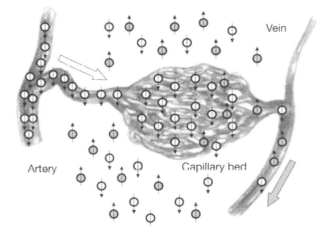

Figure 18.8 Schematic description of the principles of freely diffusible tracer theory. Inverted magnetization (white) comes from the arterial tree (white arrow) and diffuses through the capillary wall. There, spins are exchanged with the tissue magnetization (grey) and reduce its local intensity. The degree of attenuation is a direct measure of perfusion. Remaining tagged magnetization as well as exchanged water molecules flow out of the voxel of interest through the venous system (grey arrow). (Reprinted with permission from Golay et al. Top Magn Reson Imaging 2004; 15: 10–27.)

described by Edelman et al.[38] Slight T1 changes were also observed within the brain, myocardium and flowing blood, since oxygen can act as a weak intravascular contrast agent. This approach has also been employed in the kidney, where measurements with a T1-weighted inversion recovery sequence showed a significant increase in SI of the renal cortex in humans when pure oxygen was inhaled, whereas no change was observed in the medulla (Figure 18.7).[39] This technique could potentially be used to evaluate variations in cortical arterial blood flow.

Renal perfusion without contrast agents

Renal perfusion can alternatively be measured using pulsed arterial spin labelling (or spin-tagging) using endogenous water as a diffusible tracer (Figure 18.8). With this technique, a perfusion-weighted image can be generated by the subtraction of an image in which inflowing spins have been labelled from an image in which spin labelling has not been performed. Quantitative perfusion maps can then be calculated (in ml/min/100 g of tissue) when T1 of the tissue and efficiency of labelling are known. Several pulse sequence strategies have been described to tag arterial flowing spins, which can be divided into two groups (continuous or pulsed labelling) with different advantages and drawbacks as described in detail by Calamante.[40]

Continuous labelling

Methods based on continuous arterial spin-labelling[41] involve a train of RF pulses upstream (on the renal artery[42] or on the suprarenal abdominal aorta), which saturate flowing spins. Then, the labelled spins behave as a freely diffusible tracer to reduce magnetization of renal tissue water. Williams et al[43] improved the efficiency of labelling by using adiabatic inversion pulses, resulting in a two-fold increase in the difference between labelled and unlabelled states. However, these continuous labelling methods have some drawbacks. First, the method exhibits a relatively long 'transit time' between the level of labelling and the measured slice, leading to a progressive T1 relaxation of labelled spins that decreases the effect on the magnetization of tissue spins, consequently leading to an underestimation of calculated tissue perfusion. This effect may also imply that differences in blood flow between tissues could be related to differences in their transit time,[44] which may become especially important in the renal medulla as it has a very low mean transit time compared to the renal cortex. Second, repeated RF pulses can produce saturation of macromolecular spins in the blood, resulting in attenuation of free-water signal through magnetization transfer, leading also to underestimation of calculated perfusion. Third, the intravascular signal can be influenced by inflow effects, leading to an overestimation of perfusion. However, combination of delayed acquisition and flow-crushing gradients may compensate for this effect.

Pulsed labelling

Methods based on pulsed labelling are not compromised by the two major sources of error seen with continuous labelling techniques (transit time and magnetization transfer). Instead, these methods label spins with the use of a short inversion radiofrequency pulse.

Pulsed labelling can be realized as an echo planar imaging sequence with signal targeting with alternating radiofrequency (EPISTAR) that perfectly compensates for magnetization transfer effects.[45] This technique is based on four steps: (1) saturation of the imaging slice; (2) short pulse-labelling of a proximal slab (upstream) allowing the labelled flowing spins to enter the imaging plane; (3) image acquisition after a time TI; and (4) a control image with the labelling positioned distal to the imaging slice (several variants have been described for this). Next, subtraction of two images in which inflowing blood is first tagged and then not tagged yields a qualitative map of perfusion.

The flow-sensitive alternative inversion recovery (FAIR)[46] is based on two inversion recovery images, one with a slice-selective inversion (will contain flow information: T1 apparent) and one with a nonselective inversion (assuming that blood and kidney relax at the same rate, it will contain no flow information: T1). Subtraction of both images generates a value directly related to the perfusion. Extraslice spin tagging (EST), also denoted as uninverted FAIR (UNFAIR), is an alternative technique in which the flow-sensitive image is acquired following inversion of all spins outside the slice of interest, and the control image is acquired without any spin labelling. This approach is potentially more efficient than FAIR since the UNFAIR control image is entirely flow independent and need only be acquired once. Note that the transit time effects remain a concern with these pulsed labelling techniques, due to nonideal slice profile with interactions at the edges of the inversion slice with the imaging slice. Several solutions to correct these interactions have been proposed leading to variants such as sequences denoted as QUIPSS (Quantitative Imaging of Perfusion using a Single Subtraction) and QUIPSS II.[47]

Applications

The continuous labelling technique was successfully applied ex vivo using pharmacological manipulations of the intrarenal vasculature, with a decreased cortical blood flow induced by angiotensin II or an increased cortical blood flow induced by acetylcholine.[43] In an experimental transplantation model, the same authors showed that the cortical perfusion decreased during rejection and was correlated with the degree of rejection. However, this quantification of perfusion was only performed in cortex because the medullary transit time was too long.[48]

Using the EPISTAR sequence in an experimental model of renal artery stenosis in pigs, Prasad et al[49] showed that a decrease of blood flow was 100% sensitive and specific for detection of 70% renal artery stenoses. Recently, a technique associating a FAIR (flow-sensitive alternating inversion recovery) preparation and true fast imaging with free precession (True-FISP) data acquisition provided very encouraging results within the kidneys because of shorter echo time and fewer saturation effects (Figure 18.9).[50] However, these methods are complex to implement in clinical systems and have never been properly correlated to established methods. Hence, its impact in clinical practice remains uncertain.

Renal function

Glomerular filtration

Glomerular filtration rate (GFR) is the most useful quantitative index of renal function. However, standard methods for measurement of GFR, whether by measuring creatinine clearance or substances eliminated exclusively by glomerular filtration (e.g. inulin, ^{51}Cr-EDTA, ^{99m}Tc-DTPA), have certain limitations. Therefore, a reliable quantitative method based on a tracer clearance, obtained rapidly without blood and/or urine sampling, coupled with a morphological evaluation of the kidneys and the entire excretory system, would be extremely useful in the management of patients with renal disease.

Inulin or iodine contrast agents, Gd chelates such as Gd-DOTA or Gd-DTPA, all have a predominant renal

A

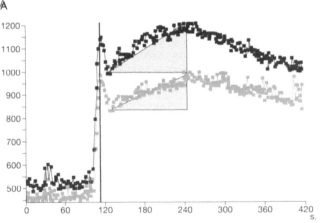

B

Figure 18.10 Signal intensity–time curves obtained in a patient with left urinary obstruction. A: anatomical image showing dilatation of the left pyelocaliceal system; B: signal intensity–time curves obtained from regions-of-interest drawn on the entire renal parenchyma (excluding pyelocaliceal system) on each side, showing three phases: a first abrupt ascending segment followed by a first peak, corresponding to the 'vascular-to-glomerular first-pass' or cortical vascular phase; a second slowly ascending segment, ended by a second peak, corresponding to the glomerulo-tubular phase; and a slowly descending segment, corresponding to the predominant excretory function and so-called 'excretory phase'. Areas under the curves have been drawn to calculate split renal function.

C

Figure 18.9 Perfusion imaging with spin-tagging method in a normal volunteer. A: Anatomical image; B: Perfusion-weighted FAIR True-Fisp image; C: Quantitative color-coded perfusion image. (Reprinted with permission from Martirosian et al. Magn Reson Med 2004; 51: 353–61.)

elimination (around 98%) by glomerular filtration without any tubular secretion or reabsorption. Therefore, these agents can conveniently be used to calculate GFR.

The sequences used for that purpose have already been mentioned. The T1-weighted dynamic sequence must have a sufficient time resolution for discrimination of vascular and filtration phases on the kidney and for sampling the AIF if quantitative measurements are required. If the time resolution of the sequence is sufficiently high, normal SI–time curve following Gd injection can be characterized by three phases (Figure 18.10): a first abrupt ascending segment followed by a first peak, corresponding to the 'vascular-to-glomerular first-pass' or 'cortical vascular phase'; a second slowly ascending segment, ended by a second peak, corresponding to the 'glomerulo-tubular phase'; and a slowly descending segment, corresponding to the predominant excretory function and so-called 'excretory phase'. If the ROI is restricted to the cortex, the slope of the second ascending segment is decreased. If the ROI is restricted to the medulla, the curve is characterized by a biphasic ascending slope, corresponding to the vascular and the uptake phases, the later segment reflects the tubular transit and progressive concentration, and is followed by the excretion phase.

Semiquantitative measurement of split renal function

Semiquantitative methods of evaluation of differential renal function are useful in assessment of patients with asymmetrical urological disease such as unilateral renal obstruction or reflux nephropathy. Here, conversion of SI into Gd concentration is not necessary. It has been shown that the functional parameters calculated from the SI–time curves obtained with a T1-weighted sequence were comparable to those derived with gamma camera scintigraphy in terms of simple parameters such as the maximum peak value, time-to-peak and the area under the curve. Although a significantly higher cortical time-to-peak value was reported in vascular nephropathies than in glomerular nephropathies,[51] its role in nephrology is not demonstrated.

Rohrschneider et al[52] demonstrated accurate calculations of the percentage of the single-kidney 'activity', referred to as split renal function, relative renal function or differential renal function.[53,54] Note, however, that measurements of these semiquantitative approaches are restricted to T1-weighted sequences in combination with a relatively small dose of contrast agent to avoid T2* effects (see above). These studies were based on a dynamic RF-spoiled gradient-echo sequence (TR = 17 ms, TE = 4 ms and RF-flipangle = 90°) with a temporal resolution of 10 s, a slice thickness including the kidney and the pyelocaliceal system and half of a standard clinically accepted dose of Gd-DTPA. An ROI is positioned around the renal parenchyma (omitting medulla and pelvis), and calculation of the relative renal function (RF) is then based on the equation:

$$RF = AUC \ (mm^2) \times S \ (mm^2)$$

where AUC corresponds to the area under the glomerulo-tubular part of the time–intensity curve (Figure 18.10) and S is the ROI area. The split renal function (SRF, in percentage) corresponds, for each kidney (SRF_R and SRF_L), to:

$$SRF_{RorL} = (RF_{RorL}/RF_R + RF_L) \times 100$$

In both an experimental study of ureteral obstruction[53] and in patients,[2,54] a high correlation between MR and renal scintigraphy was found. In addition, conversion from SI to concentration of contrast agent is not necessary, as recently demonstrated in rats with acute and chronic ureteral obstruction.[6]

Quantitative methods

Single kidney GFR (SKGFR) based on intrarenal kinetics

The requirements to quantify GFR are identical to those previously listed for perfusion measurements using T1 agents. Thus, conversion from SI to the concentration of contrast agent is necessary and, secondly, the temporal resolution of the employed sequence should be high in order to sufficiently sample the changes in SI in both arterial and renal segments following an instantaneous bolus of contrast agent. However, by introducing advanced models that take into account both the first passage of blood and the filtration part, it is possible to simultaneously calculate both RBF and SKGFR. To calculate GFR, several models have been proposed:

- The Rutland–Patlak model, which is a two-compartment model[6,55] based on the assumptions that, during the clearance (or uptake) phase, the rate of change of concentration in the kidney is constant and no significant amount of tracer leaves the kidney.[56] With MRI, the interstitial space is ignored, and Gd is considered to mix between the capillary and the glomerular compartments. This assumption may, however, fail in situations where the interstitial space is enlarged (pyelonephritis and some examples of acute renal failure), which leads to overestimation of SKGFR. The assumption that no contrast agent particles leave the ROI during the sampling period may justify the use of ROIs encompassing both cortex and medulla. The model is realized as an x–y plot (the Rutland–Patlak plot) using the ratio of the renal concentration/aortic concentration against the ratio of the integral of aortic concentration/aortic concentration. When applied to the second phase of the signal intensity–time curve (glomerulo-tubular uptake), this plot leads to a straight line, with a slope proportional to the renal clearance, and an intercept with the y-axis proportional to the cortical blood volume. 3D maps of

Figure 18.11 Example of intrarenal 3D GFR mapping after application of the Rutland–Patlak model on voxel-by-voxel basis.

GFR can now be drawn, based on 3D acquisitions and application of this model (Figure 18.11).

- *The cortical compartment model*[57] is another two-compartment model confined to the cortex, derived from the Rutland–Patlak model. This model differs firstly by the constraints that the outflow from the tubules, during the sampling period, is taken into account allowing ROIs to be drawn strictly limited to the cortex, and secondly by the fact that the aortic curve is shifted and dispersed to take into account the transit time of the contrast agent between the aorta and the kidney and the tracer dispersion in the glomeruli.[50] The residue function obtained by the deconvolution of C(t) with AIF(t), exhibits three sequential peaks (successively glomerular, proximal tubule, distal tubule). The rate constants, k_{in} and k_{out} describe the flow into and out of the proximal tubule. SKGFR can be calculated according to the following equation:

$$SKGFR = \text{maximal slope of proximal tubule peak/} C(vasc)_{max}$$

$C(vasc)_{max}$ is the ratio of the maximum of the vascular peak divided by the RBV, taking into account that the contrast agent remains in the extravascular space. The SKGFR (in ml/min) is obtained by multiplying the GFR by the volume of the renal cortex, considered to be about

70% of a healthy kidney volume.[59] This method has provided more accurate results than the Rutland–Patlak model in an experimental study in rabbits, using ^{51}Cr-EDTA as a gold standard.[58]

- A third model to calculate SKGFR is an *extensive multicompartmental model*[60] including three cortical compartments (glomerular, capillary and proximal convoluted tubules, as in the previous model), three medullary compartments (loops of Henle, distal convoluted tubules, collecting ducts) and the collecting system. Despite being complex, this model has the advantage of assessing some important tubular physiological parameters. Applied to the passage of Gd into the first two compartments, the model allows calculation of GFR.

Use, in the future, of new classes of contrast agents which are freely filtered by the glomerulus but without interstitial diffusion may improve results of modelling. The first results performed in rats are encouraging.[61]

Single kidney extraction fraction

Global renal clearance can be calculated with MRI on the basis of ex vivo T1 measurement of urine and plasma samples after IV infusion of a contrast agent,[62] according to the above-mentioned formula (GFR = U × V/P). Although accurate when compared with reference methods, this approach is not applied in clinical practice.

Recently, a quantitative method of in vivo measurement of the single kidney extraction fraction (EF) was proposed by Dumoulin et al[63] and applied to experimental studies by Niendorf et al.[64–66] This method is based on the measurement of T1 within flowing arterial and venous blood (Look and Locker method) during continuous Gd infusion whereas the steady-state equation can be used:

$$SKGFR = EF \times RBF \times (1 - Hct)$$

where RBF is the renal blood flow and Hct is the level of haematocrit in the blood. The EF is calculated from the equation:

$$EF = Ca - Cv/Ca$$

where Ca and Cv are the arterial and venous Gd concentration respectively. Because of the linear relationship between relaxation rates and concentration of Gd, EF can be expressed alternatively as:

$$EF = (1/T1a - 1/T1v)/(1/T1a - 1/T1_0)$$

where T1a is T1 in the renal artery, T1v in the vein and T1$_0$ in the blood without Gd. Once EF is calculated for each kidney, values of SKGFR can be calculated if RBF is known. Preliminary animal studies have shown consistent results compared to those calculated from inulin clearance.

Tubular function

The tubular transit and change of concentration of contrast agent in tissue can be used as indirect features of renal function. Alternatively, we can evaluate either the urinary-concentration function using the medullary T2* effect of diffusible Gd chelates during water reabsorption, or the medullary transit of macromolecular Gd chelates, based on medullary T1 effect.

Intratubular concentration of diffusible Gd chelate (T2* effect)

When using an unspoiled gradient-echo sequence (to maintain residual transverse magnetization resulting in a T1/T2* weighting), with a standard dose of Gd chelate, the high concentration of Gd reached inside the kidney is respon-

Figure 18.12 Dynamic sequence after Gd injection showing the biphasic effect of contrast agent within the kidney due to a high level of concentration within the medulla (from top-to-bottom and left-to-right): at the vascular phase, we note a T1 effect within cortex then within medulla; at the tubular phase, a T2 effect is responsible for a drop of signal within medulla then within the pyelocaliceal system.

sible for a paradoxical signal drop, observed approximately 30–40 s after the beginning of the cortical enhancement (Figure 18.12). The predominant site of signal drop is in the medulla, where the tubular concentration of Gd chelates increases (by water reabsorption), thus providing a typical medullary phase, which has been extensively described in rabbits.[67–71] The drop in SI demonstrates a centripetal progression from the cortico-medullary junction to the papilla, starting in the Henle's loop (the so-called early medullary phase), continuing into the collecting ducts (the so-called late medullary phase). However, these two medullary phases are rarely separated in humans. The strength and delay of medullary signal changes depend on sequence parameters and on physiological parameters, such as hydration and renal function, but are normally symmetrical between both kidneys. The duration between the maximal SI in the cortex and the signal drop observed in the medulla can be used to delineate a more in-depth physiological insight.[72] In experimental nephropathies with severe renal insufficiency, the signal reversal in the medulla disappeared.[73,74]

In patients, this duration has been shown as a rough estimate for SKGFR and has in fact been shown to correlate significantly with creatinine clearance.[72] This relationship may become important in kidney diseases involving unilateral impairment, such as unilateral ureteral obstruction,[75,76] renal lithotripsy[77] or renal artery stenosis.[78] In the latter case, detection of the ipsilateral functional impairment can be sensitized, as with scintigraphy, by angiotensin-converting enzyme inhibitors (ACEI).

Intratubular transit of macromolecular Gd chelate (T1 effect)

Kobayashi et al[79,80] have developed new dendrimer-based macromolecular contrast agents (<8 nm in diameter and <60 kDa molecular weight), which accumulate in the renal tubules and allow visualization of structural and functional renal damage. These agents are concentrated in proximal straight tubules in the medullary rays and outer stripe of the outer medulla. In normal mouse kidney, they reach the collecting system in 2 minutes (similar to Gd-DTPA), but differ from Gd-DTPA measurements since the parenchyma demonstrates a layered appearance with alternating light and dark bands: (1) a bright band in the subcapsular cortex; (2) a dark band in the deep cortex; (3) a bright band in the outer stripe of the outer medulla; (4) a dark band in the inner stripe of the outer medulla; and (5) a bright inner medulla. In models of renal ischaemia (cisplatin injection and ischaemia reperfusion), mildly damaged kidneys did not develop the bright band in the outer stripe and excretion was delayed, while severely damaged kidneys showed a prolonged enhancement of the superficial cortex with a low and delayed medullary enhancement. Intensity of these changes was correlated with severity or duration of ischaemia and with degree of renal dysfunction. These patterns are consis-

Figure 18.13 Renal transit time in a child with ureteral obstruction on the left side: each image is a maximum intensity projection (MIP) of dynamic volumes obtained at six time points: approximately 30 s (A), 1 min (B), 90 s (C), 2 min (D), 3 min (E) and 12 min (F) after injection. The right ureter is opacified in (E). The left ureter is opacified only lately (F). (Courtesy of Richard Jones, Emory University School of Medicine, Atlanta, USA.)

tent with the location of tubular cell injury after ischaemia (apoptosis and necrosis) in the straight proximal tubule in the outer stripe of the outer medulla.[81] Therefore, this agent could be used in animals as a biomarker of acute ischaemic disorder in pharmacological studies.

Urinary excretion and renal transit time

In acute or chronic obstruction, functional information can estimate the severity of renal impairment and help with the differentiation between nonobstructed dilated collecting system and real obstruction. Nuclear medicine techniques are routinely used for these purposes in clinical practice. MRI has the ability to associate functional data and morphological information on the renal parenchyma and collecting system.

Rorhschneider et al in an experimental model of urinary obstruction,[53] then in patients,[2,54] showed that, beside the split renal function estimation, classical criteria used in scintigraphy for obstruction could also be used with MRI. More recently, the renal transit time measured between the vascular enhancement of the cortex and the appearance of Gd within the ureter at the level of or below the lower pole of the kidney showed good agreement with scintigraphy (Figure 18.13). These methods are described in more detail in Chapter 8 about obstruction.

Angiotensin-converting enzyme inhibitor-sensitized MR renography

In the presence of significant renal artery stenosis, a drop of GFR following administration of angiotensin-converting

enzyme inhibitor can be observed with the different techniques described previously in this chapter. Details about applications of this method have been described in Chapter 16.

Other parameters of renal function

Intrarenal oxygenation

Under normal conditions, the medullary partial pressure of oxygen is low (10–20 mmHg) compared to the cortex (50 mmHg).[82] This medullary hypoxia is related to a low blood flow and high oxygen consumption due to active water and sodium reabsorption by Na^+-K^+-ATPase pumps along the thick ascending limb of the Henle's loop, located in the outer medulla. Therefore, the trade-off for an efficient urinary-concentrating mechanism seems to be the delicate balance between sufficient oxygenation and medullary hypoxia.[82] Increased tubular work such as that caused by diabetes or unilateral nephrectomy, or decreased medullary perfusion such as that induced by contrast nephropathy, can easily shift the balance towards hypoxia.

A decrease in intrarenal T2 during hypoxia using spin-echo sequences was first described by Terrier et al;[83] this predominated in the outer medulla. Then, by using T2*-weighted gradient-echo sequences, a decrease in signal intensity was demonstrated within the outer medulla during glycerol-induced renal ischaemia[84] or during hypoxia.[85] The same medullary changes were observed when a vasoconstriction was induced after L-NAME (nitric oxide inhibitor) injection.[85] These SI changes were related to variations in intrarenal oxygenation based on changes in the deoxyhaemoglobin concentration (BOLD, blood oxygen level dependent effect).

Figure 18.14 BOLD-sensitive sequence of normal rabbit kidneys before (left) and after (right) injection of L-NAME, responsible for a renal vasoconstriction: the injection produces a medullary hypoxia shown as a drop in signal intensity.

By using gradient-echo sequences with several TE values, intrarenal R2* (R2* = 1/T2*) can be quantitated.[86] This approach provides regional R2* values which appeared, in pigs, linearly correlated with measured microelectrode pO_2 values.[87] Using intrarenal R2* maps in humans, Prasad et al reported higher R2* values within the medulla than within the cortex in normally functioning kidneys due to the higher oxygen consumption in this compartment.[86] They showed that the medullary pO_2 was increased by water diuresis (at least in young individuals) and by furosemide, which inhibits active reabsorptive transport in medullary tubules.[88] Such changes could not be observed after acetazolamide injection acting on cortical proximal convoluted tubules.[89] They also showed that medullary oxygenation in rats was reduced by inhibition of the synthesis of prostaglandin[90] (Figure 18.14) and by inhibition of nitric oxide as well as by intravenous injection of radiocontrast agents.[91] Using high-resolution BOLD images of rat kidneys, we showed the highest R2* within the outer stripe of the outer medulla,[92] the compartment containing the ascending limbs of loops of Henle. Increased tubular work, due to increased GFR in experimental early diabetic nephropathy, was responsible for a decrease of oxygenation of the outer medulla.[92]

In a recent study on a pig model of unilateral dynamic renal artery stenosis, Juillard et al[93] showed that O_2 consumption decreased and R2* increased (in cortex and medulla) in proportional to the degree of reduction of renal blood flow.

Use of colour mapping of R2* has been proposed by some authors to enhance the visual conspicuity of dynamic changes in patients.[94] Higher field strength, such as 3 Teslas magnets, now available for imaging patients, provides a higher signal-to-noise ratio and a better spatial resolution.[95]

The applications of this technique to clinical conditions of intrarenal regional hypoxia have still to be established. The only clinical trial in the pathological situation published to date concerns diabetic patients without microalbuminuria, hypertension or renal insufficiency. Compared to a matched control group, these patients had no significant improvement of medullary oxygenation after water load,[96] reflecting a probable deficiency in medullary vasodilatation perhaps due to reduction of local synthesis of protaglandins, NO or other vasoactive substances.

Renal diffusion imaging

Water transport is the predominant phenomenon throughout the kidney due to its role in water reabsorption and its concentration–dilution function. These movements are mainly located within the tubular cells. Consequently, useful insights into the mechanisms of various renal diseases such as chronic renal failure, renal artery stenosis and ureteral obstruction may be obtained by measuring the diffusion characteristics of the kidney. However, diffusion imaging is a challenging technique within the kidney, due to the extreme sensitivity of diffusion-weighted sequences to several sources of artifacts.

Technical issues

In diffusion-weighted sequences, which are also T2 weighted, the SI decreases when diffusion gradients are activated according to the movements of water molecules within the tissue. Diffusion imaging is usually performed using different diffusion-weighted images with diffusion-sensitive gradients applied according to selected 'b-values', from which a map of the apparent diffusion coefficient (ADC) is made. However, the attenuation of SI observed on diffusion-weighted sequences depends on two factors. First, it depends on the molecular movements within the intra- and extracellular spaces that are determined by temperature and biological barriers present in the tissue (cellular membranes, fibres, organelles, macromolecules, etc.). Second, it depends on 'external' factors like blood perfusion, magnetic susceptibility, cardiac pulsation rate and respiratory movements.[97] Many difficulties remain patent for abdominal applications, such as susceptibility artifacts originated from bowel gas, peristaltic and respiratory movements and arterial pulsatility, which is important to consider for kidney applications because of the size of abdominal arteries and their high flow rates, especially in the renal arteries.

The effect of arterial pulsatility on SI is often neglected in abdominal diffusion imaging, probably due to the increased acquisition time imposed by cardiac triggering. However, a study by Mürtz et al[98] demonstrated that using a respiratory-triggered diffusion MRI significantly improves the accuracy and the reproducibility of ADC values in liver, spleen and kidneys, with an optimal delay in the range 500–600 ms, whereas the absence of respiratory triggering increases ADC values because of a spin-dephasing effect.

Knowledge of the tissue characteristics is important in order to choose adequate sequence parameters. For example if diffusion of water molecules is isotropic within the tissue (i.e. randomly oriented), measurement of ADC is independent of the direction of the employed diffusion-sensitive gradients, as generally presented in the liver and most tumours. In the kidney, on the other hand, the intrarenal structure generates an anisotropic water movement (i.e. predominant in one direction), especially within medulla.[99] When diffusion is anisotropic, diffusion coefficient values will depend on the direction of diffusion gradients: therefore, the only reproducible measurement is the trace of the diffusion tensor (ADC trace), which needs either to encode three or more directions of space for each b-value, or to use a single measurement with an 'isotropic diffusion preparation',[100] which is less time consuming.

The choice of employed b-values reported in the different renal studies differs markedly. High b-values improve the precision of measurements (lower standard deviation) but also increase the acquisition time. Therefore, only two separate b-values (b = 0 and b > 0) are typically used in diffusion MRI. The maximum b-value has an impact on calculated ADC values, i.e. the lower the b-value the higher the ADC because of an increased contribution of random 'external' factors that are independent of the molecular diffusion. To reduce these effects, which are most predominant for $b < 100$ s/mm^2, it is recommended to use high b-values,[101,102] knowing that they decrease the signal-to-noise ratio. A compromise must therefore be found, and in our experience three b-values between 0–400 s/mm^2 should be used for the kidney; these are relatively lower than those in brain (about 0–1000 s/mm^2).

Respiratory control is possible with breath-holding if compatible with the scan duration and whenever the cooperation of the patient is adequate. Echo planar imaging (EPI) acquisitions help in that sense. If not, respiratory compensation or navigator echoes can be used, but this method has never been compared to breath-holding. The scan duration depends on the number of slices, number of b-values, maximum b-value and number of diffusion-encoding directions.

In summary, technical constraints for diffusion MRI in the kidney are as follows: cardiac gating, breath-holding for native kidneys (not necessarily for transplants), three diffusion-encoding directions in the renal parenchyma, at least two b-values with a maximum between 500 and 800 s/mm^2, and the use of a single-shot EPI sequence[103–106] or a multishot EPI sequence (for better signal-to-noise ratio).

Applications

The many technical protocols that exist may explain the variability of reported ADC values of normal cortex and medulla in the literature. Most renal diffusion studies have measured ADC in only one direction[103,105,106] due to time constraints with the assumption that the molecular diffusion of water was isotropic. Ries et al[99] recently demonstrated that

ADC values were higher in the cortex than in the medulla and that diffusion in medulla was anisotropic (Figure 18.15). Renal ADC values are lower in neonates and increase progressively with age, with the largest increase during the

A

B

Figure 18.15 Diffusion-weighted MR imaging of normal human kidney. A: T2 weighted image of the left kidney without diffusion weighting (b = 0). B: ADC-trace map, obtained with single-shot echo-planar sequence, and showing higher ADC values within the cortex than within the medulla. Reprinted with permission from reference 99.

first years of life.[107] Hydration has been shown to increase global ADC values,[104] but the protocol was not optimized. Therefore, a new validation should be performed because a normalized hydration would be required for clinical studies.

In acute renal disease, diffusion-weighted imaging could be useful to separate cellular oedema from cellular necrosis, i.e. assessment of reversible versus nonreversible renal function as in acute brain ischaemia. In an experimental model of diabetic nephropathy, we showed that the regional ADC values decreased in the outer medulla, where ischaemic tubular cell lesions occur.[92] However, the exact role of this method in evaluating prognosis of acute renal diseases through the characterization of cell viability has still to be defined.

In chronic renal diseases, including renal artery stenosis and ureteral obstruction, a decrease of ADC was noted[104,103] and they were highly correlated with serum creatinine levels.[103] The idea that development of fibrosis in chronic renal diseases could be correlated to a restricted diffusibility of water spins and to decreased diffusion coefficients, should be explored in the future, with many potential applications such as follow-up of chronic rejection in renal transplants.

Diffusion-weighted imaging can also be used to characterize the tumours, based on structural changes. Depending on their type and their grade, tumours present with extremely variable perfusion level, cellular density, free water content, necrotic areas, i.e. a variable density of tissue barriers to water movements.[108] Therefore, rapidly growing tumours should be characterized, in viable and non-necrotic areas, by a high density of organelles and cytoskeleton, restricting water movements. A decrease of ADC in this type of tumour has been verified within the liver, where hepatocarcinomas and metastases showed lower ADC than benign tumours,[109] and within prostate[102] and kidney, where carcinomas presented with very low values of ADC.[110]

Renal sodium imaging

Intrarenal sodium distribution is characterized by a cortico-medullary gradient, essential for the urinary concentrating process. It is closely associated with renal function. In a recent study, Maril et al[111] demonstrated the three-dimensional intrarenal sodium gradient. Recording of a ^{23}Na MR signal requires specifically tuned coils. Its resonance frequency is 53 MHz at 4.7 T. By measuring the sodium R1 and R2 in vivo as well as in excised kidneys it was shown that changes in SI were directly proportional to tissue sodium concentration. In normal kidneys, sodium SI increased gradually along the cortico-medullary axis, from the edge of the cortex through to the outer part of the inner medulla (slope of 0.53 ± 0.12 relative intensity units per mm). Conversion of intensity units to tissue sodium concentration units yielded a slope of 31 ± 3 mmol/l/mm (from 60 mmol/l in the external edge of the cortex to 360 mmol/l in the inner medullary edge). Furosemide administration as well as urinary obstruction

produced marked and distinct alterations of medullary sodium profiles. The changes in sodium gradient also correlated with the extent of damage and the residual function of the kidneys. Clinical use of this technique has not yet been investigated.

Renal pH MR imaging

Tissue pH can be measured either by MR spectroscopy or by MRI, using intrinsic resonance changes related to pH variations or pH-sensitive Gd complexes, respectively. With the latter, SI changes are dependent on both pH value and agent concentration. Therefore, to measure tissue pH, it is necessary to inject sequentially two agents with the same pharmacokinetics: one is insensitive (allowing normalization) and the other sensitive to pH. Using this technique and a gadolinium-based pH-sensitive contrast agent, Gd-DOTA-4AmP[5–112] Raghunand et al[113] computed pH images of the kidney before and after acetazolamide administration. Normal kidneys showed a pH of 7.0–7.4 whereas the pixels corresponding to the papilla and calyces had a pH of 5.75–7. After administration of acetazolamide, carbonic anhydrase inhibitor which causes systemic metabolic acidosis and alkalinization of urine, pH increased significantly within medulla calyces and ureters (pH = 7.5–8) and decreased in extrarenal tissues.

Cellular MR imaging

MR imaging of intrarenal inflammation

Macrophages, virtually absent in normal kidneys, may infiltrate renal tissues in specific nephropathies such as acute proliferative types of human and experimental glomerulonephritides,[114] renal graft dysfunctions (rejection and acute tubular necrosis)[115] and nonspecific kidney diseases such as hydronephrosis.[116] This macrophagic attraction is a dynamic process under the control of chemotactic molecules (Fc fragment of immunoglobulins, TGF-β, TNF-α, etc.) and expression level of leucocyte adhesion molecules. The degree of macrophagic infiltration and proliferation is correlated with the severity of renal disease, whereas it remains unclear if macrophages produce direct renal insults or if they are a consequence of the disease in order to regulate the inflammatory response. Their role is complex, contributing to glomerular and tubulo-interstitial injury through the secretion of various cytokines and proteases which induce changes in extracellular matrix and progressive fibrotic changes (glomerulosclerosis, tubulointerstitial fibrosis).[117]

The macrophagic activity may vary, depending on the type of kidney disease and its severity. It predominates within the glomeruli (i.e. within the cortex) in glomerulonephritis, or within the interstitium (i.e. diffuse, within all kidney compartments) in interstitial nephritis or in hydronephrosis.

Today, in clinical practice, the degree of inflammatory response in the kidney can only be approached by renal biopsy. Therefore, identification of intrarenal macrophage infiltration with a noninvasive technique has great potential since it could participate in characterization of the kidney disease and its activity and monitor response to treatment.

Iron-oxide particles are used with MRI for in vivo targeting of mononuclear phagocytic system cells. Small particles of iron oxide (SPIO) are phagocytized by Kupffer cells of the liver and are already used in clinical practice.[118] Ultrasmall superparamagnetic particles of iron oxide (USPIO) are small-sized nanoparticles which have a longer half-life in the bloodstream (2 h in rats and 36 h in humans) and are avidly captured several hours after intravenous injection by extrahepatic cells with phagocytic activity, which include blood circulating monocytes and resident macrophages that are present in most tissues. The exact mechanism of iron capture is not known and may be cell specific.

Several models of experimental nephropathies in rats were used to demonstrate the detectability of intrarenal macrophagic activity in vivo. In a model of nephrotic syndrome in the rat[119] USPIO-enhanced MR images performed at 24 h demonstrated a diffuse decrease of SI predominating within the outer medulla. The degree of decrease of SI was correlated with the number of macrophages within each renal compartment and to the amount of iron within the tissue. In a model of obstructed kidney the same technique demonstrated a diffuse homogeneous decrease of SI in the three renal compartments. All obstructed kidneys demonstrated diffuse macrophagic infiltration on pathological examination.[120]

In a rat model of anti-GBM glomerulonephritis with a glomerular macrophagic infiltration similar to the human Goodpasture's syndrome, we evaluated the possibility of differentiating glomerular from interstitial macrophagic infiltration. In this model significant signal drop was observed only in the cortex where glomerular lesions were located. The intensity of signal drop was strongly correlated with the degree of proteinuria at day 2 and day 14.[120]

The same technique was also used in models of acute and chronic rejection.[121,122] In both situations, medical treatment of rejection decreased the MR SI changes. The technique also demonstrated macrophagic activity within the medulla in a model of reperfusion ischaemia of the kidney and no change was noted in the cortex.[123] This is due to a medullary infiltration by mononuclear cells, within the lumen of vasa recta, which is at a maximum between 48 h and 72 h after the ischaemic injury.[124]

In summary, these experimental results showed that MR imaging, 24 h after injection of USPIO, can demonstrate intrarenal signal variations due to iron ingestion by macrophages or by glomerular cells gaining endocytic activity, i.e. mesangial cells, and can localize precisely this endocytic

A

B

Figure 18.16 Patient with renal transplant and acute rejection. T2*-weighted MR imaging before (A) and 72 h after intravenous injection of USPIO (B) shows a decrease of signal related to inflammatory cellular infiltration in all renal compartments.

activity in the different kidney compartments. Different types of experimental renal diseases show different and reproducible types of intrarenal capture of USPIO which reflect different patterns of macrophagic infiltration and endocytic activity. Moreover, the degree of renal disease appeared to be correlated to the degree of endocytic activity, which may have significant implications in clinical practice.

The results of the first clinical study were published recently,[125] based on 12 patients. MR imaging was performed 3 days after USPIO injection (Sinerem®, Guerbet Group) to ensure the elimination of signal changes from vascular blood volume, knowing that the blood half-life of USPIO is 36 h. All patients but one with an inflammatory component on cortical biopsy showed a significant decrease of SI after USPIO injection (Figure 18.16). Patients with chronic and fibrotic disease without an inflammatory component on biopsy did not show any significant change. Three patients with acute tubular necrosis (two transplanted kidneys and one native kidney) showed a significant decrease of SI within the medulla. These preliminary clinical findings seem to corroborate experimental results and call for larger multicentre clinical trials, and evaluation of imaging at 2 days after injection to reduce delay in the diagnosis.

MR imaging of intrarenal cell therapy

Multipotent stem cells have shown great therapeutic promise because of their natural capability of regenerating damaged tissues. Noninvasive imaging techniques allowing in vivo assessment of the location of stem cells are therefore of great value for experimental studies in which these cells are transplanted. Using SPIO preparations to magnetically label cells, several groups have demonstrated the feasibility of grafting and subsequent visualization of neural progenitor cells in spine[126] and brain,[127] and mesenchymal stem cells (MSC) in myocardium.[128] MSC can be isolated from the bone marrow and expanded in vitro.[129] They can colonize many organs including liver and kidney after grafting. Recently, the possibility of differentiation of MSC into mesangial cells[130,131] and of haematopoietic stem cells (HSC) into tubular cells was demonstrated in vivo.[132]

Magnetically labelled stem cells were implanted in the heart and central nervous system, providing a high concentration of cells, with a high T2* effect. While MR imaging was able to demonstrate cell migration away from the injection site in these two organs, such a migration could not be observed within the kidney.[133] The renal distribution following intravascular administration of SPIO-labelled MSC was investigated. No renal uptake of labelled stem cells was observed in vivo after intravenous administration.[134] However, labelled MSC within kidney was observed in vivo with MRI (1.5 T) following injection into the renal artery.[133] So, this route can be used to seed cells throughout the target organ for tissue regeneration or transgene expression. It provides a means to immediately verify if the cells have indeed grafted within the target organ. Possibly, it may also allow an estimation of the number of cells that were seeded. Finally, sequential imaging studies will allow assessment of the permanence of the grafted cells over time.

Conclusion

MR imaging has a huge potential for noninvasive evaluation of multiple parameters of renal function. Semiquantitative approaches are now coming into clinical practice, mostly in the field of obstructive uropathy. Quantification of renal perfusion or glomerular filtration still requires development and validation with reference methods. Many technical issues remain to be solved including fast R1 calculation. It is possible that with higher gradient performances and perhaps higher field strengths, improvements in acquiring functional information may occur in the near future, permitting wider use of functional measurements in clinical practice.

Finally, USPIO-enhanced MR imaging of the kidney offers the possibility of identifying noninvasively the inflammatory component within the kidney which may have a major impact on subsequent development of fibrosis. Cellular labelling with these particles may also help for in vivo monitoring of renal stem cell therapies.

Acknowledgements

Acknowledgements for fruitful collaboration and discussion in many of these studies, to: C. Bos, J. Bulte, C. Combes, C. Deminière, P. Desbarat, J. Frøkiaer, I. Gordon, R. Jones, L. Juillard, C.T.W. Moonen, A. Prigent, M. Pedersen, M. Ries, J. Ripoche, B. de Senneville and H. Trillaud.

References

1. Bennett HF, Li D. MR imaging of renal function. Magn Reson Imaging Clin N Am 1997; 5: 107–26.

2. Rohrschneider WK, Haufe S, Wiesel M et al. Functional and morphologic evaluation of congenital urinary tract dilatation by using combined static-dynamic MR urography: findings in kidneys with a single collecting system. Radiology 2002; 224: 683–94.

3. Montet X, Ivancevic MK, Belenger J et al. Noninvasive measurement of absolute renal perfusion by contrast medium-enhanced magnetic resonance imaging. Invest Radiol 2003; 38: 584–92.

4. Ivancevic MK, Zimine I, Montet X et al. Inflow effect correction in fast gradient-echo perfusion imaging. Magn Reson Med 2003; 50: 885–91.

5. Pedersen M, Frokier J, Grenier N. Quantitative measurement of renal function using contrast enhanced MRI: an initial experience. In: Int Scientific Meeting Radionucl Nephr-Urol, ISCORN; 2004; La Baule; 2004. p. Poster presentation, M15.

6. Pedersen M, Shi Y, Anderson P et al. Quantitation of differential renal blood flow and renal function using dynamic contrast-enhanced MRI in rats. Magn Reson Med 2004; 51: 510–7.

7. Rusinek H, Lee VS, Johnson G. Optimal dose of Gd-DTPA in dynamic MR studies. Magn Reson Med 2001; 46: 312–6.

8. Lee JH, Li X, Sammi MK, Springer CS Jr. Using flow relaxography to elucidate flow relaxivity. J Magn Reson 1999; 136: 102–13.

9. Freeman AJ, Gowland PA, Mansfield P. Optimization of the

ultrafast Look-Locker echo-planar imaging T1 mapping sequence. Magn Reson Imaging 1998; 16: 765–72.

10. Noseworthy MD, Kim JK, Stainsby JA et al. Tracking oxygen effects on MR signal in blood and skeletal muscle during hyperoxia exposure. J Magn Reson Imaging 1999; 9: 814–20.

11. Chen Z, Prato FS, McKenzie C. T1 fast acquisition relaxation mapping (T1-FARM): an optimized reconstruction. IEEE Trans Med Imaging 1998; 17: 155–60.

12. Zheng J, Venkatesan R, Haacke EM et al. Accuracy of T1 measurements at high temporal resolution: feasibility of dynamic measurement of blood T1 after contrast administration. J Magn Reson Imaging 1999; 10: 576–81.

13. McKenzie CA, Pereira RS, Prato FS et al. Improved contrast agent bolus tracking using T1 FARM. Magn Reson Med 1999; 41: 429–35.

14. Pedersen M, Dissing T, Deding D et al. MR renography based on contrast-enhanced T1-mapping. In: Medicine ISfMRi, editor. International Society for Magnetic Resonance in Medicine; Miami; 2005. p. 526.

15. Bjornerud A, Johansson LO, Briley-Saebo K, Ahlstrom HK. Assessment of T1 and T2* effects in vivo and ex vivo using iron oxide nanoparticles in steady state – dependence on blood volume and water exchange. Magn Reson Med 2002; 47: 461–71.

16. Schoenberg SO, Rieger J, Johannson LO et al. Diagnosis of renal artery stenosis with magnetic resonance angiography: update 2003. Nephrol Dial Transplant 2003; 18: 1252–6.

17. Debatin JF, Ting RH, Wegmuller H et al. Renal artery blood flow: quantitation with phase-contrast MR imaging with and without breath holding. Radiology 1994; 190: 371–8.

18. Mustert BR, Williams DM, Prince MR. In vitro model of arterial stenosis: correlation of MR signal dephasing and transstenotic pressure gradients. Magn Reson Imaging 1998; 16: 301–10.

19. Schoenberg SO, Just A, Bock M et al. Noninvasive analysis of renal artery blood flow dynamics with MR cine phase-contrast flow measurements. Am J Physiol 1997; 272: H2477–84.

20. Schoenberg SO, Knopp MV, Bock M et al. Renal artery stenosis: grading of hemodynamic changes with cine phase-contrast MR blood flow measurements. Radiology 1997; 203: 45–53.

21. Schoenberg SO, Knopp MV, Londy F et al. Morphologic and functional magnetic resonance imaging of renal artery stenosis: a multireader tricenter study. J Am Soc Nephrol 2002; 13: 158–69.

22. Axel L. Cerebral blood flow determination by rapid-sequence computed tomography: theoretical analysis. Radiology 1980; 137: 679–86.

23. Trillaud H, Grenier N, Degreze P et al. First-pass evaluation of renal perfusion with TurboFLASH MR imaging and superparamagnetic iron oxide particles. J Magn Reson Imaging 1993; 3: 83–91.

24. Prasad PV, Cannillo J, Chavez DR et al. First-pass renal perfusion imaging using MS-325, an albumin-targeted MRI contrast agent. Invest Radiol 1999; 34: 566–71.

25. Aumann S, Schoenberg SO, Just A et al. Quantification of renal perfusion using an intravascular contrast agent (part 1): results in a canine model. Magn Reson Med 2003; 49: 276–87.

26. Weisskoff RM, Chesler D, Boxerman JL, Rosen BR. Pitfalls in MR measurement of tissue blood flow with intravascular tracers: which mean transit time? Magn Reson Med 1993; 29: 553–8.

27. Ostergaard L, Weisskoff RM, Chesler DA et al. High resolution measurement of cerebral blood flow using intravascular tracer bolus passages. Part I: Mathematical approach and statistical analysis. Magn Reson Med 1996; 36: 715–25.

28. Trillaud H, Degreze P, Mesplede Y et al. Evaluation of experimentally induced renal hypoperfusion using iron oxide particles and fast magnetic resonance imaging. Acad Radiol 1995; 2: 293–9.

29. Schoenberg SO, Aumann S, Just A et al. Quantification of renal perfusion abnormalities using an intravascular contrast agent (part 2): results in animals and humans with renal artery stenosis. Magn Reson Med 2003; 49: 288–98.

30. Vallee JP, Lazeyras F, Khan HG, Terrier F. Absolute renal blood flow quantification by dynamic MRI and Gd-DTPA. Eur Radiol 2000; 10: 1245–52.

31. Peters AM, Brown J, Hartnell GG et al. Non-invasive measurement of renal blood flow with 99mTc DTPA: comparison with radiolabelled microspheres. Cardiovasc Res 1987; 21: 830–4.

32. Dujardin M, Sourbron S, Luypaert R et al. Quantification of renal perfusion and function on a voxel-by-voxel basis: a feasibility study. Magn Reson Med 2005; In press.

33. Trillaud H, Degreze P, Combe C et al. Evaluation of intrarenal distribution of ultrasmall superparamagnetic iron oxide particles by magnetic resonance imaging and modification by furosemide and water restriction. Invest Radiol 1994; 29: 540–6.

34. Trillaud H, Degreze P, Combe C et al. USPIO-enhanced MR imaging of glycerol-induced acute renal failure in the rabbit. Magn Reson Imaging 1995; 13: 233–40.

35. Vexler VS, Berthezene Y, Clement O et al. Detection of zonal renal ischemia with contrast-enhanced MR imaging with a macromolecular blood pool contrast agent. J Magn Reson Imaging 1992; 2: 311–9.

36. Laissy JP, Benderbous S, Idee JM et al. MR assessment of iodinated contrast-medium-induced nephropathy in rats using ultrasmall particles of iron oxide. J Magn Reson Imaging 1997; 7: 164–70.

37. Laissy JP, Idee JM, Loshkajian A et al. Reversibility of experimental acute renal failure in rats: assessment with USPIO-enhanced MR imaging. J Magn Reson Imaging 2000; 12: 278–88.

38. Edelman RR, Hatabu H, Tadamura E et al. Noninvasive assessment of regional ventilation in the human lung using oxygen-enhanced magnetic resonance imaging. Nat Med 1996; 2: 1236–9.

39. Jones R, Ries M, Moonen C, Grenier N. Functional imaging of the kidneys using the inhalation of pure oxygen: a feasability study. In: Internation Society of Magnetic Resonance in Medicine; 2001; Glasgow: p. 523.

40. Calamante F, Thomas DL, Pell GS et al. Measuring cerebral blood flow using magnetic resonance imaging techniques. J Cereb Blood Flow Metab 1999; 19: 701–35.

41. Detre JA, Leigh JS, Williams DS, Koretsky AP. Perfusion imaging. Magn Reson Med 1992; 23: 37–45.

42. Roberts DA, Detre JA, Bolinger L et al. Renal perfusion in humans: MR imaging with spin tagging of arterial water. Radiology 1995; 196: 281–6.

43. Williams DS, Zhang W, Koretsky AP, Adler S. Perfusion imaging of the rat kidney with MR. Radiology 1994; 190: 813–8.

44. Alsop DC, Detre JA. Reduced transit-time sensitivity in noninvasive magnetic resonance imaging of human cerebral blood flow. J Cereb Blood Flow Metab 1996; 16: 1236–49.

45. Edelman RR, Siewert B, Darby DG et al. Qualitative mapping of cerebral blood flow and functional localization with echo-planar MR imaging and signal targeting with alternating radio frequency. Radiology 1994; 192: 513–20.

46. Kwong KK, Chesler DA, Weisskoff RM et al. MR perfusion studies with T1-weighted echo planar imaging. Magn Reson Med 1995; 34: 878–87.

47. Wong EC, Buxton RB, Frank LR. Quantitative imaging of perfusion using a single subtraction (QUIPSS and QUIPSS II). Magn Reson Med 1998; 39: 702–8.

48. Wang JJ, Hendrich KS, Jackson EK et al. Perfusion quantitation in transplanted rat kidney by MRI with arterial spin labeling. Kidney Int 1998; 53: 1783–91.

49. Prasad PV, Kim D, Kaiser AM et al. Noninvasive comprehensive characterization of renal artery stenosis by combination of STAR angiography and EPISTAR perfusion imaging. Magn Reson Med 1997; 38: 776–87.

50. Martirosian P, Klose U, Mader I, Schick F. FAIR true-FISP perfusion imaging of the kidneys. Magn Reson Med 2004; 51: 353–61.

51. Dalla-Palma L, Panzetta G, Pozzi-Mucelli RS et al. Dynamic magnetic resonance imaging in the assessment of chronic medical nephropathies with impaired renal function. Eur Radiol 2000; 10: 280–6.

52. Rohrschneider WK, Hoffend J, Becker K et al. Combined static-dynamic MR urography for the simultaneous evaluation of morphology and function in urinary tract obstruction. I. Evaluation of the normal status in an animal model. Pediatr Radiol 2000; 30: 511–22.

53. Rohrschneider WK, Becker K, Hoffend J et al. Combined static-dynamic MR urography for the simultaneous evaluation of morphology and function in urinary tract obstruction. II. Findings in experimentally induced ureteric stenosis. Pediatr Radiol 2000; 30: 523–32.

54. Rohrschneider WK, Haufe S, Clorius JH, Troger J. MR to assess renal function in children. Eur Radiol 2003; 13: 1033–45.

55. Hackstein N, Heckrodt J, Rau WS. Measurement of single-kidney glomerular filtration rate using a contrast-enhanced dynamic gradient-echo sequence and the Rutland-Patlak plot technique. J Magn Reson Imaging 2003; 18: 714–25.

56. Patlak CS, Blasberg RG, Fenstermacher JD. Graphical evaluation of blood-to-brain transfer constants from multiple-time uptake data. J Cereb Blood Flow Metab 1983; 3: 1–7.

57. Hermoye L, Annet L, Lemmerling P et al. Calculation of the renal perfusion and glomerular filtration rate from the renal impulse response obtained with MRI. Magn Reson Med 2004; 51: 1017–25.

58. Annet L, Hermoye L, Peeters F et al. Glomerular filtration rate: assessment with dynamic contrast-enhanced MRI and a cortical-compartment model in the rabbit kidney. J Magn Reson Imaging 2004; 20: 843–9.

59. Hegedus V, Faarup P. Cortical volume of the normal human kidney. Correlated angiographic and morphologic investigations. Acta Radiol Diagn (Stockh) 1972; 12: 481–96.

60. Lee VS, Rusinek H, Noz ME et al. Dynamic three-dimensional MR renography for the measurement of single kidney function: initial experience. Radiology 2003; 227: 289–94.

61. Mandry D, Pedersen M, Odille F et al. Renal functional contrast-enhanced magnetic resonance imaging: evaluation of a new rapid-clearance blood pool agent (P792) in Sprague-Dawley rats. Invest Radiol 2005; 40: 295–305.

62. Choyke PL, Austin HA, Frank JA et al. Hydrated clearance of gadolinium-DTPA as a measurement of glomerular filtration rate. Kidney Int 1992; 41: 1595–8.

63. Dumoulin CL, Buonocore MH, Opsahl LR et al. Noninvasive measurement of renal hemodynamic functions using gadolinium enhanced magnetic resonance imaging. Magn Reson Med 1994; 32: 370–8.

64. Niendorf ER, Santyr GE, Brazy PC, Grist TM. Measurement of Gd-DTPA dialysis clearance rates by using a look-locker imaging technique. Magn Reson Med 1996; 36: 571–8.

65. Niendorf ER, Grist TM, Frayne R et al. Rapid measurement of Gd-DTPA extraction fraction in a dialysis system using echo-planar imaging. Med Phys 1997; 24: 1907–13.

66. Niendorf ER, Grist TM, Lee FT Jr et al. Rapid in vivo measurement of single-kidney extraction fraction and glomerular filtration rate with MR imaging. Radiology 1998; 206: 791–8.

67. Matthaei D, Frahm J, Haase A, Hanicke W. Regional physiological functions depicted by sequences of rapid magnetic resonance images. Lancet 1985; 2: 893.

68. Pettigrew RI, Avruch L, Dannels W et al. Fast-field-echo MR imaging with Gd-DTPA: physiologic evaluation of the kidney and liver. Radiology 1986; 160: 561–3.

69. Grenier N, Barat JL, Ducassou D, Broussin J. [Intrarenal kinetics of Gd-DOTA in sequential MRI in rabbits. Reproducibility study]. Ann Radiol (Paris) 1989; 32: 186–95.

70. Carvlin MJ, Arger PH, Kundel HL et al. Use of Gd-DTPA and fast gradient-echo and spin-echo MR imaging to demonstrate renal function in the rabbit. Radiology 1989; 170: 705–11.

71. Choyke PL, Frank JA, Girton ME et al. Dynamic Gd-DTPA-enhanced MR imaging of the kidney: experimental results. Radiology 1989; 170: 713–20.

72. Krestin G, Schuhmann-Giampieri G, Huastein J et al. Functional dynamic MRI, pharmacokinetics and safety of Gd-DTPA in patients with impaired renal function. Eur Radiol 1992; 2: 16–23.

73. Carvlin MJ, Arger PH, Kundel HL et al. Acute tubular necrosis: use of gadolinium-DTPA and fast MR imaging to evaluate renal function in the rabbit. J Comput Assist Tomogr 1987; 11: 488–95.

74. Frank JA, Choyke PL, Girton ME et al. Gadolinium-DTPA enhanced dynamic MR imaging in the evaluation of cisplatinum nephrotoxicity. J Comput Assist Tomogr 1989; 13: 448–59.

75. Semelka RC, Hricak H, Tomei E et al. Obstructive nephropathy: evaluation with dynamic Gd-DTPA-enhanced MR imaging. Radiology 1990; 175: 797–803.

76. Fichtner J, Spielman D, Herfkens R et al. Ultrafast contrast enhanced magnetic resonance imaging of congenital hydronephrosis in a rat model. J Urol 1994; 152: 682–7.

77. Krestin G, Fischbach R, Vorreuther R, von Schulthess G. Alterations in renal morphology and function after ESWL therapy: evaluation with dynamic contrast-enhanced MRI. Eur Radiol 1993; 3: 227–33.

78. Tsushima Y, Murakami T, Kuruma H et al. T2*-weighted

dynamic MR imaging in renal artery or vein stenosis. AJR Am J Roentgenol 1997; 168: 1041–3.

79. Kobayashi H, Kawamoto S, Jo SK et al. Renal tubular damage detected by dynamic micro-MRI with a dendrimer-based magnetic resonance contrast agent. Kidney Int 2002; 61: 1980–5.

80. Kobayashi H, Jo SK, Kawamoto S et al. Polyamine dendrimer-based MRI contrast agents for functional kidney imaging to diagnose acute renal failure. J Magn Reson Imaging 2004; 20: 512–8.

81. Offerman JJ, Meijer S, Sleijfer DT et al. Acute effects of cis-diamminedichloroplatinum (CDDP) on renal function. Cancer Chemother Pharmacol 1984; 12: 36–8.

82. Brezis M, Rosen S. Hypoxia of the renal medulla – its implications for disease. N Engl J Med 1995; 332: 647–55.

83. Terrier F, Lazeyras F, Posse S et al. Study of acute renal ischemia in the rat using magnetic resonance imaging and spectroscopy. Magn Reson Med 1989; 12: 114–36.

84. Vexler VS, de Crespigny AJ, Wendland MF et al. MR imaging of blood oxygenation-dependent changes in focal renal ischemia and transplanted liver tumor in rat. J Magn Reson Imaging 1993; 3: 483–90.

85. Trillaud H, Delalande C, Quesson B et al. BOLD MR signal changes due to hypoxia and renal vasoconstriction in rat kidney. In: International Society of Magnetic Resonance in Medicine; 1998; Sydney: p. 396.

86. Prasad PV, Chen Q, Goldfarb JW et al. Breath-hold R2* mapping with a multiple gradient-recalled echo sequence: application to the evaluation of intrarenal oxygenation. J Magn Reson Imaging 1997; 7: 1163–5.

87. Pedersen M, Dissing T, Morkenborg J et al. Validation of quantitative BOLD MRI measurements in kidney: application to unilateral ureteral obstruction. Kidney Int 2005; 67: 2305–12.

88. Brezis M, Agmon Y, Epstein FH. Determinants of intrarenal oxygenation. I. Effects of diuretics. Am J Physiol 1994; 267: F1059–62.

89. Priatna A, Epstein FH, Spokes K, Prasad PV. Evaluation of changes in intrarenal oxygenation in rats using multiple gradient-recalled echo (mGRE) sequence. J Magn Reson Imaging 1999; 9: 842–6.

90. Prasad PV, Epstein FH. Changes in renal medullary pO_2 during water diuresis as evaluated by blood oxygenation level-dependent magnetic resonance imaging: effects of aging and cyclooxygenase inhibition. Kidney Int 1999; 55: 294–8.

91. Prasad PV, Priatna A, Spokes K, Epstein FH. Changes in intrarenal oxygenation as evaluated by BOLD MRI in a rat kidney model for radiocontrast nephropathy. J Magn Reson Imaging 2001; 13: 744–7.

92. Ries M, Basseau F, Tyndal B et al. Diffusion and BOLD-contrast imaging in the kidneys of diabetic rats. In: International Society of Magnetic Resonance in Medicine; 2001; Glasgow: p. 362.

93. Juillard L, Lerman LO, Kruger DG et al. Blood oxygen level-dependent measurement of acute intra-renal ischemia. Kidney Int 2004; 65: 944–50.

94. Zuo CS, Rofsky NM, Mahallati H et al. Visualization and quantification of renal R2* changes during water diuresis. J Magn Reson Imaging 2003; 17: 676–82.

95. Li LP, Vu AT, Li BS et al. Evaluation of intrarenal oxygenation by BOLD MRI at 3.0 T. J Magn Reson Imaging 2004; 20: 901–4.

96. Epstein FH, Veves A, Prasad PV. Effect of diabetes on renal medullary oxygenation during water diuresis. Diabetes Care 2002; 25: 575–8.

97. Schaefer PW, Grant PE, Gonzalez RG. Diffusion-weighted MR imaging of the brain. Radiology 2000; 217: 331–45.

98. Murtz P, Flacke S, Traber F et al. Abdomen: diffusion-weighted MR imaging with pulse-triggered single-shot sequences. Radiology 2002; 224: 258–64.

99. Ries M, Jones RA, Basseau F et al. Diffusion tensor MRI of the human kidney. J Magn Reson Imaging 2001; 14: 42–9.

100. Wong EC, Cox RW, Song AW. Optimized isotropic diffusion weighting. Magn Reson Med 1995; 34: 139–43.

101. Norris DG. Implications of bulk motion for diffusion-weighted imaging experiments: effects, mechanisms, and solutions. J Magn Reson Imaging 2001; 13: 486–95.

102. Issa B. In vivo measurement of the apparent diffusion coefficient in normal and malignant prostatic tissues using echo-planar imaging. J Magn Reson Imaging 2002; 16: 196–200.

103. Namimoto T, Yamashita Y, Mitsuzaki K et al. Measurement of the apparent diffusion coefficient in diffuse renal disease by diffusion-weighted echo-planar MR imaging. J Magn Reson Imaging 1999; 9: 832–7.

104. Muller MF, Prasad PV, Bimmler D et al. Functional imaging of the kidney by means of measurement of the apparent diffusion coefficient. Radiology 1994; 193: 711–5.

105. Yamada I, Aung W, Himeno Y et al. Diffusion coefficients in abdominal organs and hepatic lesions: evaluation with intravoxel incoherent motion echo-planar MR imaging. Radiology 1999; 210: 617–23.

106. Fukuda Y, Ohashi I, Hanafusa K et al. Anisotropic diffusion in kidney: apparent diffusion coefficient measurements for clinical use. J Magn Reson Imaging 2000; 11: 156–60.

107. Jones RA, Grattan-Smith JD. Age dependence of the renal apparent diffusion coefficient in children. Pediatr Radiol 2003; 33: 850–4.

108. Herneth AM, Guccione S, Bednarski M. Apparent diffusion coefficient: a quantitative parameter for in vivo tumor characterization. Eur J Radiol 2003; 45: 208–13.

109. Taouli B, Vilgrain V, Dumont E et al. Evaluation of liver diffusion isotropy and characterization of focal hepatic lesions with two single-shot echo-planar MR imaging sequences: prospective study in 66 patients. Radiology 2003; 226: 71–8.

110. Cova M, Squillaci E, Stacul F et al. Diffusion-weighted MRI in the evaluation of renal lesions: preliminary results. Br J Radiol 2004; 77: 851–7.

111. Maril N, Margalit R, Mispelter J, Degani H. Functional sodium magnetic resonance imaging of the intact rat kidney. Kidney Int 2004; 65: 927–35.

112. Zhang S, Wu K, Sherry AD. A novel pH-sensitive MRI contrast agent. Angew Chem Int Ed Engl 1999; 38: 3192–4.

113. Raghunand N, Howison C, Sherry AD et al. Renal and systemic pH imaging by contrast-enhanced MRI. Magn Reson Med 2003; 49: 249–57.

114. Cattell V. Macrophages in acute glomerular inflammation. Kidney Int 1994; 45: 945–52.

115. Grau V, Herbst B, Steiniger B. Dynamics of monocytes/macrophages and T lymphocytes in acutely rejecting rat renal allografts. Cell Tissue Res 1998; 291: 117–26.

116. Schreiner GF, Harris KP, Purkerson ML, Klahr S. Immunological aspects of acute ureteral obstruction: immune cell infiltrate in the kidney. Kidney Int 1988; 34: 487–93.

117. Erwig LP, Kluth DC, Rees AJ. Macrophages in renal inflammation. Curr Opin Nephrol Hypertens 2001; 10: 341–7.

118. Weissleder R, Cheng HC, Bogdanova A, Bogdanov A Jr. Magnetically labeled cells can be detected by MR imaging. J Magn Reson Imaging 1997; 7: 258–63.

119. Hauger O, Delalande C, Trillaud H et al. MR imaging of intrarenal macrophage infiltration in an experimental model of nephrotic syndrome. Magn Reson Med 1999; 41: 156–62.

120. Hauger O, Delalande C, Deminiere C et al. Nephrotoxic nephritis and obstructive nephropathy: evaluation with MR imaging enhanced with ultrasmall superparamagnetic iron oxide – preliminary findings in a rat model. Radiology 2000; 217: 819–26.

121. Zhang Y, Dodd SJ, Hendrich KS et al. Magnetic resonance imaging detection of rat renal transplant rejection by monitoring macrophage infiltration. Kidney Int 2000; 58: 1300–10.

122. Beckmann N, Cannet C, Fringeli-Tanner M et al. Macrophage labeling by SPIO as an early marker of allograft chronic rejection in a rat model of kidney transplantation. Magn Reson Med 2003; 49: 459–67.

123. Jo SK, Hu X, Kobayashi H et al. Detection of inflammation following renal ischemia by magnetic resonance imaging. Kidney Int 2003; 64: 43–51.

124. Ysebaert DK, De Greef KE, Vercauteren SR et al. Identification and kinetics of leukocytes after severe ischaemia/reperfusion renal injury. Nephrol Dial Transplant 2000; 15: 1562–74.

125. Hauger O, Grenier N, Deminière C et al. Late Sinerem®-enhanced MR imaging of Renal Diseases: a pilot study. In: Radiological Society of North America; 2004; Chicago: p. 512.

126. Bulte JW, Zhang S, van Gelderen P et al. Neurotransplantation of magnetically labeled oligodendrocyte progenitors: magnetic resonance tracking of cell migration and myelination. Proc Natl Acad Sci USA 1999; 96: 15256–61.

127. Hoehn M, Kustermann E, Blunk J et al. Monitoring of implanted stem cell migration in vivo: a highly resolved in vivo magnetic resonance imaging investigation of experimental stroke in rat. Proc Natl Acad Sci USA 2002; 99: 16267–72.

128. Kraitchman DL, Heldman AW, Atalar E et al. In vivo magnetic resonance imaging of mesenchymal stem cells in myocardial infarction. Circulation 2003; 107: 2290–3.

129. Jiang Y, Jahagirdar BN, Reinhardt RL et al. Pluripotency of mesenchymal stem cells derived from adult marrow. Nature 2002; 418: 41–9.

130. Imasawa T, Utsunomiya Y, Kawamura T et al. The potential of bone marrow-derived cells to differentiate to glomerular mesangial cells. J Am Soc Nephrol 2001; 12: 1401–9.

131. Ito T, Suzuki A, Imai E et al. Bone marrow is a reservoir of repopulating mesangial cells during glomerular remodeling. J Am Soc Nephrol 2001; 12: 2625–35.

132. Lin F, Cordes K, Li L et al. Hematopoietic stem cells contribute to the regeneration of renal tubules after renal ischemia-reperfusion injury in mice. J Am Soc Nephrol 2003; 14: 1188–99.

133. Bos C, Delmas Y, Desmouliere A, et al. In vivo MR imaging of intravascularly injected magnetically labeled mesenchymal stem cells in rat kidney and liver. Radiology 2004; 233: 781–9.

134. Hauger O, Frost E, Deminière C et al. MR evaluation of the glomerular homing of magnetically labeled mesenchymal stem cells in a rat model of nephropathy. Radiology 2005; In press.

19 Positron emission tomography imaging of the kidneys

Zsolt Szabo, William B Mathews

Technology

PET scanners

Positron emission tomography is a rapidly growing field of clinical nuclear medicine with most frequent applications in oncology and less frequent applications in cardiology and neurology. Recent developments have resulted in instruments that can image the whole body within 10–15 minutes, at a spatial resolution of 5 6 mm and counting sensitivities of 30 cps/Bq/ml.[1] The advantage of PET is that the images are readily corrected for radioisotope decay, radiopharmaceutical dose, tissue attenuation and scatter. The concentration of the radiopharmaceutical can be calibrated and displayed in MBq/ml, kBq/ml/MBq injected dose or mEq/ml. These properties of PET make quantification of renal blood flow and glomerular filtration rate (GFR) straightforward and also make imaging of molecular targets including enzymes and receptors of the kidneys possible. Despite the many advantages, clinical applications of PET are still in their early development.

Hybrid PET/CT imaging has the advantages that both types of images, molecular and anatomical, are immediately available, the same bed is used for both scans, which results in minimal organ movement, and, last but not least, the scans are close in time and can be displayed in a single, integrated image set.[2, 3] Of special interest would be combined imaging of a molecular target with PET and angiography with CT in renovascular hypertension, an approach that has already been tested for myocardial imaging.[4] The accuracy of CT angiography to detect renal artery stenosis is very high[5–7] but PET could provide information on tissue viability by measuring expression of proteins that are upregulated or downregulated in hypoxia and other disease states. Technical challenges, such as image distortion by respiratory motion are being addressed in studies not directly related to renal imaging.[8]

Image acquisition and processing

Imaging times in renal PET studies depend on the isotope and the study type. Renal blood flow studies carried out with O-15 labelled water, rubidium-82 or N-13 labelled ammonia can be finished in minutes[9,10] while functional studies of glomerular filtration require imaging times of 20–30 minutes.[11] Kinetic investigations of receptor binding or metabolism required 60–90 minutes of imaging time,[10,12,13] which decreases the appeal of these studies compared to FDG PET in oncology, where total body imaging can now be accomplished in as short a time as 10 minutes.[2]

Four types of PET imaging devices are being used: (a) small animal PET scanners for mice and rats; (b) dedicated PET scanners for larger animals and humans; (c) hybrid PET/CT scanners for human or animal studies; and (d) dual head gamma-camera-based coincidence detectors. Small animal scanners and dedicated PET scanners are excellent for research and the most promising clinical imaging device is hybrid PET/CT. Coincidence detectors are not suited for renal imaging studies since they offer relatively limited sensitivity and spatial resolution and do not permit acquisition of dynamic PET studies.

Iterative reconstruction[1] will have an impact on PET imaging studies of the kidneys as it can correct artifacts caused by high variance in the regional distribution of the radioligand and has the feature of modelling and minimizing tissue attenuation and scatter. The most broadly applied iterative method, called ordered-subsets expectation maximization (OSEM) algorithm was introduced in 1994 to accelerate the convergence time of iteration[14] without compromising image quality.

Imaging targets

The main advantage of PET is that the images provide quantitative information on tracer kinetics. Kinetic parameters that correlate with biologically defined processes can be calculated for the entire renal cortex or as pixel-based parametric images. Renal PET studies can be classified as functional imaging studies, metabolic imaging studies, or molecular imaging studies. Examples of functional imaging studies are determinations of renal blood flow with O-15 labelled water, Rb-82, N-13 ammonia or copper-64 PTSM. Functional imaging studies also include measurements with tracers that are eliminated by glomerular filtration such as Co-55 labelled EDTA or Ga-68 labelled DTPA. Metabolic imaging studies can be performed to assess oxidative metabolism with C-11 acetate or glucose metabolism with sugar analogues.

The renin-angiotensin system is attainable for molecular imaging; its molecular targets that have been explored include the angiotensin-converting enzyme (ACE) and the angiotensin II subtype 1 receptor (AT1R). Glucose analogues can be radiolabelled with carbon-11 or fluorine-18 and their accumulation depends not only on the degree of glucose metabolism, but also on the expression of related proteins such as the membrane glucose transporters and the hexokinase enzyme. Thus, glucose analogues can be classified both as metabolic tracers (i.e. substrates) and molecular tracers (i.e. ligands).

Functional imaging

Functional imaging of the kidneys with PET has been performed for research purposes for a long time and the images are quantitative and of excellent quality. Most important functional studies are those used for quantification of renal blood flow and for assessment of regional glomerular function.

Renal blood flow

Renal blood flow can be quantified with O-15 water ($H_2^{15}O$), rubidium-82, N-13 ammonia, copper-64 PTSM or copper-62 PTSM. These tracers are not exclusive for renal imaging, however. O-15 water has been frequently used for measurement of cerebral blood flow while Rb-82 and PTSM have been used for measurement of myocardial blood flow. Blood flow tracers can be divided into two categories: category I tracers such as O-15 water are freely diffusible between the tissue compartments; category II tracers such as Rb-82, N-13 ammonia and Cu-62 PTSM are physiologically retained in the tissue.[15]

O-15 water

The original method of renal blood flow determination with $H_2^{15}O$ was performed in experimental animals and was based on short bolus administration of the tracer into the renal artery.[16] No imaging device was available and the washout of radioactivity was measured with external probes, just like it was done previously with radioactive inert gases. Curve analysis revealed two compartments, one with a flow rate of 370 ml/min/100 g and another with 55 ml/min/100 g. The faster component was explained by blood flow in the renal cortex and the slower component was explained by blood flow in the medulla and remaining tissues. Assuming a parallel connectivity model, the compartmental distribution was 55% for the fast and 45% for the slower component.

With present high-resolution PET scanners, individual time–activity curves can be obtained from the cortical and medullary volume elements (voxels) and fitted with individual monoexponential impulse response functions. The tracer is administered into a peripheral vein rather than the renal artery and therefore an input function has to be determined to estimate renal blood flow by numerical solution of a convolution integral.

After intravenous injection, O-15 water is transported through the cardiopulmonary vasculature and reaches the kidney via the renal artery. Due to a laminary flow in the large vessels, mixing and delay in cardiac chambers and arborization in the pulmonary blood vessels, the radioactive bolus becomes largely distorted before it reaches the renal parenchyma, but the fraction of radioactivity that reaches the kidneys during the first pass via the renal arteries will remain proportional to the distribution of the cardiac output. Due to nearly complete parenchymal extraction and rapid diffusion, O-15 water will enter all tissue partition within a short period of time so that its accumulation can be quantified both by a dynamic washin–washout model and a static autoradiographic model. Both models will yield the renal blood flow. A dynamic PET study consisting of a sequence of 5-s images is acquired over a period of at least 60 seconds. For the autoradiographic method the imaging time must be long enough to allow distribution of the radiotracer in the kidneys but short enough to avoid tracer washout. Since 20% of water is glomerularly filtered during its renal transit, the measurement should also be short enough to minimize the counts arising from the tubular lumen. The autoradiographic method is based on determination of tissue activity. A practical solution is to include in the integration a time interval that starts with tracer onset and ends with peak organ activity. Advantage of the autoradiographic method is that the amount of activity that enters the kidney depends on renal blood flow and is not influenced by glomerular filtration, tubular extraction or reuptake of the tracer from tubuli into parenchyma and the renal veins. The dynamic tracer kinetic model of O-15 water is based on the assumptions that all activity is extracted by the parenchyma, extraction is very rapid, and tubular transport has not started or is insignificant at a level that does not influence the calculation of renal blood flow.

Renal blood flow PET studies have potential applications in physiology and pharmacology. Using O-15 water, in pigs the average renal blood flow was determined to be 220 ml/min/100 g.[17] After treatment with ACE inhibitors renal blood flow increased by 22% while the effective renal plasma flow (ERPF) increased only by 15%.

PET imaging with O-15 labelled water has also been used for quantification of renal blood flow in human subjects with normal renal function and chronic renal disease.[9] The images were of exceptional quality (Figure 19.1). Human PET studies were obtained after intravenous injection of 1110–1850 MBq (30–50 mCi) O-15 water dissolved in 1 ml

Figure 19.1 Renal blood flow images obtained with O-15 water. Reprinted with permission from reference 9.

saline. The dynamic PET study consisted of 30 frames, 3 seconds each. Parametric images were obtained on a pixel basis using an arterial input function obtained noninvasively from a 1 cm circular region of interest (ROI) drawn in the centre of the abdominal aorta. The diameter of the aorta was obtained by sonography and the aorta was modelled as a long cylinder. A partial volume correction table was developed for cylinders of various diameters using a point spread function that was obtained using a two-dimensional Gaussian filter based on the full width at half maximum (FWHM) of the PET scanner. A recovery coefficient was derived from these correction maps and was used to correct the activity estimated in the aorta. The renal blood flow of the kidneys measured with this method was 340 ± 40 ml/min/100 g in healthy individuals, and was equal in the two kidneys. Renal blood flow was not influenced by probenecid, an antagonist of the organic anion transporter[9] that, on the other hand, significantly affected effective renal plasma flow (ERPF) in the same subjects. In a group of patients with renal dysfunction renal blood flow was 210 ± 110 ml/min/100 g.[9]

The microsphere model

Determination of renal blood flow with radioactive or colour-coded microspheres, although a very accurate method, is not applicable in human subjects since it may cause ischaemic damage of vital organs. The microsphere model is discussed here since it has been used for quantification of the renal blood flow with category II radiotracers.[15] This group includes tracers with very high extraction fraction such as gallium-68 macroaggregated human serum albumin,[18] carbon-11 methylalbumin microspheres,[19,20] and Ga-68 microspheres[21] or with moderately high extraction fraction such as copper PTSM and Rb-82.

In experimental animals, blood flow determination with microspheres is based on injection of microspheres into the left atrium or left ventricle.[22,23] Upon mixing with the blood, the microspheres are ejected into the bloodstream and dispersed in the circulation according to the distribution of the cardiac output. A reference blood sample is collected over 2–3 minutes from a femoral artery using a Harvard pump at speed F_{rel} (in ml/min). The total blood collection time is not important as long as it is longer than the time needed for complete distribution of the microspheres. Cardiac output (CO) in ml/min is calculated from the following equation:

$$CO = F_{rel} \frac{A_{tot}}{A_{bl}}$$

where, A_{tot} represents the counts of total injected activity and A_{bl} represents the activity measured in the blood withdrawn with the Harvard pump. If radioligands with longer half lives are used, the animal is sacrificed and the kidneys are removed to measure tissue activity. If positron emitters such as Ga-68 or C-11 are used, tissue activity can be measured with PET. Renal blood flow is calculated from the counts in the kidney (A_k) as follows:

$$RBF = F_{rel} \frac{A_k}{A_{bl}}$$

If the counts for the entire organ are included in the calculation, the resulting parameter will represent blood flow per kidney; division by the weight of the organ will yield blood flow parameter (or perfusion) in ml/min/g.

Rb-82

Rubidium-82 is a generator-produced potassium analogue with a physical half life of 75 seconds. Advantages of rubidium-82 are a high extraction (> 80%) and slow washout in the kidneys.[24]

The operational equation for determination of renal blood flow with Rb-82 is:

$$C_T \backslash C_A = \frac{FE}{\dfrac{FE}{p} + \lambda}$$

where C_T and C_A represent tissue and arterial activities, F is flow, E is extraction fraction, p is the tissue blood partition coefficient and λ is the physical decay constant. $C_a(t)$ can be obtained by sequential blood sampling. $C_a(t)$ can also be estimated from a time–activity curve derived from the abdominal aorta in which case it has to be corrected for partial volume effects. If the tracer is administered by continuous infusion rather than bolus injection, an equilibrium state is reached and the tissue/blood activity is used to assess renal blood flow. This simplified method requires only one blood sample and is useful for serial measurements. It has been applied in animal models of renal artery obstruction, occlusion and reperfusion. However, it resulted in a nonlinear correlation with the true renal blood flow measured with microspheres.[25]

Copper-PTSM

Copper(II)-pyruvaldehyde bis (n-4-methylthiosemicarbazone) or Cu-PTSM is a typical category II tracer. It is radiolabelled with positron-emitting isotopes Cu-64 or Cu-62. Cu-64 is a cyclotron product with a half life of 12.7 h; Cu-62 is a generator product with a half life of 9.8 min. Extraction fraction of Cu-PTSM is high and its tissue clearance is slow, therefore the modified microsphere model is applicable. Renal blood flow measured with Cu-PTSM is 229 ml/min/100 g in rats and correlates well with the renal blood flow obtained with radioactive microspheres.[26,27] The most simple model that has been used is the 'trapped' tracer model which is basically the microsphere model modified for the extraction fraction of the tracer:

$$F = \frac{F_{ref} Q_{tiss}}{Q_{ref} E_{tiss}}$$

where, F represents tissue blood flow, F_{ref} is the arterial sample flow rate in ml/min, Q_{tiss} is tissue activity, Q_{ref} is integrated arterial sample activity and E_{tiss} is the flow-dependent tissue extraction fraction. In rats, comparison with renal blood flow measurements obtained with Co-57 labelled 15 μm microspheres resulted in an apparent renal extraction fraction value of 93% while the apparent extraction in the myocardium was 62%.[28] Both values were higher than the extraction fraction values measured during first pass (hence expressing the apparent extraction fraction) which indicated that extraction was probably not instantaneous and some recirculation of the tracer had occurred. In the brain the apparent extraction fraction of Cu-PTSM is even higher than 100%. In dogs, renal cortical blood flow determined with Cu-PTSM is 300–550 ml/min/100 g and correlates well with the microsphere method.[27] Correlation between flow values determined with Cu-PTSM and microspheres is much better in the renal cortex than the medulla, an effect which can result not only from the inaccuracy of the PET technique but also from the documented underestimation of medullary flow by microspheres.[27]

N-13 ammonia

Renal blood flow measurements with N-13 labelled ammonia are based on a compartmental model which consists of a reversible binding compartment that is serially connected with a second, irreversible binding compartment.[29] Parametric images are obtained with the pixel based Gjedde–Patlak plot.[30,31] The slope of the linear portion of this plot is equivalent to renal blood flow, when the effective extraction from blood to reversible compartment is close to 100%.[29] Linearity of the plot is achieved when plasma and tissue activity are at equilibrium. This requirement is typically fulfilled before the tracer reaches the tubular lumen. Renal blood flow measured with N-13 ammonia in dogs is 400 ml/min/100 g and correlates well with renal blood flow values estimated with O-15 water.[29]

Using N-13 ammonia a mean baseline value of 316 ml/min/100 g kidney was obtained in pigs. Four conditions known to affect renal blood flow were studied. (1) Kidneys were subjected to varying durations of warm ischaemia, demonstrating a progressive decrease in renal blood flow with increasing ischaemic insult. Return to normal values was impaired in animals exposed to the greatest degree of ischaemia (180 minutes rather than 150 or 120 minutes ischaemia). (2) Allograft rejection was produced by cross-transplantation of kidneys between animals and the resulting decrease in renal blood flow failed to normalize. (3) In unilateral nephrectomy renal blood flow increased two-fold in the remaining kidney by 7 days due to compensatory renal hypertrophy. (4) Lastly, there was an inverse, linear relationship between toxic cyclosporine levels and renal blood flow, indicative of vascular-mediated cyclosporine nephrotoxicity. Thus PET provided quantitative data on the renal blood flow in several multiple important physiologic models.[10]

Glomerular filtration

Tracers that can be used to depict glomerular filtration with PET include gallium-68 EDTA and cobalt-55 EDTA. Cobalt-55 is a positron-emitting radioisotope produced by proton irradiation of iron with a T½ of 18 h. Wistar rats were imaged with PET using this tracer[11] and chromium 51 labelled EDTA was used as a reference. Sequential PET images were processed with regions of interest to calculate tissue time–activity curves. In animals with normal kidneys the time–activity curves were symmetrical. Unilateral kidney function was reduced by cooling the organ and the time–activity curves showed reduced amplitudes in these organs.

The half life of Co-55 is relatively long but it is balanced by a short biological half life so that the radiation dose can be kept low in normal renal function or moderate renal dysfunction. Human studies with Co-55 EDTA have not been reported.

Metabolism

C-11 acetate

Carbon-11 ([^{11}C] acetate) acetate has been developed as a tracer of myocardial metabolism. After uptake in the cell, acetate is converted to acetyl-CoA and enters the Krebs cycle, releasing the radiolabel as [^{11}C] CO_2. There is a direct relationship between oxygen consumption and washout of radioactivity from the myocardium.[32] Renal uptake of [^{11}C] acetate is prompt and high target-to-background ratios are achieved even if renal function is markedly reduced. The metabolic product of carbon-11 acetate is carbon dioxide dissolved in plasma which is cleared from the renal parenchyma by way of circulation. Renal uptake of [^{11}C] acetate is reduced in parenchymal renal disease and haemodynamically significant renal artery stenosis.[12]

The kinetic model of C-11 acetate is relatively simple with only one exponential component in the impulse response function. Its renal uptake depends on blood flow and extraction of the tracer which is 20–25%. Since (similarly to F-18 FDG) the extraction fraction is not the limiting step of uptake, C-11 acetate cannot be used as a flow tracer.[12] However, since its renal release largely depends on oxidative metabolism C-11 acetate is a tracer of oxidative metabolism.

Nearly linear correlation between the renal uptake and release has been described in subjects with normal kidney and in patients with renal artery stenosis, diabetic nephropathy, hypertensive nephropathy and membranous glomerulonephritis. Marked disassociation of the two parameters (release decreased to larger degree than uptake) has been found in renal cell carcinoma (rate constant of release 0.1465 in normal kidney and 0.024 in cancer) which resulted in increasing tumour to nontumour ratios and excellent delineation of the tumour from the normal kidney.[12]

An important advantage of C-11 acetate is that it is not excreted into urine, for this reason it has been used for imaging of prostate cancer. Diagnostic accuracy of [^{11}C] acetate PET in prostate cancer is higher than the accuracy of [^{18}F] FDG PET[33] and similar to the accuracy of [^{11}C] choline PET.[34]

Sugar analogues

Glucose is an important energy resource for the kidneys and glucose analogues are discussed in this section as metabolic agents although they could also be discussed in the section on molecular imaging since their accumulation in the tissues largely depends on the expression and function of membrane transporters and metabolizing enzymes.

Glucose transporters (GLUTs) represent a family of facilitative transporters which catalyse the transport of glucose down its concentration gradient and into cells of target tissues. GLUT1 is ubiquitously expressed with particularly high levels in human erythrocytes and in endothelial cells lining the blood vessels of the brain. GLUT3 is found in neurons. GLUT2 is present in liver, intestine, kidney, and pancreatic beta cells and functions as part of the glucose sensor system.[35]

Several glucose transporters have been identified in glomeruli including the isoforms GLUT1, 3 and 4, and the sodium-dependent glucose transporter subtype 1. GLUTs 1,

3 and 4 are high-affinity, low-capacity proteins. A different class of transporters, the sodium-dependent glucose transporter (SGLT) is also a high-affinity low-capacity transporter. Both transporter types can be saturated under normal glucose conditions.[36] Polymorphisms of the glucose transporters have been indicated in the increased susceptibility of the kidneys to the development of nephropathy in noninsulin dependent diabetes mellitus.[37–39]

GLUT1 is the predominant glucose transporter in mesangial cells. In hypertensive Dahl salt-sensitive (S) rats there is an 80% upregulation of glomerular GLUT-1 protein expression. These studies suggest a link between haemodynamic and metabolic factors that may cooperate in inducing progressive glomerular injury in conditions characterized by glomerular hypertension.[40] Both angiotensin II and epithelial growth factor (EGF) are involved in the regulation of GLUT1 expression.[41]

Glucose analogue radioligands have the potential to investigate the following important scientific questions: (a) what is the expression of glucose transporters and their relationship to the development of nephropathy in diabetes; (b) which drugs can be used to reduce the activity of glucose transporters to prevent high glucose-induced diabetic glomerulosclerosis. Fluorine-18 labelled FDG is the most important substrate of the GLUT transporter family but it is not an appropriate tracer for imaging glucose uptake in the kidneys because it is excreted into the tubular lumen and accumulated in the renal collecting system.

In the healthy human kidney, there are at least three different human renal Na^+-glucose cotransporters, SGLT1, SGLT2 and SGLT3.[42] A new class of antidiabetic drugs, derivatives of phlorizin, are inhibitors of SGLT. Phlorizin derivatives inhibit glucose uptake in the small intestine and enhance glucose excretion in the kidneys by blocking the reuptake.[43] These drugs may become an important tool for imaging the SGLT. A glucose analogue that is substrate of the SGLT but not of the GLUT, methyl-D-glucoside has been recently radiolabelled with carbon-11 by methylation of glucose (Figure 19.2). Beta-methyl-D-glucoside is accumulated in the kidneys to a higher extent than the alpha-anomer. Autoradiography showed that methyl-D-glucoside was distributed throughout the renal cortex, suggesting that both sodium-D-glucose cotransporters expressed in kidney, SGLT1 and SGLT2, were involved in ligand binding. Electrical

Figure 19.2 Chemical structure of methylglucoside.

Figure 19.3 Renal accumulation of methylglucosides. Ex vivo autoradiographic images of mouse kidney slices were obtained 30 min after injection of 2'-[^{18}F]fluoroethyl-beta-D-glucoside (A = transverse slice; B = coronal slice) or [^{11}C]-methyl-alpha-D-glucoside (D = coronal slice). Section C represents the same section as A after staining with haematoxylin–eosin. C = cortex; OS = outer stripe of outer medulla; IS = inner stripe of outer medulla; IZ = inner zone of medulla. Bar = 1 mm. Reprinted with permission from reference 45.

measurements in *Xenopus* oocytes revealed that alpha-methyl-D-glucoside and beta-methyl-D-glucoside were transported by the human SGLT1 transporter.[44]

[^{11}C]-methyl-α-D-glucoside is mainly accumulated in the renal cortex that contains S1 and S2 segments of renal proximal tubules. No accumulation of [^{11}C]-methyl-α-D-glucoside has been observed in the outer stripe of the outer medulla because most [^{11}C]-methyl-α-D-glucoside is cleared from the glomerular filtrate in the S1 and S2 segments (Figure 19.3). Another glucoside, 2'-[^{18}F] fluoroethyl-beta-D-glucoside accumulates in the outer part of the outer medulla, a kidney region that contains the S3 segments of renal proximal tubules where SGLT1 is found. Experimental data suggest that the activity of SGLT1 in humans can be visualized by 2'-[^{18}F] fluoroethyl-beta-D-glucoside, whereas the activity of both SGLT1 and SGLT2 can be visualized by [^{11}C]-methyl-α-D-glucoside.[45]

Molecular imaging targets

Molecular imaging targets can be either proteins that are expressed in the organ of interest or molecules from the genetic machinery such as messenger RNA (mRNA).

Function of membrane transport proteins such as the organic anion transporter have been successfully imaged with ligands such as ^{99m}Tc MAG3 for a long time. Other proteins with functional importance in the kidneys are enzymes, receptors and components of the signal transduction cascades.

Enzymes

Angiotensin-converting enzyme

A deletion/insertion (D/I) polymorphism of the human angiotensin-converting enzyme ACE gene is related to 14–50% of the interindividual variance in serum ACE activity.[46] D/I polymorphism has been implicated in the pathogenesis of a variety of cardiovascular disorders, including diabetic and IgA nephropathy.

In patients with nondiabetic renal disease decline of glomerular filtration rate is faster in the DD homozygotes than in ID heterozygotes or II homozygotes and patients with the DD genotype are resistant to commonly advocated renoprotective therapy.[47] An association has also been established between I/D polymorphism and salt-sensitive hypertension. Hypertensive patients with II and DI genotypes have significantly higher prevalence of salt sensitivity than hypertensive patients with the DD genotype.[48,49] On the other hand, myocardial hypertrophy in response to exercise (studied only in healthy individuals) is stronger in DD and ID carriers than in II homozygotes.[50] Hormones, such as oestrogen can modulate tissue ACE activity and alter ACE mRNA concentrations.[51] PET studies would permit measurement of the organ density of the ACE and the dependence of enzyme density on genetic polymorphisms, sex hormone levels or dietary sodium. PET could also be used to study the role of tissue ACE in the development of arterial hypertension, renal or cardiovascular diseases.

The first radioligand introduced for PET imaging of the ACE was [^{18}F] fluorocaptopril. It showed high uptake in organs with high ACE concentrations such as the lung, kidney and aorta. When different amounts of unlabelled 4-*cis*-fluorocaptopril were coinjected in rats, a dose of greater than 5 µg/kg decreased the lung uptake by one-half while only 1 µg/kg decreased the kidney uptake by one half. In general, the binding was saturable with the expected capacity. [^{18}F] fluorocaptopril administered to a human also resulted in a displaceable uptake in the lung and kidney.[52] A compartmental receptor-binding model has been designed to quantify binding of [^{18}F] fluorocaptopril[53,54] and a study has been carried out in humans to determine the dose of ACE inhibitor required to specifically block ACE. The combined forward rate constant for [^{18}F] fluorocaptopril, which is proportional to the ACE is reduced in primary pulmonary hypertension. Low doses of ACE inhibitors were needed to block the effects of ACE on vascular remodelling in this disease.[55]

More recently a second ACE inhibitor, (4S)-1-[(S)-3-mercapto-2-methylpropanoyl]-4-phenylthio-L-proline (zofenoprilat), the active metabolite of the potent ACE inhibitor zofenopril calcium, was labelled with carbon-11 achieving a radiochemical yield of 5–10% and specific radioactivity from 0.5–1.5 Ci/μmol (18.5–55.5 GBq/μmol). Preliminary in vivo human evaluation of the radioligand showed that the drug accumulated in organs with high ACE levels such as the lungs and kidneys, and in organs involved in drug metabolism such as the liver and gall bladder.[56]

Farnesyl transferase

Cellular proliferation is the major characteristic of renal diseases. The *ras* represents a class of regulatory proteins with implications in proliferative renal diseases with particular involvement in cell differentiation, proliferation, apoptosis and fibrogenesis. The activity of *ras* depends on its anchor to the cellular membrane through a farnesyl link.

Farnesylation of the *ras* is mediated by the enzyme farnesyl protein transferase (FPT) which can be blocked by farnesyl transferase inhibitors (FTIs). FTIs have been proposed as chemotherapeutic agents since they have the potential effect to deactivate the *Ras* protein.[57] Farnesyl transferase inhibitors are also being investigated for the treatment of proliferative glomerular diseases.[58] The farnesyl transferase inhibitor, (S)-1-(3-fluoromethyl-5-iodophenyl)-4-[1-(4-cyanobenzyl)-5-imidazoyl]-5-[([11C]-methanesulfonyl)-ethyl]-2-piperazinone has been radiolabelled with carbon-11 for imaging the kidneys.[59] Specific binding was very high, 75–99%.

Angiotensin receptors

Two major receptor subtypes, AT1R and AT 2R have been identified in humans. In rodents there are three subtypes, AT1aR, AT1bR and AT2R. In humans the AT1R gene is located on chromosome 3 and the receptor is found in the kidney glomeruli with high focal density. The receptor is also present in the inner stripe of the outer medulla with a more diffuse distribution.[60] The AT 2R receptor gene is located on chromosome X. The role of this receptor is less well understood in the adult organism but it may be involved in the regulation of arterial blood pressure with an antagonistic effect to the AT1R.

AT1R mediates most of the physiological effects of angiotensin II including renal blood flow, glomerular filtration, sodium and water reabsorption, myocardial contractility and aldosterone secretion. Expression of the receptor is modulated by many factors, including angiotensin II, dietary sodium, testosterone, oestrogens, stress hormones, ACE inhibitors, thyroid hormones and renal hypoperfusion. PET is well suited for in vivo examination of AT1R regulation and effects of some of the mentioned factors have already been investigated using animal models.[61,62] Significance of human studies would be among others that they could provide important insights into the regulation of the AT1R by sex hormones or into the contribution of AT1R regulation to sodium sensitivity hypertension.

In arterial hypertension AT1R may be upregulated or may become hyper-responsive by another mechanisms.[63] Thus, hypertension could result from multiple regulatory alterations of the renin-angiotensin system: (a) increased total number of receptors; (b) increased number of physiologically active receptors; (c) inappropriate upregulation of receptors in response to sodium intake, stress or altered hormone levels; (d) increased concentration of circulating renin and angiotensin II. These multiple possibilities of receptor dysregulation prompt the design of three PET imaging paradigms: (1) solitary PET measurements to assess the receptor status in health and disease; (2) same day repeat PET measurements with short-term pharmacological or physiological interventions to assess the occupancy and availability of the receptor; and (3) long-term, longitudinal PET measurements to study receptor up- or downregulation. All three types of experiment have been performed in experimental animals.[61,62,64]

AT1R antagonists are an important resource for the development of radioligands for PET. Nonpeptide, small molecular AT1R antagonists have been subsequently developed based on imidazole derivatives. One class of AT1R antagonists (Figure 19.4) has a biphenyltetrazole moiety in its structure.[65]

Losartan   **Valsartan**   **Irbesartan**   **Candesartan**

Figure 19.4 Biphenyltetrazole AT1R antagonists.

Figure 19.5 Radiosynthesis of [^{11}C] L-159,884. L-159,884 is a high-affinity ligand with an IC$_{50}$ of 0.08 nM in rabbit aorta tissue.[74]

Figure 19.6 Unmetabolized [^{11}C] L-159,884 in dog plasma (left), urine (middle) and kidney (right) at 30, 60 and 90 minutes postradioligand injection. Dashed line shows measurements in dogs on low-sodium diet and dotted line shows measurements in dogs on high-sodium diet.

Radioligand development

Multiple drugs known to have high selectivity and affinity for the AT1R have been radiolabelled for PET imaging. These radioligands include MK-996 (formerly designated L-159,282), L-162,574 and L-159,884. Of these methoxy-substituted analogues of MK-996, [^{11}C] L-159,884 demonstrated the most favourable biodistribution, radiation dosimetry and a lack of urinary excretion (Figure 19.5).

Biodistribution studies in mice show rapid radioligand uptake in the kidneys, lungs and heart and a rapid plasma clearance and high and sustained uptake in the kidneys. Specific binding in mouse kidney is 70%. Pretreatment of mice with an AT 2R-specific antagonist or adrenergic antagonists confirmed the selectivity of [^{11}C] L-159,884 for the AT1R.

In dogs, clearance of unmetabolized [^{11}C] L-159,884 and its replacement by metabolites is very rapid. Essentially all activity found in the urine is in the form of metabolites. Despite the rapid accumulation and excretion of radioactive metabolites, 85–90% of the tissue radioactivity is unmetabolized [^{11}C] L-159,884 (Figure 19.6), which is favourable for PET studies.

Recently a new radioligand [^{11}C] KR-31173 has been developed for imaging the AT1R with PET (Figure 19.7). KR-31173 is a derivative of the potent AT1R antagonist SK-

1080.[66,67] In biodistribution studies performed in mice, this radioligand did not accumulate in the brain but other organs showed excellent tissue-to-blood activity ratios with highest accumulation in the adrenals, followed by kidneys, liver, lungs and heart. Specific binding of the radioligand in the adrenals, kidneys, lungs and heart was 90% and was inhibited both with MK-996 and with unlabelled KR-31173.[68] PET imaging studies of mice, dogs and baboons demonstrated high organ uptake and specific binding. [^{11}C] KR-31173 is a promising radioligand for human applications.

PET studies

PET studies with [^{11}C] L-159,884 have been performed in mice, dogs, pigs and baboons with an injected dose of 370–740 mBq (10–20 mCi) at a specific activity of higher than 74 GBq/μmol (2000 mCi/μmol). The injected mass of the drug is always less than 5 μg. A typical dynamic PET study lasts 90–100 minutes and images of increasing scan times (first scans 15 s, last scans 10 min) are acquired to compensate for the physical decay of carbon-11. Monitoring of vital signs demonstrates no changes after injection of any of the AT1R-specific PET radioligands.

Both kidneys and the left adrenal are clearly visualized on coronal images of dogs obtained after 50 minutes but high

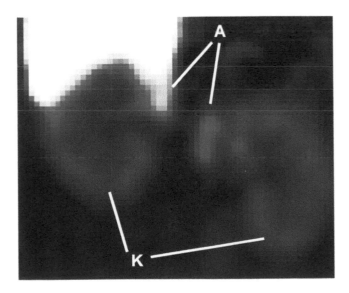

$^{11}CH_3I$, 80°C
NaH, THF

HCl
80°C

SK-1080
IC_{50} = 1.01 nM (Human)
IC_{50} = 11.6 nM (Rat Liver)

[^{11}C] KR31173
IC_{50} = 3.27 nM (Rat Liver)

Figure 19.7 Radiolabelling of KR-31173 with carbon-11 and comparison to SK-1080.

liver uptake may interfere with the upper pole of the right kidney and the right adrenal (Figure 19.8). In humans it is expected that the adrenals will also be easily visualized and hybrid PET/CT imaging will help localize the adrenals and separate them from the kidneys and liver.

Imaging studies were performed in dogs before and after pretreatment with 1 mg/kg of the specific AT1R antagonist MK-996 to estimate specific binding. The effectiveness of MK-996 in blocking AT1 receptors was tested by an angiotensin II challenge test. After 1 mg/kg MK-996, no pressure effect of Ang II was detected, suggesting complete occupancy of AT1R.

Renal time–activity curves derived from the dynamic PET studies by means of regions of interest (ROI) analysis revealed radioactivities in the kidney cortices at 90–100 min postinjection of 110 and 40 Bq/cc/MBq (100 and 40 nCi/cc/mCi) injected tracer for the control and inhibition studies, respectively. This difference corresponded to a displaceable binding of 60%.

Dissociation of [^{11}C] L-159,884 from AT1R in vivo is very slow and the drug appears to be insurmountable. Time–activity curves derived from the renal cortex have

Figure 19.8 Coronal images of the kidneys (K) and adrenals (A) obtained in a dog 55–95 minutes after intravenous administration of [^{11}C] L-159,884.

$$\int_0^T C_p(t)dt / C_p(T)$$

Figure 19.9 'Gjedde–Patlak' plot of [^{11}C] L-159,884 in the dog renal cortex calculated from a control and a post-MK-996 study. Significant reduction of the slope from 0.03 to 0.01 illustrates inhibition of radioligand binding due to blockade of AT$_1$ receptors by MK-996.

been analysed both by the 'Gjedde–Patlak plot'[30,31] to obtain the influx rate constant and by Logan analysis[69] to calculate the distribution volume and binding potential. Pretreatment with MK-996 reduced the influx rate constant of the radioligand from 0.03 to 0.01, consistent with a specific binding component of 67% suitable for quantitative PET studies of the AT$_1$R (Figure 19.9). In dogs, intravenous administration of 0.1, 0.01 and 0.001 mg/kg of unlabelled L-159,884 coinjected with the radioactive ligand, results in a reduction in specific binding of 70%, 50% and no change, respectively. These observations have important implications. When injected at high specific activity (0.1 μg/kg), [^{11}C] L-159,884 will not saturate specific binding sites and kinetic parameters of the tracer using compartmental models will be applicable. On the other hand, binding of the radioligand is saturable and displaceable, consistent with the concept of receptor–ligand interaction.

Imaging receptor regulation

Longitudinal PET experiments in dogs showed that dietary sodium is a major physiologic stimulus of AT$_1$R regulation. Paired dynamic PET studies with [^{11}C] L-159,884 and H$_2$^{15}O were performed in beagle dogs. In the first group of L-H animals ($n = 7$), the first PET study was performed after 2 weeks of low sodium diet (10 mEq NaCl/day); then, a second PET study was performed after 2 weeks on a high sodium diet (300 mEq NaCl/day). This group imitated high switching diet to high-sodium intake. In the second group of H-L animals ($n = 7$), the opposite schedule was applied to mimic elimination of sodium from the diet. Renal cortical blood flow (RBF), determined by H$_2$^{15}O/PET, did not differ significantly between animals on low- and high-sodium diets.

Binding of [^{11}C] L159,884 (expressed as BP), was 54% higher in animals on the L-H diet compared to those on the H-L regimen. Dietary sodium loading increased glomerular as well as renal cortical AT$_1$R by 40–60% compared to levels in the glomeruli and cortex in dogs maintained on a sodium-restricted diet. Quantitative RT PCR revealed an 18% increase in AT1 receptor mRNA in the renal cortex from dogs on the high-salt diet compared to dogs on a low-salt diet and the in vitro parameters B$_{max}$ and mRNA expression correlated positively with the binding potential of [^{11}C] L159,884 determined by PET. Thus, increased binding in vivo and in vitro occurred concurrently with increased expression of AT$_1$R mRNA, consistent with receptor upregulation at the transcriptional level. On the other hand, the magnitude of increased receptor density was more pronounced than the magnitude of the mRNA upregulation, suggesting that post-transcriptional amplification mechanisms may also play a role in receptor regulation. These experiments underscore the value of PET as a tool with which the physiologically effective concentration of the receptor can be measured in vivo.

PET studies and in vitro binding experiments and mRNA determinations were confirmed by autoradiography which also demonstrated that the majority of AT receptors in the cortex of the dog kidney was of the AT$_1$R subtype and was located in the glomeruli.[61]

Parameters of AT$_1$R expression were in an inverse relationship with plasma renin activity, angiotensin II and aldosterone levels. The dog kidney, which has only one AT$_1$R subtype like in humans, represents a clinically more relevant model than rodents for studying renal AT$_1$R regulation. Renal PET images of [^{11}C] L-159,884 predominantly reflect changes in glomerular AT$_1$R and may prove to be an instrumental tool to investigate mechanisms of human hypertension and other kidney-related diseases.

Hypertension

Human imaging studies of the AT$_1$R have not yet been performed since [^{11}C] L-159,884 is not successful in human studies (Szabo et al. unpublished data) but other studies indicate the possible role of the AT$_1$R in the development of arterial hypertension. One of the best correlations in vivo investigated so far was found between plasma renin activity, plasma angiotensin II or aldosterone levels on one hand and AT$_1$R mRNA levels on the other in peripheral blood cells (platelets and mononuclear leucocytes) of primary and secondary hypertension, such as primary hyperaldosteronism and renovascular disease.[70]

Preliminary PET studies have been performed in dogs with renal artery stenosis and [^{11}C] L-159,884 binding measured by the binding potential was found to be increased (Figure 19.10). The binding potential normalized after 3 months. Subsequent autopsy revealed extensive collaterals in the area of the capsular arteries of the stenotic kidney that could

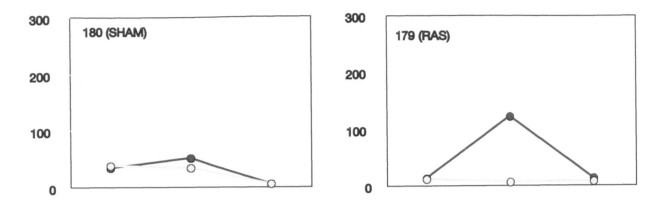

Figure 19.10 Effect of renal artery stenosis on the binding potential of [^{11}C] L-159,884 in the operated kidney (red) and contralateral kidney (yellow) of a sham-operated animal (animal # 180) and of an animal with renal artery stenosis (animal # 179). Graphs are calibrated for a maximum of 300 unitless dimensions since the binding potential is calculated from the ratio of k_3/k_4 and k_3 and k_4 have identical dimensions. For each animal, the first measurement was performed at baseline, the second measurement 3 weeks after surgery and the third measurement 3 months after surgery. In the sham-operated animal the binding potential was similar for the right and left kidney and reproducible at the three time points. In the animal with renal artery stenosis radioligand binding was very high 3 weeks after surgery and returned to normal 3 months after surgery. Normalization of the binding potential in this animal is explained by development of extensive collateral blood vessels to the kidney.

explain the compensatory increase in perfusion of the stenotic kidneys and normalization of ATI receptor expression. This finding could be of particular significance for similar studies performed in humans with renovascular hypertension since it indicates that: (1) the ATIR may be a sensitive probe of renal ischaemia; and (2) if an equilibrium between organ oxygen demand (atrophy) and blood supply (collaterals) develops ATIR protein expression may return to normal levels.

Aldosterone-producing adenomas are another cause of secondary hypertension. Aldosterone secretion in most patients with aldosterone-producing adenomas is typically unresponsive to angiotensin II stimulation. In some patients, however, plasma aldosterone increases in response to angiotensin II stimulation. This differential aldosterone responsiveness has been shown to be related to the levels of ATIR in the adenoma.[71,72] ATIR is expressed in aldosterone-producing adenomas but its density (which is already high in the normal gland) is not significantly higher than in nontumorous adrenal cortex. In Cushing's disease, phaeochromocytomas and cortical carcinomas ATIR are reduced.[73]

Requirements for clinical PET imaging of the kidneys

Rapid spread of PET and PET/CT imaging in oncology can be explained by the rapid development of treatment options that are based on molecular pharmacology and the variance of individual tumours in their response to therapy that can be predicted from these imaging studies. FDG PET provides images of cancer of very high quality and its sensitivity for even relatively small cancer foci is very good. On the other hand, specificity of FDG PET scans for cancer detection is quite limited if one takes into consideration the normal variants of FDG distribution and many diseases, foremost inflammations, that can result in accumulation of the radiopharmaceutical and complicate interpretation of images. Of great help is inclusion of the anatomical information obtained from MRI or CT to improve interpretation of the PET scans. It is important to emphasize that not only the need for imaging has increased but also the PET technology has experienced rapid improvement.

The success of FDG PET is derived from multiple factors including: (1) increased clinical need; (2) improved imaging technology; and (3) availability of a widely applicable radiopharmaceutical. We have to consider these three points if we want to understand why spread of PET technology into nuclear nephro-urology has been so slow until now. First, the present techniques apparently suffice to meet the need which is focused on measurement of renal function, specifically on determination of GFR or quantitative imaging of tubular function. Multiple imaging modalities are available including MRI, MRA and CT that can provide functional images of the kidneys with high spatial resolution and excellent image quality.

For PET imaging to strive in nephro-urology, its necessity has to be established. The technology of image acquisition and processing is already available. To minimize competition with other imaging modalities such as CT or MRI, renal imaging must focus on molecular mechanisms. FDG, which is the magical bullet for oncological PET is not the right tracer for the kidneys. Its accumulation in renal parenchyma is poorly understood and is unpredictable even in renal cell cancer. Delineation of the renal parenchyma is insufficient since the tracer is excreted into the urine. (In contrast to other organs, in the kidneys FDG does not follow the kinetics of glucose completely; it is not a substrate of the SGLT and is not reabsorbed from the tubular lumen.)

An important issue is PET imaging time. It is necessary to develop radioligands either with very rapid or with very slow dissociation from molecular targets. In the first case rapid dynamic studies, in the second delayed single images would be performed. For accurate assessment of split renal function such as the GFR, a dynamic study of very short duration of only 5 minutes could be sufficient if initiated with radioligand injection. Delayed single images could be more useful to measure receptor regulation in renovascular hypertension or transplant rejection. Both early postinjection dynamic studies and late postinjection static studies could be obtained in 5 minutes which is the goal of diagnostic PET imaging.

References

1. Tarantola G, Zito F, Gerundini P. PET instrumentation and reconstruction algorithms in whole-body applications. J Nucl Med 2003; 44: 756–69.

2. Townsend DW. Physical principles and technology of clinical PET imaging. Ann Acad Med Singapore 2004; 33: 133–45.

3. Koepfli P, Hany TF, Wyss CA et al. CT attenuation correction for myocardial perfusion quantification using a PET/CT hybrid scanner. J Nucl Med 2004; 45: 537–42.

4. Slomka PJ. Software approach to merging molecular with anatomic information. J Nucl Med 2004; 45: 36S–45S.

5. Kaatee R, Beek FJ, de Lange EE et al. Renal artery stenosis: detection and quantification with spiral CT angiography versus optimized digital subtraction angiography. Radiology 1997; 205: 121–7.

6. Kim TS, Chung JW, Park JH et al. Renal artery evaluation: comparison of spiral CT angiography to intra-arterial DSA. J Vasc Interv Radiol 1998; 9: 553–9.

7. Carlos RC, Axelrod DA, Ellis JH et al. Incorporating patient-centered outcomes in the analysis of cost-effectiveness: imaging strategies for renovascular hypertension. AJR Am J Roentgenol 2003; 181: 1653–61.

8. Goerres GW, Burger C, Schwitter MR et al. PET/CT of the abdomen: optimizing the patient breathing pattern. Eur Radiol 2003; 13: 734–9.

9. Alpert NM, Rabito CA, Correia DJ et al. Mapping of local renal blood flow with PET and $H_2^{15}O$. J Nucl Med 2002; 43: 470–5.

10. Killion D, Nitzsche E, Choi Y et al. Positron emission tomography: a new method for determination of renal function. J Urol 1993; 150: 1064–8.

11. Goethals P, Volkaert A, Vandewielle C et al. 55Co-EDTA for renal imaging using positron emission tomography (PET): a feasibility study. Nucl Med Biol 2000; 27: 77–81.

12. Shreve P, Chiao PC, Humes HD et al. Carbon-11-acetate PET imaging in renal disease. J Nucl Med 1995; 36: 1595–601.

13. Szabo Z, Kao PF, Burns HD et al. Investigation of angiotensin II/AT1 receptors with carbon-11-L-159,884: a selective AT1 antagonist. J Nucl Med 1998; 39: 1209–13.

14. Hudson H, Larkin R. Accelerated image reconstruction using ordered subsets of projection data. IEEE Trans Med Imag 1994; 14: 61–72.

15. Hutchins GD. What is the best approach to quantify myocardial blood flow with pet? J Nucl Med 2001; 42: 1183–4.

16. Peters JE, Ter-Pogossian MM, Rockoff ML et al. Measurement of renal blood flow by means of radioactive water labeled with oxygen 15. In: Blaufox MD, Funck-Brentano JL, eds, Radionuclides in Nephrology. New York: Grune and Stratton. 1971; 27–36.

17. Juillard L, Janier MF, Fouque D et al. Dynamic renal blood flow measurement by positron emission tomography in patients with CRF. Am J Kidney Dis 2002; 40: 947–54.

18. Even GA, Green MA. Gallium-68–labeled macroaggregated human serum albumin, ^{68}Ga-MAA. Int J Rad Appl Instrum B 1989; 16: 319–21.

19. Brooks DJ, Frackowiak RS, Lammertsma AA et al. A comparison between regional cerebral blood flow measurements obtained in human subjects using 11C-methylalbumin microspheres, the $C^{15}O_2$ steady-state method, and positron emission tomography. Acta Neurol Scand 1986; 73: 415–22.

20. Turton DR, Brady F, Pike VW et al. Preparation of human serum methyl-[^{11}C]methylalbumin microspheres and human serum methyl-[^{11}C]methylalbumin for clinical use. Int J Appl Radiat Isot 1984; 35: 337–44.

21. Mintun MA, Ter-Pogossian MM, Green MA et al. Quantitative measurement of regional pulmonary blood flow with positron emission tomography. J Appl Physiol 1986; 60: 317–26.

22. Chin A, Radhakrishnan J, Fornell L, John E. Effects of tezosentan, a dual endothelin receptor antagonist, on the cardiovascular and renal systems of neonatal piglets. J Pediatr Surg 2001; 36: 1824–8.

23. Heyman M, Payne B, Hoffmann J, Rudolph A. Blood flow measurements with radionuclide-labelled particles. Prog Cardiovasc Dis 1997; 10: 55–79.

24. Mullani NA, Ekas RD, Marani S et al. Feasibility of measuring first pass extraction and flow with rubidium-82 in the kidneys. Am J Physiol Imaging 1990; 5: 133–40.

25. Tamaki N, Rabito CA, Alpert NM et al. Serial analysis of renal blood flow by positron tomography with rubidium-82. Am J Physiol 1986; 251: H1024–30.

26. Young H, Carnochan P, Zweit J et al. Evaluation of copper(II)-pyruvaldehyde bis (N-4-methylthiosemicarbazone) for tissue blood flow measurement using a trapped tracer model. Eur J Nucl Med 1994; 21: 336–41.

27. Shelton ME, Green MA, Mathias CJ et al. Assessment of regional myocardial and renal blood flow with copper-PTSM and positron emission tomography. Circulation 1990; 82: 990–7.

28. Young H, Carnochan P, Zweit J et al. Tissue blood flow estimation with copper(II)-pyruvaldehyde bis (N-4 methylthiosemicarbazone) and PET. J Nucl Biol Med 2002; 38: 89–91.

29. Nitzsche EU, Choi Y, Killion D et al. Quantification and parametric imaging of renal cortical blood flow in vivo based on Patlak graphical analysis. Kidney Int 1993; 44: 985–96.

30. Gjedde A. Compartmental analysis. In: Wagner HNJ et al, eds, Principles of Nuclear Medicine. Philadelphia: Saunders. 1995; 451–61.

31. Patlak CS, Blasberg RG, Fenstermacher JD. Graphical evaluation of blood-to-brain transfer constants from multiple-time uptake data. J Cereb Blood Flow Metab 1983; 3: 1–7.

32. Klein LJ, Visser FC, Knaapen P et al. Carbon-11 acetate as a tracer of myocardial oxygen consumption. Eur J Nucl Med 2001; 28: 651–68.

33. Oyama N, Miller TR, Dehdashti F et al. 11C-acetate PET imaging of prostate cancer: detection of recurrent disease at PSA relapse. J Nucl Med 2003; 44: 549–55.

34. Kotzerke J, Volkmer BG, Glatting G et al. Intraindividual comparison of [11C] acetate and [11C] choline PET for detection of metastases of prostate cancer. Nuklearmedizin 2003; 42: 25–30.

35. Watson RT, Pessin JE. Intracellular organization of insulin signaling and GLUT4 translocation. Recent Prog Horm Res 2001; 56: 175–93.

36. Heilig CW, Brosius FC 3rd, Henry DN. Glucose transporters of the glomerulus and the implications for diabetic nephropathy. Kidney Int Suppl 1997; 60: S91–9.

37. Grzeszczak W, Moczulski DK, Zychma M et al. Role of GLUT1 gene in susceptibility to diabetic nephropathy in type 2 diabetes. Kidney Int 2001; 59: 631–6.

38. Baroni MG, Oelbaum RS, Pozzilli P et al. Polymorphisms at the GLUT1 (HepG2) and GLUT4 (muscle/adipocyte) glucose transporter genes and non-insulin-dependent diabetes mellitus (NIDDM). Hum Genet 1992; 88: 557–61.

39. Tao T, Tanizawa Y, Matsutani A et al. HepG2/erythrocyte glucose transporter (GLUT1) gene in NIDDM: a population association study and molecular scanning in Japanese subjects. Diabetologia 1995; 38: 942–7.

40. Gnudi L, Viberti G, Raij L et al. GLUT-1 overexpression: Link between hemodynamic and metabolic factors in glomerular injury? Hypertension 2003; 42: 19–24.

41. Nose A, Mori Y, Uchiyama-Tanaka Y et al. Regulation of glucose transporter (GLUT1) gene expression by angiotensin II in mesangial cells: involvement of HB-EGF and EGF receptor transactivation. Hypertens Res 2003; 26: 67–73.

42. Wright EM. Renal Na(+)-glucose cotransporters. Am J Physiol Renal Physiol 2001; 280: F10–18.

43. Tsujihara K, Hongu M, Saito K et al. Na(+)-glucose cotransporter inhibitors as antidiabetics. I. Synthesis and pharmacological properties of 4'-dehydroxyphlorizin derivatives based on a new concept. Chem Pharm Bull (Tokyo) 1996; 44: 1174–80.

44. Bormans GM, Van Oosterwyck G, De Groot TJ et al. Synthesis and biologic evaluation of [11C]-methyl-d-glucoside, a tracer of the sodium-dependent glucose transporters. J Nucl Med 2003; 44: 1075–81.

45. de Groot TJ, Veyhl M, Terwinghe C et al. Synthesis of 18F-fluoroalkyl-beta-D-glucosides and their evaluation as tracers for sodium-dependent glucose transporters. J Nucl Med 2003; 44: 1973–81.

46. Ivanovic V, McKusick MA, Johnson CM 3rd et al. Renal artery stent placement: complications at a single tertiary care center. J Vasc Interv Radiol 2003; 14: 217–25.

47. van Essen GG, Rensma PL, de Zeeuw D et al. Association between angiotensin-converting-enzyme gene polymorphism and failure of renoprotective therapy. Lancet 1996; 347: 94–5.

48. Giner V, Poch E, Bragulat E et al. Renin-angiotensin system genetic polymorphisms and salt sensitivity in essential hypertension. Hypertension 2000; 35: 512–17.

49. Poch E, Gonzalez D, Giner V et al. Molecular basis of salt sensitivity in human hypertension. Evaluation of renin-angiotensin-aldosterone system gene polymorphisms. Hypertension 2001; 38: 1204–9.

50. Montgomery HE, Clarkson P, Dollery CM et al. Association of angiotensin-converting enzyme gene I/D polymorphism with change in left ventricular mass in response to physical training. Circulation 1997; 96: 741–7.

51. Gallagher PE, Li P, Lenhart JR et al. Estrogen regulation of angiotensin-converting enzyme mRNA. Hypertension 1999; 33: 323–8.

52. Hwang DR, Eckelman WC, Mathias CJ et al. Positron-labeled angiotensin-converting enzyme (ACE) inhibitor: fluorine-18-fluorocaptopril. Probing the ACE activity in vivo by positron emission tomography. J Nucl Med 1991; 32: 1730–7.

53. Markham J, McCarthy TJ, Welch MJ, Schuster DP. In vivo measurements of pulmonary angiotensin-converting enzyme kinetics. I. Theory and error analysis. J Appl Physiol 1995; 78: 1158–68.

54. Schuster DP, McCarthy TJ, Welch MJ et al. In vivo measurements of pulmonary angiotensin-converting enzyme kinetics. II. Implementation and application. J Appl Physiol 1995; 78: 1169–78.

55. Qing F, McCarthy TJ, Markham J, Schuster DP. Pulmonary angiotensin-converting enzyme (ACE) binding and inhibition in humans. A positron emission tomography study. Am J Respir Crit Care Med 2000; 161: 2019–25.

56. Matarrese M, Salimbeni A, Turolla EA et al. C-11 radiosynthesis and preliminary human evaluation of the disposition of the ACE inhibitor [11C] zofenoprilat. Bioorg Med Chem 2004; 12: 603–11.

57. Gibbs JB, Kohl NE, Koblan KS et al. Farnesyltransferase inhibitors and anti-Ras therapy. Breast Cancer Res Treat 1996; 38: 75–83.

58. Khwaja A, O'Connolly J, Hendry B. Prenylation inhibitors in renal disease. Lancet 2003; 355: 741–4.

59. Szabo Z, Ravert HT, Mathews WB et al. kinetic modeling of a farnesyl transferase specific PET radiotracer. J Nucl Med 1999; 40: 228P.

60. Johnson HA. Diagnosis by the bit: a method for evaluating the diagnostic process. Ann Clin Lab Sci 1989; 19: 323–31.

61. Szabo Z, Speth RC, Brown PR et al. Use of positron emission tomography to study AT1 receptor regulation in vivo. J Am Soc Nephrol 2001; 12: 1350–8.

62. Owonikoko T, Fabucci M, Brown P et al. In vivo investigation of estrogen regulation of adrenal and renal angiotensin (AT1) receptor expression by PET. J Nucl Med 2003; 45: 94–100.

63. Goodfriend TL. Angiotensin receptors: history and mysteries. Am J Hypertens 2000; 13: 442–9.

64. Aleksic S, Szabo Z, Scheffel U et al. In vivo labeling of endothelin receptors with [(11)C] L-753,037: studies in mice and a dog. J Nucl Med 2001; 42: 1274–80.

65. de Gasparo M, Catt KJ, Inagami T et al. International union of pharmacology. XXIII. The angiotensin II receptors. Pharmacol Rev 2000; 52: 415–72.

66. Hong KW, Kim CD, Lee SH, Yoo SE. The in vitro pharmacological profile of KR31080, a nonpeptide AT1 receptor antagonist. Fundam Clin Pharmacol 1998; 12: 64–9.

67. Lee BH, Seo HW, Kwon KJ et al. In vivo pharmacologic profile of SK-1080, an orally active nonpeptide AT1-receptor antagonist. J Cardiovasc Pharmacol 1999; 33: 375–82.

68. Mathews WB, Yoo SE, Lee SH et al. A novel radioligand for imaging the AT1 angiotensin receptor with PET. Nucl Med Biol 2004; 31: 571–4.

69. Logan J, Fowler JS, Volkow ND et al. Graphical analysis of reversible radioligand binding from time-activity measurements applied to [N-^{11}C-methyl]-(−)-cocaine PET studies in human subjects. J Cereb Blood Flow Metab 1990; 10: 740–7.

70. Shibata H, Suzuki H, Murakami M et al. Angiotensin II type 1 receptor messenger RNA levels in human blood cells of patients with primary and secondary hypertension: reference to renin profile. J Hypertens 1994; 12: 1275–84.

71. Chen YM, Wu KD, Hu-Tsai MI et al. Differential expression of type 1 angiotensin II receptor mRNA and aldosterone responsiveness to angiotensin in aldosterone-producing adenoma. Mol Cell Endocrinol 1999; 152: 47–55.

72. Tanabe A, Naruse M, Arai K et al. Gene expression and roles of angiotensin II type 1 and type 2 receptors in human adrenals. Horm Metab Res 1998; 30: 490–5.

73. Opocher G, Rocco S, Cimolato M et al. Angiotensin II receptors in cortical and medullary adrenal tumors. J Clin Endocrinol Metab 1997; 82: 865–9.

74. Hamill TG, Burns HD, Dannals RF et al. Development of [^{11}C] L-159,884: a radiolabelled, nonpeptide angiotensin II antagonist that is useful for angiotensin II, AT1 receptor imaging. Appl Radiat Isot 1996; 47: 211–18.

Urinary tract infection in children

20 Introduction

Isky Gordon

Urinary tract infection (UTI) in children has been the subject of debate and controversy for many decades. As data are emerging, so well-held beliefs are thrown into doubt. Imaging has been one of the major cornerstones in the investigation of children with a proven UTI. This has arisen because there was a widely held belief that a UTI in a child identified a susceptible population of children in whom active treatment often including surgery could alter the natural history. However the advent of routine prenatal ultrasound examinations of the fetus coupled with the introduction of ^{99m}Tc DMSA scintigraphy and the results of a few longitudinal studies have caused serious rethinking of the role of imaging, of what kind of imaging should be undertaken and in which children.

The following issues will be discussed in the following chapters.

Why should we image these children?

Hypertension

The development of hypertension in later life in children with a damaged kidney has been accepted as a fact. There are few long-term longitudinal studies to evaluate this belief, however sustained systemic hypertension in children over one year of age is most commonly due to renal disease. There is only one true long-term epidemiological study[1] that shows no difference in the blood pressure of children with a UTI when comparing those with scars from those without scars. However, what is clear is that those children with severe scarring had a higher blood pressure than those with less severe degrees of scarring. Other workers[2] also suggest that it is the severe loss of renal parenchyma that leads to hypertension rather than a focal scar. Data presented by Hansson (Chapter 23) showed that a scarred kidney does not predispose the child to hypertension. During the discussion at the La Baule symposium, there was reluctance of the participants to disregard the importance of hypertension. However should public health measures include the measurement of blood pressure in annual school medicals of all children, then the detection of renal parenchymal abnormalities in children with a UTI would not be necessary from the point of later-onset hypertension.

Renal failure

The incidence of UTI in children is high, yet the frequency of renal failure is very low. This suggests that chronic renal failure is a very rare complication of UTI and cannot be the rationale for the imaging of children with a UTI.

Pre-eclampsia

Another clinical indication in the past for imaging girls with a UTI, is the suggested higher incidence of pre-eclampsia in those with scarred kidneys compared to those with normal kidneys. Hansson (Chapter 23) presents data that do not support this teaching. Furthermore, in most of Europe the majority of pregnant women attend antenatal clinics where blood pressure is routinely measured and urine is tested, so that the development of pre-eclampsia is detected at an early stage.

There was general agreement that the primary goal of investigation of children with UTI is to identify patients at risk (see below), prevent further infections and prevent progressive renal damage.

Which children should we image?

The current teaching in many institutions is that one should investigate every child with the first UTI. However, every paediatrician knows that UTI is not a homogeneous condition. Under the umbrella of UTI is included the older girl with dysuria and frequency; the very ill child who requires hospital admission and intravenous antibiotics; the septic infant and the infant who is off his feeds, is febrile and has a positive urine culture. Some institutions then divided children on an age basis, with the children under 2 years of age being the most difficult diagnostic problem and so receiving more aggressive investigations. The challenge of the healthcare professionals is to identify that group who do require imaging. In children with a UTI, Rossleigh (Chapter 22) points out the difficulty of identifying clinically those with and those without renal involvement suggesting a ^{99m}Tc DMSA scan is the only way forward. However if a renal parenchymal defect has little or no long-term consequence, then why identify it?

The importance of an underlying malformation, the need for surgical intervention and the prevention of morbidity remain the goals for imaging. To avoid over-investigation of many for the discovery of the few who need medical intervention, the concept of the child at risk or the susceptible child was introduced by Hansson (Chapter 23). The identification of the susceptible child is dependent on the clinical team, the features are any one of the following:

- Recurrent UTI;
- Bacteraemia;
- Sick infant (hospitalized);
- Unusual organism (non E. coli);
- Clinical signs (poor stream/palpable kidneys);
- Slow response to treatment;
- Prenatal ultrasound diagnosis of a renal/urinary tract abnormality;
- Recurrent cystitis in a girl (usually over 3 years of age).

Thus there is now a strong move in many institutions to identify this subgroup of children who require imaging and move away from imaging all children with a proven UTI. It is within this subgroup of children that one will find the children with obstructive uropathies, calculus disease, the congenital malformed kidneys and the children with bladder abnormalities.

What role does VUR play in UTI?

The teaching from the 1960s has been that UTI and VUR lead to renal damage, thus VUR became the villain of paediatric nephrology. Despite numerous publications showing that renal damage may occur in children with UTI without VUR, nevertheless there is a strong desire to hold on to the belief that VUR is the major pathology in acquired pyelonephritic scarring. The evidence that VUR is seen in 30% of most cohorts of children with a UTI studied – yet many of these kidneys are shown to be normal on DMSA scintigraphy – is ignored by many clinicians.

In Chapter 23, Hansson presents data that support the fact that dilating VUR is associated with damaged kidneys, however he also presents data where boys with VUR (median age 0.3 years) had more renal damage than girls (median age 2.8 years). This strongly suggests that the boys are highly likely to have congenitally malformed kidneys associated with VUR rather than acquired pyelonephritic scarring. Prenatal ultrasound has shown that a group of children (mainly boys) are being detected who have both an abnormal kidney and vesico-ureteric reflux (VUR). Thus highlighting the fact that many children previously considered to have acquired reflux nephropathy were likely to have had congenitally malformed kidneys associated with VUR, the so-called congenital reflux nephropathy.

Although it has been suggested, in a recent article from Hoberman et al[3] that micturating cystourethrography (MCUG) is a first-line imaging test, strong arguments against this statement were presented by Hansson and approved by the audience at the La Baule meeting. However, although we have downgraded the importance of VUR, we must not let the pendulum swing to the other extreme and ignore all VUR. VUR remains important in children with recurrent UTI, and since there is a high chance of bladder dysfunction in this group, renal damage may develop with this combination of features. Progressive renal damage may occur in the child with a prenatal diagnosis of hydronephrosis who has both VUR and UTIs. MCU also has an important role when the ultrasound detects a bladder or lower ureteric abnormality.

What is the impact of prenatal ultrasound diagnosis on imaging children with a UTI?

Early prenatal ultrasound examinations up to 20–24 weeks of pregnancy may not detect any abnormality. However late prenatal ultrasound (after 32 weeks gestation) will detect most major congenital malformations, but this test is not universally undertaken. When a prenatal abnormality has been detected, this child then fits into the 'child at risk' group. There is a need to distinguish between the most commonly found abnormality, i.e. isolated renal pelvic dilatation or pelvi-ureteric junction dilatation, that very rarely presents with a UTI from intermittent dilatation, small bright kidney, big bladder of oligohydramnios, all of which require follow-up.

When should we image?

If the clinician accepts the responsibility of identifying children with a UTI who are at risk, then imaging should start very soon after the diagnosis is made. The only exception to this is the child with recurrent symptomatic UTIs where imaging can be delayed till the infection has been cleared especially as this is usually in the older girl.

How should we image?

There was agreement that the primary goal of investigation of children with UTI is to prevent further infections and prevent progressive renal damage. This dictates the imaging strategy that one may adopt. There was little debate on the advantages and disadvantages of the different imaging techniques. The strengths and limitations are well described by Dacher and Rossleigh (Chapters 21 and 22).

A strategy suggested by Dacher (Chapter 21) was positively considered by the audience at the La Baule symposium. Ultrasound should be the first imaging test as this will identify hydronephrosis, hydroureter, thick-walled bladder, renal and bladder calculi as well as the small kidney and a renal abscess. The limits of ultrasound are however in the detection of a renal parenchymal defect. This is the role of the DMSA scan. For those children identified as 'at risk' a DMSA scan is then required in addition to the ultrasound. In the presence of a normal ultrasound and DMSA no further imaging is required.

With an abnormal kidney on ultrasound but no hydronephrosis, a DMSA scan and a MCUG are required to assess individual renal function, parenchymal defects and the presence of VUR.

In the presence of uretero-hydronephrosis, a diuretic renogram and a MCUG are required, while in cases of isolated hydronephrosis on ultrasound, a diuretic renogram without MCUG is required.

References

1. Wennerstrom M, Hansson S, Hedner T et al. Ambulatory blood pressure 16–26 years after the first urinary tract infection in childhood. J Hypertens 2000; 18: 485–91.

2. Patzer L, Seeman T, Wuhl E et al. Day- and night-time blood pressure elevation in children with higher grades of renal scarring. J Pediatr 2003; 142: 117–22.

3. Hoberman A, Charron M, Hickey RW et al. Imaging studies after a first febrile urinary tract infection in young children. N Engl J Med 2003; 348: 195–202.

21 The point of view of the radiologist

Jean-Nicolas Dacher

Introduction

Several imaging modalities are available for the evaluation of children with urinary tract infection (UTI). They mainly include ultrasound (grey scale, colour and power Doppler), ^{99m}Tc-dimercaptosuccinic acid scintigraphy (DMSA scan) and reflux studies. Intravenous urography (IVU), enhanced CT and MRI were also considered useful evaluation tools.

Imaging can be performed: (1) during the acute phase of infection; (2) at the end of antibiotic treatment; and (3) several months after the acute infection to search for scarring.

The most common management of a young child with UTI is as follows:

- ultrasound at the acute phase to detect a cause or complication;
- voiding cystourethrography (VCUG) to eliminate vesicoureteric reflux;
- delayed DMSA scan to detect scarring.

There remains an ongoing debate regarding the optimal imaging strategy to apply in children with UTI. For example, the utility of ultrasound during the acute phase of infection has recently been questioned.[1] Some authors have advocated DMSA scintigraphy during acute infection. Several different examination strategies have been proposed to diagnose vesicoureteric reflux.

The general objective of this review was to assess each of the available studies, as well as the most recent technical knowledge, in order to suggest a reasonable, cost-effective and efficient evaluation using the lowest possible amount of ionizing radiation while limiting invasive procedures.

Which objectives for imaging?

The objectives for imaging children with UTI could be: (1) Identify and treat patients with a life-threatening condition (particularly in the case of neonates). (2) Prevent renal and bladder damage, arterial hypertension and eclampsia. (3) Detect children with underlying disease (reflux, voiding dysfunction, obstruction). (4) Avoid unnecessary follow-up examinations in children who did not have acute pyelonephritis (APN) (particularly in under-3-year-olds).

Which children should be investigated?

There are many different subsets of children with UTI and not all require the same imaging management. Among the factors to be considered when deciding whether or not to perform imaging are: fetal US, age, gender, previous medical history, physical signs, voiding dysfunction, renal function and course of the disease under treatment.

Although the question remains difficult, some basic rules should be considered.

- Neonates and infants with fever and a positive urinary culture should be imaged during the acute infection to detect those with severe disease (abscess, pyohydronephrosis or acute pyelonephritis). The high rate of complications justifies imaging, and US is particularly effective in thin patients.
- The high prevalence of congenital vesicoureteric reflux in under-3-year-old children with an initial proven febrile UTI justifies a reflux test. Congenital reflux predominates in male infants, and in cases of positive family history.
- Acute phase imaging could be avoided in children or adolescents with typical uncomplicated acute pyelonephritis. Imaging could be limited to children with an unusual course of treatment, or infected with uncommon bacteria.
- At least, if one considers that UTI could present a risk of late complication (hypertension, eclampsia, renal failure, etc.); a delayed DMSA scan should be performed in children with a previous medical history of proven acute pyelonephritis to evaluate renal contours and function.

Imaging children with acute infection: ultrasound or not?

Recently, the role of US in the evaluation of UTI in children was critically evaluated.[1] Hoberman et al reported a 12%

Figure 21.1 Typical US pattern of acute pyelonephritis. Hyperechoic focus of the enlarged lower pole of the left kidney. Mild dilatation of the adjacent calyces.

rate of sonographic abnormalities in a population of children with UTI. Moreover, the authors claimed that fetal US should be enough to detect all children with urinary tract malformation in developed countries. Hence they concluded that, in a child with UTI who had normal prenatal scans, US would not be relevant.

This point of view should be weighted by the following considerations:

1. It has been demonstrated that prenatal US alone should not be used to evaluate children with congenital vesicoureteric reflux, the most frequent malformation associated with UTI.[2–4]
2. Hydronephrosis as a consequence of uretero-pelvic junction (UPJ) obstruction can be diagnosed at any age of life (even in patients who had normal prenatal sonograms) and can become complicated with severe infection.
3. Even in developed countries, communication between pre- and postnatal medical teams remains defective.[5]

4. Ultrasound is an efficient means of diagnosing infectious emergencies such as renal abscess, pyohydronephrosis with or without kidney stone.
5. Ultrasound technique varied among the different published studies in regard to acute pyelonephritis.[1,6–10] Not all studies used high frequency scanning and colour or power Doppler. These tools can detect subtle abnormalities which have been described in association with acute pyelonephritis. Sonography signs were divided into two categories: I. Signs of pyelitis include mild dilatation, thickened pelvic wall (nonspecific for APN), and increased echogenicity of the renal sinus.[11] II. Signs of nephritis include nephromegaly, triangular hyperechogenicity (Figure 21.1) or rounded hypoechoic area. A decreased perfusion on colour/power Doppler (spontaneously or after IV infusion of microbubbles) is frequent (Figure 21.2).[6,7]
6. In school-age girls with UTI and voiding dysfunction, bladder US completes the flowmetry examination (or urodynamics) to search for residual urine.[12]
7. At the least, ultrasound scanning is absolutely noninvasive, feasible at the bedside, does not deliver ionizing radiation, and remains relatively inexpensive.

As previously stated, the sensitivity of ultrasound for the diagnosis of APN varies greatly among series and institutions since the operators (expert paediatric radiologists interested in the subject in some studies vs residents or sonographers in others), the techniques (prone and supine position scanning, use of colour/power Doppler, sedation, injection of contrast medium, high-frequency scanning) and equipment are widely varied. Even under optimal technical conditions, the diagnostic accuracy of colour Doppler US for APN ranged from 80–90%[9,10] and remained below that of DMSA scintigraphy, enhanced CT or MRI (Figure 21.3).

We still believe, in spite of a recent study,[1] that US could remain the first-line examination in children with UTI. Moreover, follow-up examinations could be conditioned by the US results. The following strategies could be considered:

Figure 21.2 Grey scale, power and colour Doppler US of the left kidney in a 1-year-old girl with typical left acute pyelonephritis. Grey scale US showed hyperechoic undifferentiated upper pole of the left kidney. Power and colour Doppler showed decreased flow.

Figure 21.3 Five-year-old girl with acute pyelonephritis. Excellent correlation between power Doppler ultrasound (decreased flow) and DMSA scan (decreased uptake) at the upper pole of the right kidney. Both examinations were performed during the acute phase of infection.

Figure 21.4 Eight-year-old girl with acute pyelonephritis. Colour Doppler ultrasound showed decreased flow at the upper pole of the left duplicated kidney (top left). The upper pole ureter was slightly dilated and followed down to its vesical implantation (bottom left). No ureterocele was found. VCUG showed reflux into the upper pole ureter which was confirmed to be ectopic on cystoscopy (right).

Figure 21.5 Cyclic VCUG in a 1-month-old baby boy who had UTI. The first filling of the bladder did not show reflux. Right then bilateral reflux were found on second and third fillings.

1. If optimal US scanning is completely normal in a child with febrile UTI, a DMSA scan could be considered in order to definitely eliminate or assess the diagnosis of APN. In the absence of any abnormality on both US and DMSA scan, VCUG is not necessary. This idea is based on the excellent negative predictive value of acute DMSA scintigraphy regarding renal scarring.[10] The only exception to that rule would be the case of a child with recurrent infection.

2. When US shows dilatation (of the pelvis, ureter or both) or any other sign of urinary tract malformation (dupli-cated ureter, ureterocele), VCUG is extremely important to assess the anatomy and micturition (see section on hydronephrosis) (Figure 21.4).

3. If US revealed APN, acute DMSA does not seem necessary.[13] VCUG could be considered on an age and gender basis.

    a. In an under-3-year-old child with a first episode of febrile UTI, we would recommend VCUG rather than any other reflux test to detect congenital reflux (Figure 21.5). The anatomy (urethra in boys) and bladder sphincter function (micturition) are well

cystographie 1   cystographie 2

Avant traitement   **Après traitement**

débimétrie 1   débimétrie 2

Figure 21.6 Follow-up of voiding dysfunction in a young girl. Evaluation of the child with associated VCUG and flowmetry. Left; pretreatment examinations. VCUG showed typical spinning top urethra. Low grade left reflux was present as well as a right bladder diverticulum. Micturition (upper curve) was dampened, and perineal floor EMG (bottom curve) was abnormally active. Right; post-treatment examinations. Treatment included diet and biofeedback. Clinical symptoms had disappeared as well as reflux and bladder diverticulum. Flowmetry had normalized.

defined by VCUG. In our experience, isotopic or sonographic reflux detection techniques (less or nonradiating at all) should be employed for follow-up.

b. In the particular case of school-age girls with APN, it is extremely important to diagnose voiding dysfunction (oriented interview, flowmetry) and to detect scarring by DMSA.[14] The frequently associated reflux is the consequence of a long-standing high-pressure bladder. In most cases VCUG, which is not well tolerated in this subset of children, is of limited interest.

Concurrent studies have been proposed to evaluate children with acute UTI. Gadolinium-enhanced inversion recovery sequences of MRI[15] appeared extremely interesting but availability of equipment has limited their use in research studies. Enhanced CT[6] is also effective but it delivers radiation, requires iodine injection and sometimes sedation. Hence, it cannot be widely recommended in such a frequent disease. Patients presenting with renal abscess, stone and 'pseudo tumour' (all detected on US) particularly require CT as well as children with an unusual course of antibiotic treatment.

In the setting of acute UTI, US (or CT) can be used to guide the placement of a percutaneous nephrostomy tube when pyohydronephrosis or a renal or pararenal abscess has been diagnosed.

Voiding cystourethrography (VCUG)

Although several concurrent studies were recently reported, VCUG remains the gold standard examination. It permits a quick and effective detection of vesicoureteric reflux (when performed with the cyclic method). It clearly illustrates the male urethra. In addition, VCUG can show micturition and help diagnose bladder instability or dysfunctional voiding.

However, VCUG delivers radiation and requires either an indwelling catheter or a suprapubic puncture. For these reasons, VCUG should be considered on an individual basis and limited in its use and indications. Retrograde or suprapubic approaches are no different in terms of sensitivity. While the retrograde route is usually considered more invasive, it does not require preliminary bladder ultrasound.

After vesicoureteric reflux is detected, it is necessary to classify it as congenital or secondary. Over recent years, prenatal diagnosis of congenital reflux has become a common situation.

Congenital reflux, a consequence of ureteral meatus malformation, mainly occurs in boys. In the recent past, prenatal diagnosis of congenital reflux became the most common diagnostic condition. Among under-1-year-old children, UTI predominates in boys, but reflux is frequently absent when prenatal US is normal. The grade of that frequently bilateral reflux is usually high at the time of diagnosis and tends to decrease with growth. The rate of children who can be managed conservatively is inversely proportional to the grade at the time of diagnosis. After 3 years of age, congenital reflux in a previously well child becomes a questionable diagnosis.

Secondary reflux can be the consequence of bladder sphincter complex dysfunction. Neurogenic bladder should be considered and eliminated, but the most frequent cause of this type of reflux is voiding dysfunction. Children with voiding dysfunction (usually girls) do not require repeated invasive procedures. Imaging should be limited to bladder US to search for residual urine after micturition and DMSA scintigraphy since the association between voiding dysfunction and UTI presents a high risk of scarring. US can be performed after noninvasive flowmetry (Figure 21.6).[16] The challenge in

Figure 21.7 Enhanced CT scan showing a scarred left kidney in a child with a history of pyelonephritis.

those children is to preserve the kidneys (preventing recurrent infections) and the bladder sphincter function (education, diet, biofeedback, physiotherapy, etc.).

Detection of scarring

Acute pyelonephritis can lead to renal scars. However, the role of APN in the development of hypertension, eclampsia or chronic renal failure was not supported by recent studies.[17] Detection of scarring is based on DMSA scintigraphy. Intravenous urography should no longer be performed in that indication.

DMSA is a cortical marker labelled with technetium 99m that provides both morphological and functional information.[18] A scar is defined as a defect in the renal outline with little or no DMSA uptake. The main difficulty is to differentiate acute infection and genuine renal scarring. It is generally considered that 6 months after the last episode of infection, the scar only is responsible for a persisting defect. However, there is a continuing debate on this point.[19]

CT and MR can also show renal scars (Figure 21.7); however, those techniques have limitations which have been previously discussed.

In conclusion, there is no consensus on the optimal way to image and follow-up children with UTI. However, ongoing dynamic research continues to be performed throughout the world and fewer questions remain unaddressed. It is likely that too much importance has been given to vesicoureteric reflux in the past. Efforts should now be made to assess the best way to detect children who require treatment, to prevent APN renal complications and to preserve the bladder sphincter complex function.

Acknowledgement

The authors thank Richard Medeiros, Rouen University Hospital Medical Editor, for his advice in editing the manuscript.

References

1. Hoberman A, Charron M, Hickey RW et al. Imaging studies after a first febrile urinary tract infection in young children. N Engl J Med 2003; 348: 195–202.
2. Moorthy I, Joshi N, Cook JV, Warren M. Antenatal hydronephrosis: negative predictive value of normal postnatal ultrasound – a 5-year study. Clin Radiol 2003; 58: 964–70.
3. Phan V, Traubici J, Hershenfield B et al. Vesicoureteral reflux in infants with isolated antenatal hydronephrosis. Pediatr Nephrol 2003; 18: 1224–8.
4. Anderson NG, Wright S, Abbott GD et al. Fetal renal pelvic dilatation – poor predictor of familial vesicoureteral reflux. Pediatr Nephrol 2003; 18: 902–5.
5. Nishisaki A. Imaging studies after a first febrile urinary tract infection in young children (comment). N Engl J Med 2003; 348: 1812.
6. Dacher JN, Pfister C, Monroc M et al. Power Doppler sonographic pattern of acute pyelonephritis in children. AJR 1996: 166; 1451–5.
7. Riccabona M, Fotter R. Urinary tract infection in infants and children: an update with special regard to the changing role of reflux. Eur Radiol 2004; 14: L78–L88.
8. Alon US, Ganapathy S. Should renal ultrasonography be done routinely in children with urinary tract infection? Clin Pediatr 1999; 38: 21–5.
9. Morin D, Veyrac C, Kotzki PO et al. Comparison of ultrasound and DMSA scintigraphy changes in acute pyelonephritis. Pediatr Nephrol 1999; 13: 219–22.
10. Hitzel A, Liard A, Vera P et al. Color and Power Doppler sonography versus DMSA scintigraphy in acute pyelonephritis and in prediction of renal scarring. J Nucl Med 2002; 43: 27–32.
11. Dacher JN, Avni EF, François A. Renal sinus hyperechogenicity in acute pyelonephritis: description and pathological correlation. Pediatr Radiol 1999; 29: 179–82.
12. Dacher JN, Savoye-Collet C. Urinary tract infection and functional bladder sphincter disorders in children. Eur Radiol 2004; 14: L101–6.
13. El Hajjar M, Launay S, Hossein-Foucher C et al. Power

Doppler sonography and acute pyelonephritis in children: comparison with Tc-DMSA scintigraphy. Arch Pediatr 2002; 9: 21–5.

14. Naseer SR, Steinhardt GF. New renal scars in children with urinary tract infections, vésico-urétéral reflux and voiding dysfunction: a prospective evaluation. J Urol 1997; 158: 566–8.

15. Lonergan GJ, Pennington DJ, Morrison JC et al. Childhood pyelonephritis: comparison of gadolinium enhanced MR imaging and renal cortical scintigraphy for diagnosis. Radiology 1998; 207: 377–84.

16. Pfister C, Dacher JN, Gaucher S et al. The usefulness of minimal urodynamic evaluation and pelvic floor biofeedback in children with chronic voiding dysfunction. Br J Urol 1999; 84: 1054–7.

17. Goldraich NP, Goldraich IH. Update on DMSA renal scanning in children with urinary tract infection. Pediatr Nephrol 1995; 9: 221–6.

17. Wennerstrom M, Hansson S, Hedner T et al. Ambulatory blood pressure 16–26 years after the first urinary tract infection. J Hypertens 2000; 18: 485–91.

18. Ditchfield MR, Grimwood K, Cook DJ et al. Persistent renal cortical scintigram defects in children 2 years after urinary tract infection. Pediatr Radiol 2004; 34: 465–71.

22 The point of view of the paediatric nuclear medicine physician

Monica A Rossleigh

Introduction

Urinary tract infection (UTI) is a common problem. In children, 3–5% of girls and 1–2% of boys have had a symptomatic UTI.[1] In Australia, UTI accounts for 1.2% of all family physician–patient encounters.[2] UTI may be complicated or uncomplicated. Complicated UTIs are those that occur in the presence of other factors such as obstruction, calculi, vesicoureteric reflux, or systemic disease, e.g. diabetes. While in adults imaging in UTI only occurs if there is a suspicion of complicated UTI, it is widely recommended that imaging be undertaken in children after their first UTI.[3]

There is widespread but not universal agreement that ultrasound examination should be the initial investigation when a child presents with a UTI.[4,5] Ultrasound examination is undertaken to exclude the presence of hydronephrosis or obstruction, to exclude structural abnormalities such as small kidneys and ureteroceles and to exclude the presence of renal calculi.

There is currently debate in the literature whether cystograms should be undertaken for the detection of vesicoureteric reflux (VUR). It is well documented that approximately 30% of children with UTI have VUR and that VUR may predispose to upper tract involvement with infection. However, it has been confirmed by a number of workers that UTI frequently occurs in the absence of demonstrable reflux.[6–8]

Acute pyelonephritis in the absence of demonstrable reflux is common. Rosenberg found VUR in only 24% of children with DMSA scan evidence of acute pyelonephritis.[6] Majd found VUR in only 37% of patients with acute pyelonephritis.[7] Ditchfield found VUR in 39% of children with acute pyelonephritis demonstrated on acute renal cortical scintigraphy.[8] Conversely, 53% of children with VUR did not have upper tract involvement with the acute UTI. The correlation between the incidence of renal cortical scarring and the grade of VUR has been debated. Farnsworth evaluated 113 infants less than 1 year of age at risk of renal scarring.[9] He demonstrated that there was a markedly significant increase in the incidence of renal cortical scarring detected on the DMSA study in children with high-grade VUR when compared to lower grades. Conversely there was also a statistically significant absence of renal cortical abnormalities on the DMSA study in children with low-grade VUR when compared to the higher grades. Stockland investigated 303 children with UTI before 2 years of age and found that there was a significantly increased risk of renal damage on the DMSA scan in children with dilating, i.e., high-grade VUR.[10] On the other hand, in two systematic reviews and meta-analyses, it was difficult to convincingly show a relationship between VUR and renal damage in children with UTI.[11,12] What are possible explanations for these opposing findings? It appears clear that on an acute DMSA study performed at the time of UTI, there appears to be no relationship between the presence of VUR and acute pyelonephritis and that on a late scan performed at least 3 months from a UTI, the incidence of renal cortical scarring is related to the grade of VUR. In the reviews and meta-analysis of the literature, a clear distinction may not have been made between data obtained from acute studies and information obtained from late scans obtained distant from the UTI. Another possible source of error is that in a significant number of publications, DMSA findings are correlated with the presence of VUR, without taking into account the grade of VUR.

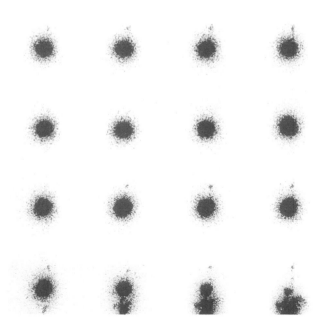

Figure 22.1 Direct radionuclide cystogram revealing VUR into the right kidney on both filling and voiding.

A

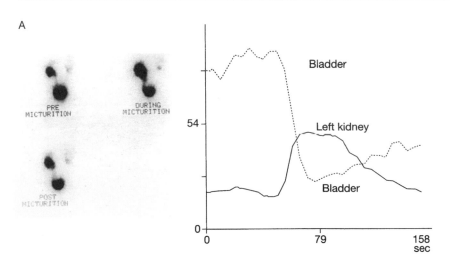

Figure 22.2 A: Indirect radionuclide cystogram revealing VUR into a lower pole moiety of a left duplex kidney on voiding. B: Indirect radionuclide cystogram revealing bilateral VUR on voiding far more marked on the left. C: Indirect radionuclide cystogram detecting VUR on the right in the last eight frames of the acquisition (starting just before micturition). On the left side, the kidney is clearly visualized on all images: this can be left VUR during natural bladder filling, but marked stasis could be another explanation and should be carefully excluded.

B

The radiological cystogram gives excellent anatomical definition and the grade of reflux can be determined using the international classification for VUR.[13] It is essential in the first UTI in a male to assess the urethra and to exclude the presence of posterior urethral valves. However, the radiation dose from a radiological cystogram is in general higher than the radiation dose from a radionuclide cystogram.

Radionuclide cystograms can be performed in three ways: direct, indirect and suprapubic.

Direct radionuclide cystogram

Bladder catheterization is required as with a radiological cystogram. A small amount of radioactivity, e.g. 20 MBq technetium 99m-sulphur colloid, DTPA or pertechnetate is instilled into the urinary bladder via a bladder catheter and

C

Figure 22.3 A: Normal DMSA study. The top row shows anterior and posterior planar views and the bottom row shows oblique posterior as well as posterior pinhole images. B: Normal DMSA pinhole views of the kidneys with prominent columns of Bertin, which vary in shape and number. C: Normal DMSA posterior planar images with a prominent splenic impression. D: Normal posterior planar DMSA images. The image on the left has movement artefact as evidenced by blurred renal outlines which are not present on re-imaging on the right, when no movement has occurred. E: Normal posterior planar DMSA image with hypoactive poles, which is a normal variant and is recognized as a classical pitfall.

normal saline gently heated to body temperature is infused into the bladder until voiding occurs. Ten-second dynamic images are obtained during filling and voiding and the sequence can be repeated while the bladder catheter remains in situ (Figure 22.1). The advantage of the direct radionuclide cystogram over a contrast cystogram is not only the lower radiation dose associated but the ability for a longer observation time when compared to the radiological cystogram. It should be noted that VUR is an intermittent and variable phenomenon and that repeat filling of the bladder may demonstrate VUR which is not evident on the first fill.[14]

Post ratios
Left kidney – 53.03%
Right kidney – 46.96%

Geometric mean ratios
Left kidney – 50.41%
Right kidney – 49.59%

Distance: 9.9485

Distance cm: 8.7140

Nomograms of renal
length versus age
weight and height.
Mean +/– SD shown.

+ Lt kidney
+ Rt kidney

Figure 22.4 Computer analysis of DMSA study with differential renal function calculation, renal length measurement and normograms for renal length at varying age, height and weight.

Indirect radionuclide cystogram

The advantage of this technique in that a bladder catheter is not required but the disadvantage of this technique is that the child must be toilet trained. The target group for the detection of VUR and the subsequent prevention of reflux nephropathy is children under 3 years of age.[15] The indirect radionuclide cystogram cannot be applied in this group because of their inability to void on demand. With this technique, VUR can only be detected in the older age group in which reflux nephropathy is most likely already established or excluded.

This technique requires the intravenous administration of technetium 99m MAG 3. Dynamic renal imaging can be obtained. When the child is ready to void approximately 30–60 minutes postinjection, the child sits with their back to the gamma camera and 5-second frame dynamic imaging is acquired commencing 30 seconds before voiding until micturition is complete (Figure 22.2).

Suprapubic cystography

This has recently been described using both the radiological approach with the instillation of contrast or by the instillation of radionuclide. Oswald and co-workers described the use of the instillation of contrast into the bladder by a suprapubic

puncture.[16] They reported that the mean pain score was lower in the suprapubic group compared to children examined using the transurethral route. In the group of children who underwent transurethral cystography the pain score increased with age, whereas in the group where a suprapubic puncture was used, the pain score decreased with age. Their conclusions were that in children older than 24 months, the suprapubic approach was preferred. Wilkinson described the application of percutaneous direct radionuclide cystography in children.[17] He applied this technique to 103 toilet-trained children aged between 2.1 and 15.6 years. Most children preferred the percutaneous suprapubic injection when compared to an intravenous injection. He found the images easy to interpret and the detection of reflux more reliable as it avoided the doubt as to whether the activity in the renal areas was due to reflux or excretion when comparing this technique to the indirect radionuclide cystogram.

Despite these two papers encouraging the use of this technique, this method of the detection of VUR has not been widely accepted.

Renal cortical imaging utlizing technetium 99m dimercaptosuccinic acid (DMSA)

DMSA is an excellent renal cortical imaging agent and is the radiopharmaceutical of choice. Approximately 40% of the

Figure 22.5 A: Unifocal pyelonephritis or acute lobar nephronia involving the upper pole of the left kidney (upper row) which resolved on the follow-up DMSA study performed 3 months later (lower row). B: Unifocal pyelonephritis of the upper pole of the right kidney on the left image which resolved on the follow-up scan performed 9 months later on the right image. Reprinted from Nuclear Medicine in Clinical Diagnosis and Treatment, 3rd edition, Ell and Gambir (eds), copyright 2004 with permission from Elsevier.

Figure 22.6 A: Multifocal pyelonephritis of the left kidney which resolved on follow-up studies. B: Multifocal pyelonephritis of both kidneys on the acute study on the left which resolved on the follow-up study on the right. Reprinted from Nuclear Medicine in Clinical Diagnosis and Treatment, 3rd edition, Ell and Gambir (eds), copyright 2004 with permission from Elsevier.

administered dose accumulates in the distal tubular cells, providing excellent visualization of the renal cortex, after background activity has cleared. Dynamic tracers with high excretion rates such as ^{99m}Tc-mercaptoacetyltriglycine (MAG3) give less accurate information on renal cortical abnormalities and constitute only second-choice tracers. Guidelines have been published for the performance of this investigation.[18,19] The recommended minimum dose is 15–20 MBq with a maximum adult dose of 100–110 MBq. The administered dose should be scaled on a body surface basis. Images should be acquired 2–3 h after tracer injection but if significant hydronephrosis exists, late images (4–24 h) or frusemide injection may be helpful. Images should include at least a posterior view acquired for a minimum of 200 000 counts or 5 min using a high-resolution parallel-hole collimator, and both posterior oblique views. Many experts advocate the addition of pinhole images using a 2–4 mm aperture insert. Pinhole views are acquired for 100 000–150 000 counts or for 10 min.

Some workers add SPECT which may provide useful information but can increase the number of false-positive results and is more technically demanding during both acquisition and analysis. Motion artefact constitutes a problem in SPECT related to the long acquisition time. Pinhole imaging is more easily repeated than is a SPECT study. Several workers recommend the addition of either pinhole or SPECT imaging to the planar studies to increase the level of certainty with which renal cortical scintigraphy is interpreted.

A normal DMSA study exhibits homogeneous cortical uptake throughout the kidneys except for a lower concentration in the region of the collecting system (Figure 22.3). The consensus report confirmed the variety that can be found in normal images including flattening of the superolateral aspect of the upper pole of the left kidney due to splenic impression and prominent cortical columns of Bertin resulting in heterogeneous uptake.[18] Differential function calculation can be undertaken on the posterior planar view and depth correction using geometric mean data from the anterior view may also be obtained, although the need for depth correction has been questioned.[18] Renal length measurements can also be obtained and normal ranges have been established (Figure 22.4).[20]

DMSA studies are utilized either early to make the diagnosis of acute pyelonephritis or late to detect the presence of renal cortical scarring. If the DMSA study is undertaken to assess for the presence of chronic damage following UTI, the study should not be performed less than 3 months from the time of UTI. There is much debate in the literature as to the time period between UTI and scanning. The minimum period is 3 months, although some workers have advocated waiting 6 months or 12 months to ensure that all reversible findings due to resolving infection have occurred.[18] The accuracy of the DMSA study in the diagnosis of acute pyelonephritis and chronic renal cortical scarring have been established in the piglet model. Rushton and Majd from Washington Children's Hospital confirmed that the changes present on the DMSA study at the time of acute pyelonephritis do correspond to acute infective foci histologically using the piglet model.[21] Their findings were soon confirmed by Parkhouse and co-workers who also validated the sensitivity of the DMSA study in the detection of acute pyelonephritis using the piglet model.[22]

There are three patterns of DMSA scan abnormality identified at the time of acute pyelonephritis – unifocal or acute lobar nephronia (Figure 22.5), multifocal (Figures 22.6 and 22.7) and diffuse (Figure 22.8). Scan features to suggest acute changes include focal decreased or absent cortical uptake without cortical or volume loss, in which the renal cortical contour remains intact.

Rosenberg et al undertook a prospective study evaluating UTI in children by DMSA scintigraphy.[6] The clinicians were asked to assess whether children were likely to have upper tract involvement with infection on the basis of clinical findings or were considered to have lower tract infection. The children were classified into two groups. The septic group were systemically unwell and had persistent high fever of greater than 38.5°C. These children were considered to be likely to have acute pyelonephritis. The nonseptic group

Figure 22.7 A: Multifocal pyelonephritis of both kidneys in a neonate following a cystogram, demonstrating the importance of antibiotic propylaxis when catheterizing a neonate with high-grade VUR. B: Multifocal pyelonephritis of the left kidney.

were those children with a lower fever who were only mildly ill. These children were thought to have lower tract infection only. Fifteen of 20 children categorized as a septic presentation had an abnormal DMSA study, five had a normal scan ($P = 0.015$). On the other hand, of the 45 children with a nonseptic presentation 19 had an abnormal DMSA study and 26 had a normal DMSA study, i.e. no significant difference. It was concluded that when the child was assessed as having a septic presentation clinically, upper tract involvement with infection was likely. However, the converse was not true as a nonseptic presentation clinically could not reliably exclude upper tract involvement with infection.

ACUTE

8/12 FU

13/12 FU

PLANAR

PINHOLE

Figure 22.9 DMSA study in the pig revealing a scarred left kidney and normal right kidney, on planar and pinhole images. Reprinted with permission from reference 26.

Figure 22.8 Diffuse pyelonephritis of the right kidney (top row), resulting in residual permanent damage on the 13-month follow-up DMSA study (bottom row), as evidenced by a small right kidney with reduced relative function within it. (Reprinted from Nuclear Medicine in Clinical Diagnosis and Treatment, 3rd edition, Ell and Gambir (eds), copyright 2004 with permission from Elsevier.)

Figure 22.10 Normal right kidney of the pig confirming the normal scan appearance.

Figure 22.11 Extensively scarred left kidney of the pig corresponding to the scarring seen on the DMSA study. Reprinted with permission from reference 26.

In some centres, the acute DMSA study is undertaken to determine antibiotic therapy for UTI. An abnormal DMSA study will require the child to have more intensive antibiotic therapy. This approach has not been adequately validated in the literature although there is some evidence to support it. Levtchenko assessed the efficiency of 7 days of intravenous antibiotics compared to 3 days of intravenous antibiotics, both followed by an oral agent in children with acute pyelonephritis.[23] In children treated for 7 days with intravenous antibiotics, the percentage of patients with chronic renal cortical scarring on the delayed DMSA study was the same whether the children presented early or the diagnosis and treatment was delayed for more than 1 week. However, in the group treated for 3 days with intravenous antibiotics, there was a significantly higher incidence of sequelae with renal cortical scarring on the delayed DMSA study in the group of children with a delay in diagnosis and treatment of more than 1 week.

In approximately 10% of children of any age with a clinical diagnosis of acute pyelonephritis, urine cultures are found to be either equivocal or negative.[24] In this group of children, the acute DMSA study can be undertaken to confirm the clinical diagnosis and result in an appropriate management plan. Without the DMSA study, the child would remain with the diagnosis of a fever of unknown origin.

A number of centres are using the acute DMSA study to determine whether a cystogram is required for the detection of VUR.[25] If the DMSA study is abnormal, a cystogram is required whereas if the DMSA study is normal, there has not been upper tract involvement with infection and the child can be discharged from follow-up. While this approach has been advocated by a number of workers, it has still not been validated.

Figure 22.12 A: Chronic renal cortical scarring of the lower pole of the right kidney, with localized deformity of the normal renal outline and associated volume loss seen on the DMSA study. B: Renal cortical scar of upper pole of left kidney, which is detected on the posterior planar image on the left but is better delineated on the pinhole image (right panel).

Figure 22.13 Extensive scarring of the upper pole of the left component of a horseshoe kidney seen on the DMSA study.

Some workers utilize DMSA studies to assess for chronic sequelae once acute infective changes have resolved in the kidney. The utility of DMSA scintigraphy in the detection of chronic renal cortical scarring has been validated in the literature.[26]

Using the pig model, the DMSA findings of chronic scarring were confirmed histologically (Figures 22.9–22.11). The features that suggest chronic scarring on a DMSA study are defects in uptake associated with cortical thinning and volume loss resulting in a localized deformity of the renal outline (Figures 22.12 and 22.13).

The investigation of UTI is still controversial. Many workers advocate an acute DMSA study to determine future treatment and investigations. It is established that clinical and biological data are insufficient for the correct diagnosis of acute pyelonephritis[4,6] and that the DMSA study is a sensitive technique in the diagnosis of acute pyelonephritis and this has been confirmed in the animal model. Furthermore in the 10% of children with equivocal or negative urine cultures at presentation with clinical acute pyelonephritis, the diagnosis can be confirmed on the acute DMSA study.[24] A number of workers have confirmed that the risk for late sequelae for an abnormal early DMSA study ranges from 15–40%.[6,7,27] If the DMSA study is normal the risk of sequelae at 6 months is 0%. Hoberman's recent publication in which he advocates urine cultures and cystograms alone as the only investigations to determine whether antibiotics or antimicrobial prophylaxis is prescribed is not an approach supported by other workers in the field.[28]

References

1. Fidler K, Hyer W. A strategy for UTI in children. Practitioner 1998; 242: 538–41.
2. The BEACH Study. General practice activity in Australia 1999–2000. Australian Institute of Health and Welfare, 2000.
3. Report of a Working Group of the Research Unit, Royal College of Physicians. Guidelines for the management of urinary tract infection in childhood. J R Coll Physicians Lond 1991; 25: 36–42.
4. American Academy of Pediatrics, Committee on Quality Improvement, Subcommittee on Urinary Tract Infection. The diagnosis, treatment and evaluation of the initial urinary tract infection in febrile infants and young children. Pediatrics 1999; 103: 843–52.
5. Gelfand MJ, Barr LL, Abunko O. The initial renal ultrasound examination in children with urinary tract infection: the prevalence of dilated uropathy has decreased. Pediatr Radiol 2000; 30: 665–70.
6. Rosenberg AR, Rossleigh MA, Brydon MP et al. Evaluation of acute urinary tract infection in children by dimercaptosuccinic acid scintigraphy: a prospective study. J Urol 1992; 148: 1746–9.
7. Majd M, Rushton HG, Jantausch B, Wiedermann BL. Relationship among vesicoureteral reflux, P-fimbriated Escherichia coli, and acute pyelonephritis in children with febrile urinary tract infection. J Pediatr 1991; 119: 578–85.
8. Ditchfield MR, de Campo JF, Cook DJ et al. Vesicoureteral reflux: an accurate predictor of acute pyelonephritis in childhood urinary tract infections? Radiology 1994; 190: 413–15.
9. Farnsworth RH, Rossleigh MA, Leighton DM et al. The detection of reflux nephropathy in infants by [99m]Technetium dimercaptosuccinic acid studies. J Urol 1991; 145: 542–6.
10. Stokland E, Hellstrom M, Jacobsson B et al. Evaluation of DMSA scintigraphy and urography in assessing both acute and permanent renal damage in children. Acta Radiol 1998; 39: 447–52.
11. Gordon I, Barkovics M, Pindoria S et al. Primary vesicoureteric reflux as a predictor of renal damage in children hospitalized with urinary tract infection: a systematic review and meta-analysis. J Am Soc Nephrol 2003; 14: 739–44.
12. Wheeler D, Vimalachandra D, Hodson EM et al. Antibiotics and surgery for vesicoureteric reflux: a meta-analysis of randomised controlled studies. Arch Dis Child 2003; 88: 688–94.
13. International Reflux Study in Children. International system of radiographic grading of vesicoureteric reflux. Pediatr Radiol 1985; 15: 105–9.
14. Jequier S, Jequier JC. Reliability of voiding cystourethrography to detect reflux. AJR 1989; 153: 807–10.
15. Vernon SJ, Coulthard MG, Lambert HJ et al. New renal scarring in children who at age 3 and 4 years had had normal scans with dimercaptosuccinic acid: follow up study. BMJ 1997; 315: 905–8.
16. Oswald J, Riccabona M, Lusuardi L et al. Voiding cystourethrography using the suprapubic versus transurethral route in infants and children: results of a prospective pain scale orientated study. J Urol 2002; 168: 2586–9.
17. Wilkinson AG. Percutaneous direct radionuclide cystography in children: description of technique and early experience. Pediatr Radiol 2002; 32: 511–17.
18. Piepsz A, Blaufox MD, Gordon I et al. Consensus on renal cortical scintigraphy in children with urinary tract infection. Semin Nucl Med 1999; 29: 160–74.
19. Piepsz A, Colarinha P, Gordon I et al. Guidelines for ^{99m}Tc-DMSA scintigraphy in children. Eur J Nucl Med 2001; 28: BP 37–41.
20. Sisayan RM, Rossleigh MA, Mackey DWJ. Normograms of renal length in children obtained from DMSA scintigraphy. Clin Nucl Med 1993; 18: 970–3.
21. Rushton HG, Majd M, Chandra R, Yim D. Evaluation of technetium-99m-dimercaptosuccinic acid renal scans in the detection and localization of experimental acute pyelonephritis in piglets. J Urol 1988; 140: 1169–74.
22. Parkhouse HG, Godley ML, Cooper J et al. Renal imaging with ^{99m}Tc-labelled DMSA in the detection of acute pyelonephritis: an experimental study in the pig. Nucl Med Commun 1989; 10: 63–70.
23. Levtchenko E, Lahy C, Levy J et al. Treatment of children with acute pyelonephritis: a prospective randomized study. Pediatr Nephrol 2001; 16: 878–84.

24. Levtchenko EN, Lahy C, Levy J et al. Role of Tc-99m DMSA scintigraphy in the diagnosis of culture negative pyelonephritis. Pediatr Nephrol 2001; 16: 503–6.
25. Goldraich NP, Goldraich IH. Update on dimercapto-succinic acid renal scanning in children with urinary tract infection. Pediatr Nephrol 1995: 9: 221–6.
26. Rossleigh MA, Farnsworth RH, Leighton DM et al. Technetium-99m dimercaptosuccinic acid scintigraphy studies of renal cortical scarring and renal length. J. Nucl Med 1998; 39: 1280–5.
27. Ditchfield MR, Grimwood K, Cook DJ et al. Persistent renal cortical scintigram defects in children 2 years after urinary tract infection. Pediatr Radiol 2004; 34: 465–71.
28. Hoberman A, Charron M, Hickey RW et al. Imaging studies after a first febrile urinary tract infection in young children. N Engl J Med 2003; 348: 195–202.

23 The point of view of the paediatric nephrologist

Sverker Hansson

Epidemiology of urinary tract infections in children

Urinary tract infection (UTI) is one of the most common bacterial diseases in children. In a study from Göteborg, Sweden, of children who were born in 1975, the cumulative incidence of symptomatic UTI at 7 years of age was 7.8% for girls and 1.6% for boys.[1] In half of the children, the UTI had been associated with high fever, according to the original records from hospital or outpatient clinics, and in most of these, a diagnosis of acute pyelonephritis was supported by laboratory tests.

The incidence of first-time UTI is highest during the first year of life. This is most obvious for boys but also apparent for girls. Infections diagnosed during the first years of life are mostly acute pyelonephritis. A first-time UTI classified as acute cystitis occurs especially in girls of 2–6 years of age.

Figure 23.1 shows the difference in UTI incidence between boys and girls during the first two years of life. These children were part of a national UTI study in Sweden during the years 1993–95.[2,3] There were many more boys than girls during the first months of life; after 6 months of age girls dominated. UTI without high fever occurred mainly during the first few months of life. From this study the minimal incidence of UTI during the first 2 years of life was estimated and the cumulative incidence was 2.2% and 2.1% in boys and girls, respectively.[3]

Changing concepts

The primary goal of investigation of children with UTIs is to identify risk factors (such as malformations, vesicoureteral reflux (VUR), established renal damage) and also to prevent

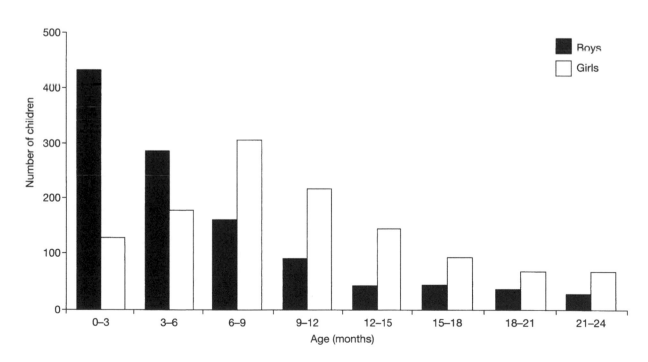

Figure 23.1 Age distribution of 2309 children with first-time UTI diagnosed before 2 years of age.

further infections and progressive renal damage. For many years the policy for investigation has been debated.[4–8] There is a wide variation from the traditional policy to investigate every child with UTI to no investigation at all. Our concepts are being changed as new techniques evolve and new knowledge is added. In this chapter, three important areas concerning childhood UTI will be discussed: the role of VUR and its treatment, the pathogenesis of renal damage and its long-term consequences, and the indications for imaging and which techniques to use.

The role of VUR

Spontaneous resolution

VUR is a common finding in children with UTI. In the large series from the Swedish UTI study 1993–95, 24% of the boys and 36% of the girls had VUR (Table 23.1).[2] The children in that study who had dilating VUR (grades III–V) were studied separately and followed for a median of 5

Table 23.1 VUR in 1953 children below 2 years of age investigated after UTI

VUR	Girls (%)	Boys (%)
None	64	76
Grade I	4	3
Grade II	14	9
Grade III	13	7
Grade IV	4	3
Grade V	1	2

A

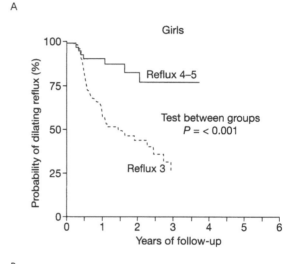

B

Figure 23.2 Spontaneous resolution of dilating reflux grade III versus grades IV–V in boys (A) and in girls (B).

years.[9] The overall chance of spontaneous regression was good and occurred in more than half of the patients. Resolution was significantly faster in boys than in girls and in children with VUR grade III compared with those with grades IV–V. It is of interest to note the low frequency of spontaneous regression in girls with the most severe grades of VUR (Figure 23.2A, B). The explanation for this is not known, but bladder dysfunction may play an important role.

VUR versus renal damage

The role of VUR in the pathogenesis of renal damage has been questioned. The term 'reflux nephropathy' was formulated in the 1970s in the belief that VUR was responsible for almost all kidney damage seen in children with urinary tract infections. Using DMSA scintigraphy it has been shown that renal damage often occurs without the presence of VUR,[10,11] and in two systematic reviews and meta-analyses it was difficult to convincingly show a relationship between VUR and renal damage in children with UTI.[12,13]

Nevertheless, a close association between VUR and renal damage has been demonstrated repeatedly over many years. In an unselected population of children with first-time acute pyelonephritis in Göteborg during the 1970s, the severity of reflux was significantly related to the frequency of scarring on urography.[14] In a recently published study of 303 children with UTI before 2 years of age, there was also a significantly increased risk for renal damage on the DMSA scan in both boys and girls with dilating VUR.[11] Besides, when the extent of scarring assessed by DMSA scintigraphy was considered (not published) the relationship between renal damage and grade of VUR was very clear and highly significant (Figure 23.3).

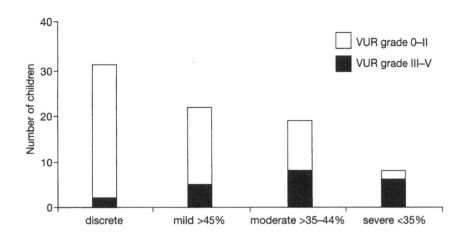

Figure 23.3 Grade of VUR in relation to extent of renal damage assessed by DMSA scintigraphy (discrete, mild, moderate and severe).

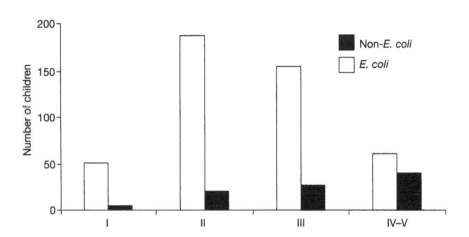

Figure 23.4 Vesicoureteric reflux in relation to bacterial species.

VUR versus bacterial species

UTI in childhood is mostly caused by *E. coli*. However, patients with malformation or dysfunction of the urinary tract may become infected by other bacterial species despite low virulence for the urinary tract. In the Swedish UTI study[2] there was a direct correlation between presence and severity of VUR and the proportion of non-*E. coli* bacteria causing the first known UTI. Thus the frequency of non-*E. coli* was 7% in children with VUR grade I, 10% in those with grade II, 15% in those with grade III and 40% in those with VUR grades IV–V (Figure 23.4). These findings are in agreement with previous publications.[11,15]

VUR versus recurrences of UTI

Children with dilating VUR are highly susceptible to recurrent UTI. In the previously mentioned Swedish UTI study pyelonephritic recurrences occurred in 18% of the boys and in 28% of the girls with VUR grade III, while the corresponding figures for children with VUR grades IV–V were 45% and 70%.[9] In view of the high incidence of recurrent pyelonephri-

tis it can be questioned whether the present practice of giving antibacterial prophylaxis to almost all children with dilating VUR is rational. In fact, no controlled study has demonstrated the efficacy of prophylaxis compared to placebo in preventing pyelonephritis or permanent renal damage.

Management of VUR

There have been several studies comparing surgical treatment and long-term prophylaxis.[16] Today reimplantation has been almost completely replaced by endoscopic subureteric injection. However, there are still many unanswered questions concerning the management of children with dilating VUR. What are the indications for the endoscopic procedure? Does it prevent recurrences? Does it prevent kidney damage? What is the value of prophylaxis? Is it good clinical practice just to observe these children starting prompt antibacterial treatment in cases of UTI recurrence? Studies addressing these questions are needed. An ongoing study, the Swedish Reflux Study, with three treatment alternatives (endoscopic injection, prophylaxis and a nontreatment observation group) was set up to answer some of these questions.

The endpoints after 2 years of follow-up are renal status according to DMSA scintigraphy, number of recurrent UTIs and reflux status.

Pathogenesis of renal damage

UTI is associated with permanent renal damage. The frequency with which damage is found in children who have had febrile UTI depends on the sensitivity of the imaging technique used to reveal the damage, and also on the timing of the investigation. This can be illustrated by a study of 157 children (median age 0.4 years, range 5 days to 5.8 years) assessed at the time of their first symptomatic UTI and one year later by DMSA scintigraphy as well as urography.[10] At the time of the UTI 68 (43%) of the children had abnormal findings on scintigraphy and 10 (6%) on urography. One year later the corresponding figures were 59 (38%) and 18 (11%). It is evident that DMSA scintigraphy has a higher sensitivity to detect renal damage, but also that some of the early uptake defects will disappear. Urography will reveal more cases with damage after one year than at the time of the UTI as the scarring process progresses.

Congenital versus acquired renal damage

Permanent damage may have developed in utero (congenital) or be acquired as a sequel of renal infection. When permanent renal damage is detected in older children and adults it is usually not possible to distinguish between congenital and acquired damage, especially when there have been recurrent UTIs. Although this distinction is difficult, there are some important differences. Risdon pointed out that among those with permanent renal damage detected in the early postnatal period there was a preponderance of boys, there was a close association with gross reflux, and damaged kidneys tended to be small with smooth outlines rather than segmentally scarred.[17,18] These results were corroborated in a study of an unselected group of 1221 children prospectively followed from their first symptomatic UTI.[19] In this cohort, 74 children were ultimately found to have permanent renal damage by urography (renal scarring). There were significant differences between the 21 boys and 53 girls with damage. The median age at the first UTI was 0.3 years in the boys and 2.8 years in the girls. Damage was already present at the first urography in 18 of the 21 boys and the damage was generalized in 15. VUR with dilatation was seen in 12 of the boys with damage on the first urography. Damage was seen on the first urography in 16 of the 53 girls and was generalized in six.

VUR with dilatation was seen in only three of the girls with damage on the first urography. Thus the damage was congenital in the majority of the boys whereas it was acquired in most girls. Furthermore, the most important factor associated with development of renal scarring in the girls was the number of attacks of febrile UTI.

There is also a gender difference with a male predominance among infants with primary reflux detected after a prenatal diagnosis of hydronephrosis.[20,21] Yeung et al, in children with antenatally diagnosed hydronephrosis, found that boys had dilated reflux and renal damage whereas girls had mild reflux but normal kidneys.[22]

Long-term complications of renal damage

Although most children with UTIs have an excellent long-term prognosis, there is a risk of serious complications in a small group. There may be impaired renal function, sometimes leading to renal insufficiency and even end-stage renal disease, hypertension and complications of pregnancy. However, in children without congenital renal damage, i.e. children with exclusively acquired damage due to pyelonephritis, this risk may be considerably smaller than previously assumed, at least in societies with a good medical healthcare system with a high detection rate of infants and small children with UTI.

Impairment of renal function

In a Swedish survey (total population 9 million) no child with a glomerular filtration rate below 30 ml/min/1.73 m^2 because of UTI was detected during the years 1986–94.[23] It is important to note that in this study all children with hypoplasia or dysplasia were classified in the malformation group.

In Göteborg a follow-up study was performed 16–26 years after the first recognized UTI in childhood in 57 with renal damage and 51 matched patients with normal kidneys.[24] They were a subgroup of an unselected cohort of 1221 cases with first-time UTI in the community during the years 1970–1979. The median glomerular filtration rate (GFR) measured by chromium[51]-edetic acid clearance was 99 ml/min/1.73 m^2 in both groups. There were eight individuals with GFR below 80 ml/min/1.73 m^2 and the lowest value was 69 ml/min/1.73 m^2. In patients with unilateral scarring the total GFR remained unchanged over the years whereas the individual GFR of the scarred kidneys declined significantly from 46 to 39 ml/min/1.73 m^2. In seven patients with bilateral scarring GFR was significantly lower at follow-up than in those with unilateral scarring, 84 and 101 ml/min/1.73 m^2, respectively. Thus, the renal function was well preserved and the risk of renal impairment in these young adults was lower than previously described, most likely as a consequence of early detection and close supervision during childhood.

Hypertension

Development of hypertension has been found in 10–30% of children and young adults with pyelonephritic renal scarring.[25–26] The risk seems to correlate with the extent of damage. However, there is reason to believe that the frequency of hypertension in these studies is higher than would be found in unselected cases of childhood UTI treated according to principles used during recent decades. In a population-based study from Göteborg, 54 women with renal scarring were followed continuously for a median of 23 years from the 1950s and 1960s; three (6%) developed hypertension.[27] In the follow-up study from Göteborg described above,[24] we also performed ambulatory 24-hour blood pressure monitoring 16–26 years after the first UTI in childhood.[28] There was no difference between the two groups with and without renal scarring, not even when patients with more extensive or bilateral scarring were analysed separately. These promising results indicate that at least from the perspective of 20 years from childhood, good care may be effective in minimizing long-term risks.

Pregnancy complications

Women who had a tendency to recurrent UTIs as girls also have an increased risk of new infections during pregnancy.[29 31] Women with renal scarring have a significant rise of blood pressure during pregnancy. In women with severe reflux nephropathy, most pregnancies are complicated.[32 33] Female patients with renal scarring should be followed carefully into adulthood and through the reproductive period.

Imaging

The traditional examinations used during the 1970s and the 1980s were intravenous urography and VCU (Table 23.2). Since pyelonephritic renal scarring is a slow process it usually takes 1–2 years until a scar becomes visible on urography.[34] This means that urography is often inconclusive as a primary tool for risk evaluation. Since the presence of VUR was a well-known risk factor it is easy to understand why VCU became a standard screening test to identify children at risk. With the development of new techniques, renal involvement is visualized directly by DMSA scintigraphy.[35] VCU may no longer be needed as a screening test. In a retrospective analysis we suggested that DMSA scintigraphy may replace VCU as

Table 23.2 Policy for investigation after childhood UTI over time

1970–1980s	Urography, VCU
1990s	Ultrasound, VCU, DMSA scintigraphy
2000s	Ultrasound, DMSA scintigraphy
Future	?

part of the primary work-up of children with UTI.[11] There were seven children who had a normal DMSA scan despite dilating VUR. All these seven children had VUR grade III and the follow-up was uneventful without recurrent UTI and with spontaneous regression of VUR. Based on these results, it can be argued that with a normal DMSA scintigraphy, VCU is not necessary. Such a policy has also been proposed by other authors previously.[36] However, this may be controversial since some authors claim that VUR should be looked for in all children with UTI irrespective of age or character of infection. Others advocate a more selective approach such as performing VCU in all infants with UTI but not in older children. We are now addressing this issue in a prospective study aimed at a simple and straightforward model.

In a recent paper, Hoberman et al argue for a radical change of policy for investigating children with UTI but with a completely different approach.[8] Their opinion is that renal ultrasonography and renal scanning at the time of the acute illness are of limited value, because they do not provide information that modifies management. This is based on the assumption that ultrasound is performed during late pregnancy (gestational weeks 30–32) so that significant abnormal findings will be identified prenatally. The use of VCU to identify children with VUR was recommended under the so far unproven assumption that continuous prophylactic antimicrobial therapy is effective in reducing the incidence of reinfection and renal scarring. However, prenatal ultrasound during late pregnancy is not a routine investigation in many parts of the world including Sweden. Another weakness is that the study was not designed to answer general questions about indications for various imaging techniques. The most severe objection concerns selection of patients; children with Gram-positive bacteria, i.e. risk patients (my comment), were excluded, as were patients < 1 month of age, severely ill children and also those with abnormalities of the urinary tract.

Conclusions

UTI is common in infants and children. A protocol for recommended investigations after UTI should be adjusted to local traditions and available resources. The timing of investigations also depends on several factors such as clinical presentation, age, response to treatment, type of bacteria and also on the availability of and experience in various imaging techniques. The challenge today is to find a simple and safe model for the primary work-up of all children with UTI including infants. Our recommendation in Göteborg today is to have a detailed family history (urinary tract abnormalities or reflux), an ultrasound and DMSA scintigraphy. The significance of VUR has been confirmed in several ways such as increased risk of renal damage, increased susceptibility to microorganisms with low virulence, and increased risk of recurrent infections. VCU is recommended in children <2 years of age with DMSA abnormalities but should also be considered in cases with unusual organisms and when there are recurrences.

The pathogenesis of renal damage has been reconsidered and it is evident that there are other mechanisms besides VUR, such as maldevelopment (congenital) and damage due to pyelonephritis. Today, much focus is on the inflammatory response and the mechanisms involved in these processes.

References

1. Hellström A, Hanson E, Hansson S et al. Association between urinary symptoms at 7 years old and previous urinary tract infection. Arch Dis Child 1991; 66: 232–4.

2. Hansson S, Bollgren I, Esbjörner E et al. Urinary tract infections in children below two years of age: a quality assurance project in Sweden. Acta Paediatr 1999; 88: 270–4.

3. Jakobsson B, Esbjörner E, Hansson S. Minimum incidence and diagnostic rate of first urinary tract infection. Pediatrics 1999; 104: 222–6.

4. Koff SA. A practical approach to evaluating urinary tract infection in children. Pediatr Nephrol 1991; 5: 398–400.

5. Haycock GB. A practical approach to evaluating urinary tract infection in children. Pediatr Nephrol 1991; 5: 401–2.

6. Stark H. Urinary tract infections in girls: the cost-effectiveness of currently recommended investigative routines. Pediatr Nephrol 1997; 11: 174–7.

7. Kass EJ, Kernen KM, Carey JM. Paediatric urinary tract infection and the necessity of complete urologic imaging. BJU Int 2000; 86; 94–6.

8. Hoberman A, Charron M, Hickey RW et al. Imaging studies after a first febrile urinary tract infection in young children. N Engl J Med 2003; 348: 195–202.

9. Esbjörner E, Hansson S, Jakobsson B. Management of children with dilating vesico-ureteric reflux in Sweden. Acta Paediatr 2004; 93: 37–42.

10. Stokland E, Hellström M, Jacobsson B et al. Evaluation of DMSA scintigraphy and urography in assessing both acute and permanent renal damage in children. Acta Radiol 1998; 39: 447–52.

11. Hansson S, Dhamey M, Sigström O et al. Dimercaptosuccinic acid scintigraphy instead of voiding cystourethrography for infants with urinary tract infection. J Urol 2004; 172: 1071–3.

12. Gordon I, Barkovics M, Pindoria S et al. Primary vesicoureteric reflux as a predictor of renal damage in children hospitalized with urinary tract infection: a systematic review and meta-analysis. J Am Soc Nephrol 2003; 14: 739–44.

13. Wheeler D, Vimalachandra D, Hodson EM et al. Antibiotics and surgery for vesicoureteric reflux: a meta-analysis of randomised controlled studies. Arch Dis Child 2003; 88: 688–94.

14. Jodal U. The natural history of bacteriuria in childhood. Infect Dis Clin North Am 1987; 1: 713–29.

15. Jantunen ME, Siitonen A, Ala-Houhala M et al. Predictive factors associated with significant urinary tract abnormalities in infants with pyelonephritis. Pediatr Infect Dis J 2001; 20: 597.

16. Jodal U, Hansson S, Hjälmås K. Medical or surgical management for children with vesicoureteric reflux? Acta Paediatr 1999 Suppl 431: 53–61.

17. Risdon RA. The small scarred kidney of childhood. A congenital or an acquired lesion? Pediatr Nephrol 1987; 1: 632–7.

18. Risdon RA. The small scarred kidney in childhood. Pediatr Nephrol 1993; 7: 361–4.

19. Wennerström M, Hansson S, Jodal U, Stokland E. Primary and acquired renal scarring in boys and girls with urinary tract infection. J Pediatr 2000; 136: 30–4.

20. Najmaldin A, Burge DM, Atwell JD. Reflux nephropathy secondary to intrauterine vesicoureteric reflux. J Pediatr Surg 1990; 25: 387–90.

21. Gordon AC, Thomas DFM, Arthur RJ et al. Prenatally diagnosed reflux: a follow up study. Brit J Urol 1990; 65: 407–12.

22. Yeung CK, Godley ML, Dhillon HK et al. The characteristics of primary vesicoureteric reflux in male and female infants with pre-natal hydronephrosis. Brit J Urol 1997; 80: 319–27.

23. Esbjörner E, Berg U, Hansson S. Epidemiology of chronic renal failure in children: a report from Sweden 1986–1994. Pediatr Nephrol 1997; 11: 438–42.

24. Wennerström M, Hansson S, Jodal U et al. Renal function 16–26 years after the first urinary tract infection in childhood. Arch Pediatr Adolesc Med 2000; 154: 339–45.

25. Wallace DMA, Rothwell DL, Williams DI. The long-term follow-up of surgically treated vesicoureteric reflux. Brit J Urol 1978; 50: 479–84.

26. Goonasekera CD, Shah V, Wade AM et al. 15-year follow-up of renin and blood pressure in reflux nephropathy. Lancet 1996; 347: 640–3.

27. Martinell J, Lidin-Janson G, Jagenburg R et al. Girls prone to urinary infections followed into adulthood. Indices of renal disease. Pediatr Nephrol 1996; 10: 139–42.

28. Wennerström M, Hansson S, Hedner T et al. Ambulatory blood pressure 16–26 years after the first urinary tract infection in childhood. J Hypertens 2000; 18: 485–91.

29. Sacks SH, Roberts R, Verrier-Jones K et al. Effect of symptomless bacteriuria in childhood on subsequent pregnancy. Lancet 1987; 2: 991–4.

30. Martinell J, Jodal U, Lidin-Janson G. Pregnancies in women with and without renal scarring after urinary infections in childhood. Brit Med J 1990; 300: 840–4.

31. Mansfield JT, Snow BW, Cartwright PC, Wadsworth K. Complications of pregnancy in women after childhood reimplantation for vesicoureteral reflux: an update with 25 years followup. J Urol 1995; 154: 787–90.

32. Kincaid-Smith P, Becker GJ. Reflux nephropathy in the adult. In: Hodson J, Kincaid-Smith P, eds. Reflux nephropathy. New York: Masson, 1979; 21–8.

33. Jungers P, Houillier P, Chauveau D et al. Pregnancy in women with reflux nephropathy. Kidney Int 1996; 50: 593–9.

34. Filly R, Friedland GW, Govan DE, Fair WR. Development and progression of clubbing and scarring in children with recurrent urinary tract infections. Radiology 1974; 113: 145–53.

35. Rushton HG. The evaluation of acute pyelonephritis and renal scarring with technetium 99m-dimercaptosuccinic acid renal scintigraphy: evolving concepts and future directions. Pediatr Nephrol 1997; 11: 108–20.

36. Rosenberg AR, Rossleigh MA, Brydon MP et al. Evaluation of acute urinary tract infection in children by dimercaptosuccinic acid scintigraphy: a prospective study. J Urol 1992; 148: 1746–9.

Index

T - #0575 - 071024 - C27 - 279/216/12 - PB - 9780367391270 - Gloss Lamination